Management of Hematological Cancer in Older People

Ulrich Wedding • Riccardo A. Audisio
Editors

Management of Hematological Cancer in Older People

Springer

Editors
Ulrich Wedding
Department of Palliative Care
University Hospital Jena
Jena, Thüringen
Germany

Riccardo A. Audisio
St Helens Teaching Hospital
University of Liverpool
St Helens
United Kingdom

ISBN 978-1-4471-6971-0 ISBN 978-1-4471-2837-3 (eBook)
DOI 10.1007/978-1-4471-2837-3
Springer London Heidelberg New York Dordrecht

Printed on acid-free paper

Springer is part of Springer Science+Business Media (www.springer.com)

Contents

Contributors

Riccardo A. Audisio, MD, FRCS St Helens Teaching Hospital, University of Liverpool, St Helens, UK

Lodovico Balducci, MD H. Lee Moffitt Cancer Center and Research Institute, University of South Florida College of Medicine, Tampa, FL, USA

Angelina Beumer, MD Department of Oncology, Deventer Ziekenhuis, Ziekenhuis, The Netherlands

Angelina Beumer-Grootenhuis, RN Department of Oncology, Deventer Ziekenhuis, Deventer, The Netherlands

Carolien Burghout, RN, M ANP Department of Haematology, Jeroen Bosch Hospital, 's-Hertogenbosch, The Netherlands

Christian Buske, MD Comprehensive Cancer Center Ulm, Institute of Experimental Cancer Research, University Hospital Ulm, Ulm, Germany

Camille Chakiba, MD Department of Medical Oncology, Institut Bergonié, Bordeaux Cedex, France

Site de Recherche Intégrée sur le Cancer, BRIO (Bordeaux Recherche Intégrée Oncologie), Bordeaux Cedex, France

Barbara Deschler, MD Interdisciplinary Clinical Trials Office, Comprehensive Cancer Center Mainfranken, University Hospital Würzburg, Würzburg, Germany

Department of Hematology/Oncology, University of Freiburg Medical Center, Freiburg, Germany

Martin Dreyling, MD, PhD Department of Medicine III, University Hospital Großhadern/LMU München, Munich, Germany

Corien M. Eeltink, RN, MA, ANP Department of Haematology, VU University Medical Center, Amsterdam, Netherlands

Martine Extermann Moffitt Cancer Center, University of South Florida, Tampa, FL, USA

Simone Ferrero, MD Division of Hematology, Department of Molecular Biotechnologies and Health Sciences, University of Torino, Torino, Italy

Paul Fields, MD Department of Haematology, Guy's and St Thomas', and Kings College Hospitals, Kings Health Partners AHSC, London, UK

Valentin Goede, MD German CLL Study Group (GCLLSG), Department of Internal Medicine, Center of Integrated Oncology Cologne-Bonn, University Hospital Cologne, Cologne, Germany

Department of Geriatric Medicine and Research, St. Marien Hospital and University of Cologne, Cologne, Germany

Michael Hallek, MD, PhD German CLL Study Group (GCLLSG), Department I of Internal Medicine, Center of Integrated Oncology Cologne-Bonn, University of Cologne, Cologne, Germany

Cluster of Excellence 'Cellular Stress Responses in Aging Associated Diseases' (CECAD), University of Cologne, Cologne, Germany

Claire Harrison, MD, DM, FRCP, FRCPath Department of Haematology, Guy's and St Thomas' NHS Foundation Trust, Great Maze Pond, London, UK

Andreas Hochhaus, Prof. Dr Abteilung Hämatologie/Onkologie, Klinik für Innere Medizin II, Universitätsklinikum Jena, Jena, Germany

Berit Jordan, MD Department of Neurology, University Hospital Halle (Saale), Halle (Saale), Germany

Karin Jordan, MD Department of Hematology/Oncology, Universitätsklinikum Halle (Saale), Halle (Saale), Germany

Youlia M. Kirova, MD Radiation Oncology, Institut Curie, Paris, France

Heidi D. Klepin, MD, MS Department of Internal Medicine, Section on Hematology and Oncology, Wake Forest School of Medicine, Winston-Salem, NC, USA

Camilla Leithold, MSc Department of Hematology and Oncology, University Hospital Halle (Saale), Halle (Saale), Germany

Roberto Lillini, PHD, AIRTUM Working Group IRCCS Azienda Ospedaliera Universitaria San Martino – IST Istituto Nazionale per la Ricerca sul Cancro, Genoa, Italy

Department of Sociology, University of Milan-Bicocca, Milan, Italy

Anne-Sophie Michallet, MD Department of Hematology, Hôpital Lyon-Sud, Hospices Civils de Lyon, Lyon, France

Roberto Mina, MD Myeloma Unit, Division of Hematology, University of Torino, Azienda Ospedaliera Città della Salute e della Scienza di Torino, Torino, Italy

Antonio Palumbo, MD Myeloma Unit, Division of Hematology, University of Torino, Azienda Ospedaliera Città della Salute e della Scienza di Torino, Torino, Italy

Timothy S. Pardee, MD, PhD Department of Internal Medicine, Section on Hematology and Oncology, Wake Forest School of Medicine, Winston-Salem, NC, USA

Alberto Quaglia†, MD Liguria Region Cancer Registry, Descriptive Epidemiology Unit, IRCCS Azienda Ospedaliera Universitaria San Martino – IST Istituto Nazionale per la Ricerca sul Cancro, Genoa, Italy

Jörn Rüssel, MD Department of Hematology and Oncology, University Hospital Halle (Saale), Halle (Saale), Germany

Susanne Saussele, MD III. Medizinische Universitätsklinik, Medizinische Fakultät Mannheim, der Universität Heidelberg, Mannheim, Germany

Farah Shariff, MD, MBBS, BSc (Hons), MRCP Department of Haematology, Guy's and St Thomas' NHS Foundation Trust, Great Maze Pond, London, UK

Pierre Soubeyran, MD Department of Medical Oncology, Institut Bergonié, Bordeaux Cedex, France

Site de Recherche Intégrée sur le Cancer, BRIO (Bordeaux Recherche Intégrée Oncologie), Bordeaux Cedex, France

Université Bordeaux, Segalen, France

Reinhard Stauder, MD, MSc Department of Internal Medicine V (Haematology and Oncology), Innsbruck Medical University, Innsbruck, Austria

Marina Vercelli, PHD Department of Health Sciences, University of Genoa, Genoa, Italy

Andreas Viardot, MD Department of Internal Medicine III, Universitätsklinikum Ulm, Ulm, Germany

Ulrich Wedding, MD Department of Palliative Care, University Hospital Jena, Jena, Thüringen, Germany

Nils Winkelmann, MD Department of Internal Medicine II, Department of Hematology and Medical Oncology, Jena University Hospital, Jena, Germany

Chapter 1
Hematological Malignancies in the Elderly: The Epidemiological Perspective

Alberto Quaglia[†], Marina Vercelli, and Roberto Lillini, AIRTUM Working Group

[†]Deceased

AIRTUM Working Group: R.T. Alto Adige (Guido Mazzoleni), R.T. Trento (Silvano Piffer), R.T. Friuli-Venezia Giulia (Diego Serraino), R.T. Veneto (Sandro Tognazzo), R.T. Mantova (Paolo Ricci), R.T. ASL Milano (Luigi Bisanti), R.T. Lombardia – Varese (Paolo Crosignani), R.T. Brescia (Michele magoni), R.T. Como (Gemma Gola), R.T. Sondrio (Maria Eugenia Sanoja Gonzalez), R.T. Piemonte – Torino (Roberto Zanetti), R.T. Piemonte – Biella (Adriano Giacomin), R.T. Liguria – Genova (Marina Vercelli), R.T. Parma (Maria Michiara), R.T. Reggio Emilia (Lucia Mangone), R.T. Modena (Massimo Federico), R.T. Ferrara (Stefano Ferretti), R.T. Romagna (Fabio Falcini), R.T. Toscano (Adele Caldarella), R.T. Macerata (Susanna Vitarelli), R.T. Umbria (Francesco La Rosa), R.T. Latina (Fabio Pannozzo), R.T. Sassari (Ornelia Sechi), R.T. Nuoro (Mario Usala), R.T. Salerno (Luigi Cremone), R.T. Catanzaro (Antonella Sutera Sardo), R.T. Palermo (Francesco Vitale), R.T. Trapani (Giuseppina Candela), R.T. Catania-Messina (Salvatore Sciacca), R.T. Siracusa (Francesco Tisano), R.T. Ragusa (Rosario Tumino)

M. Vercelli, PHD (✉)
Department of Health Sciences, University of Genoa, Italy, Genoa, Italy
e-mail: marina.vercelli@unige.it

R. Lillini, PHD
IRCCS Azienda Ospedaliera Universitaria San Martino – IST Istituto Nazionale per la Ricerca sul Cancro, Genoa, Italy

Department of Sociology, University of Milan-Bicocca, Milan, Italy

U. Wedding, R.A. Audisio (eds.), *Management of Hematological Cancer in Older People*, DOI 10.1007/978-1-4471-2837-3_1

Abstract In the more developed countries the total number of new cases with a hematological tumour was 415,433 for all ages, whilst 188,654 occurred in people aged 70 or more years, representing the 45 % of total cases, equally divided into two sexes. The most these malignancies is closely linked to age and incidence rates increased exponentially after 50 years of age.

Aetiology of hematological tumours is largely unknown. However the basic causal mechanism could be a decline in adaptive immunity, strongly related with individual age. In addition to such immunodeficiency, some specific risk factors have been found: viral infections, overweight and obesity (particularly for non-Hodgkin's lymphomas – NHL), ionising radiation and chemical compounds (particularly for leukemia). Moreover, it must to be taken into account that mortality and survival, more specifically in the elderly, are influenced negatively by socio-economic deprivation.

Considering geographical distribution, substantial variations in incidence and mortality across the world were observed. Incidence of younger and older adults was for all hematological malignancies higher in more developed countries. As regards mortality, younger people showed rates higher in developing countries, while the elderly in Western and developed areas.

The epidemic growth of NHL incidence was not finished in the first decade of 2000, even if in Italian and US old populations the rates started leveling off. Unlike incidence, mortality was descending in the elderly. Leukemia incidence trends were very often stable or weakly growing, without any tendency to decrease, but for leukemia mortality it was possible to highlight an encouraging general picture with rates often decreasing.

The elderly had always survival rates lower than those of middle aged adults. The prognostic disadvantage was larger at 1 than 5 years from diagnosis. The gap was smaller for NHL and acute myeloid leukemia, whereas the difference in survival was much larger for chronic myeloid leukemia and Hodgkin's lymphoma. Summarizing, elderly patients had a marked prognostic disadvantage with respect younger adults. However, if an elderly subject survives the first period immediately after detection and overcomes the first difficulties of access to healthcare, experiences a prognosis similar to that of a younger patient.

Keywords Hematological tumours • Aetiology • Descriptive epidemiology • Elderly • Incidence • Mortality • Survival • Trend

Introduction

Hematological malignancies are a heterogeneous group of tumours arising from lymphatic system and bone marrow. They are divided into three groups: leukaemia, lymphomas and plasma cells malignancies (multiple myeloma) and in 2008 in the world they accounted for 7 % of overall newly diagnosed cases and deaths, considering both sexes [1].

In the more developed countries for all ages the total number of new cases diagnosed with a hematological neoplasm was 415,433, whilst 188,654 occurred in people aged 70 or more years, representing 45 % of total hematological tumours, equally

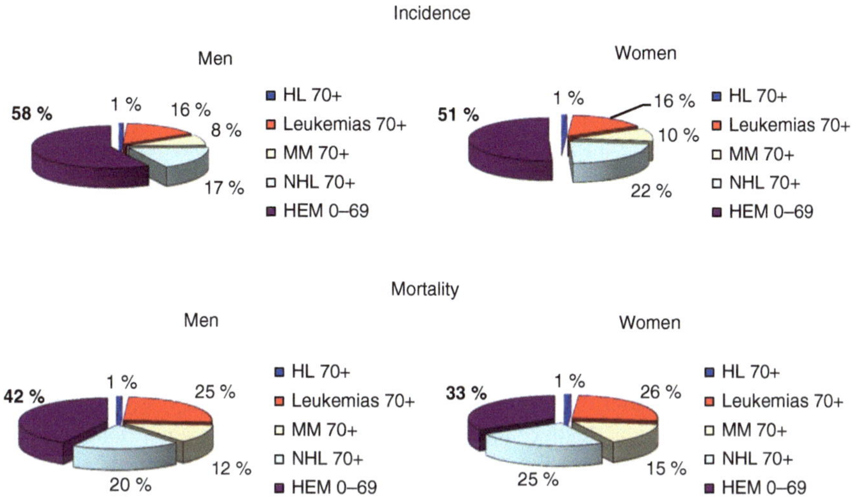

Fig. 1.1 Hematopoietic system cancers: incidence and mortality in the aged 70 years and more vs. the less than 70 years ones by site and gender (proportion per 100). *HL* Hodgkin's Lymphoma, *MM* Multiple Myeloma, *NHL* Non - Hodgkin Lymphomas, *HEMO* Hematological Tumours

divided into two sexes. As most cancers also some tumours of this group of malignancies is closely linked to age and its incidence rates increase exponentially after 50 years of age. In the more developed macro-areas, considering all the hematological tumours the number of incident cases in the elderly (≥70 years) accounted for 7 % in men and 6 % in women. Figure 1.1 show the incident cases of hematological tumours by broad age groups: in younger men (0–69 years) the yearly diagnosed new cases were 58 %, while the single entities for elderly accounted for 17, 16, 8 and 1 % in NHL, leukaemia, MM and HL respectively; in women the same values were 51 % for the younger, with the single entities accounting for 22, 16, 10 and 1 %.

The percentages of haematopoietic tumours increased strikingly in the elderly moving to mortality: 42 % of deaths occurred in younger men, 58 % in elderly men, while 33 % in younger women and even 67 % in elderly ones. In older men the single entities accounted for 25, 20, 12 and 1 % in leukaemia, NHL, MM and HL respectively, while in women the same values were 26, 25, 15 and 1 % [1].

Aetiology

Development of Hematological Tumours Is Favoured by Aging Process

Aetiology of hematological tumours is up to now largely unknown. Several risk factors have been found in epidemiological studies and some associations have been identified and assessed, even if the etiologic factors do not account for a great number of incident cases. Moreover, it must be remind to distinguish the natural history of hematological tumours occurring during childhood, adulthood, especially in the elderly. At this regard it is important to consider the latency time between the exposure to carcinogen, or more generally to the risk, and the cancer development. In any case, for most cases of hematological tumours it is impossible to find a precise genetic or environmental cause. In fact, several genetic disorders or environmental situations have been identified as risk factors, but they constitute only a small proportion of all hematological cases in the elderly [2, 3].

Leukaemia and lymphomas, like other cancers, start to grow up owing to the combination of environmental risk factors acting along with genetic susceptibilities. The most general mechanism which lead to the development of hematopoietic tumours is the lack of the equilibrium between the renewal and death of blood cells. During the lifespan, after the early development of hematological system, a balance between the renewal and death of blood cells begins. However, even if bone marrow is the tissue with the highest frequency of proliferation of stem cells, as other tissues, it must undergo ageing and its negative effects.

The balance between cell progenitors and differentiated elements has the tendency to go off during aging, because, B lymphocytes in particular decrease their production [4, 5]. It is probably that the mechanism of senescence lead to a decline in B cell production, as a phenomenon already fixed in blood cells progenitors. In addition, hematopoietic cells begin to age and lose their physiological functions, with the alterations of the expression of some genes devoted to check the healthy status of DNA. Summarising, bone marrow and hematological system lose their capability to check for homeostasis and to repair DNA damages owing to ageing [6]. The impairment of progenitors involves principally the lymphoid compartment and, to a lesser extent, the proliferation of the myeloid cell line.

In addition to the lost ability of cells to differentiate, some authors have found that also the environment of bone marrow, where the progenitors develop, changes its physiological conditions. Owing to the close relationship between haematic cells and the support tissue where they proliferate and differentiate, the physiological status is completely dependent by the stromal elements of bone marrow. All these hematological shortcomings lead to a decline in adaptive immunity and are strongly related with the individual's age [7–9].

Immunosuppression

Both quantitative (the decrease of differentiated lymphocytes) and qualitative (compromised quality of stromal functions) defects cause a decline of all immune system [10, 11]. Such immunosuppression has been confirmed by some analyses which have studied in wide cohort of patients the correlation between immunodeficiency (congenital or acquired) and the probability to develop hematological cancers. At this proposal, is of particular interest a study which has shown that about

25 % of patients suffering from congenital immunodeficiency will develop cancers, particularly non Hodgkin lymphoma (50 % of the tumours in excess) [12]. Furthermore, in literature it is well known that transplants, through immunosuppression, cause especially hematological tumours of myeloid cells such as acute myeloid leukaemia (AML) [13].

These marked alterations, principally affecting the lymphocytic line, influence both the development of lymphomas and leukaemia in elderly patients. More precisely, the main occurrence of hematological malignancies is made up by lymphatic cells in childhood and myeloid cells in adulthood, especially in old people. Another evidence is provided by a Dutch population-based study. It is an innovative investigation based on the relationships between autoimmune disorders and lymphoproliferative tumours. The authors found that the prevalence of autoimmune and chronic inflammation was significantly associated with newly diagnosed lymphoproliferative malignancies. In particular, the positive correlation with some lymphoma subtypes was striking [14].

Viral Infections

The aforementioned analysis showed as, in addition to the immune system impairment, related to aging, also the infections directly could be considered an important risk factor for hematological tumours, particularly in the elderly. De va schans determined that infective agents can cause mainly lymphomas through three action mechanisms. First, virus interacts directly with lymphocytes, as for Epstein-Barr virus. Second, other viruses, such as HIV, give rise to an acquired immunosuppression syndrome [14]. It is well known that the NHL is closely linked to HIV positive infection and now is decreasing in incidence also thanks to the introduction in the mid-1990s of antiretroviral therapy. A third mechanism concerns some viruses and autoimmune diseases, like rheumatoid arthritis: the lymphomas could be caused by a chronic immune stimulation which leads to a too much intense and deregulated cell lymphatic proliferation [15].

The viral hypothesis was confirmed by a meta-analysis dealing with NHL and HCV-positive persons that found a pooled relative risk very high (around 2.0–2.5) [16]. As regards HBV, a recent study performed in South Korea showed that there was an association between chronic hepatitis B virus infection and higher risk of developing NHL: HBsAg-positive subjects developed easier NHL than general population [17]. It is difficult to assess the existence of an association between HCV and HBV and other hematological tumours, due to the small number of cases enrolled in the studies, however, weaker associations were found also with Hodgkin's lymphoma (HL) and multiple myeloma (MM) [16].

The EBV is a viral risk factor that produces tumours principally in two ways. In a first case EBV acts as a cofactor together with immunosuppression (HIV infection, transplants). Second, EBV is present in the total cases of Burkitt's lymphomas and, outside the endemic areas, it is detected in some sporadic lymphomas [18].

Focusing the attention on the single types of leukaemia, it is difficult to individuate specific viral agents able to influence the incidence of such tumours. Nevertheless, it would seem that could exist an association between AML and parvovirus B19 [19]. Another virus affecting the haematic system is an endemic retrovirus (HTLV type-1, type-2) spread in Japan, Caribbean and South-Eastern US, which causes some rare forms of hematological malignancies, such as T-cell leukaemia/lymphoma [20]. The low incidence and the long latency period suggest the participation of a multistep pattern with multiple genetic mutations to observe the onset of the disease, which occurs more frequently in adults and elderly people [21].

Overweight and Obesity

The prevalence of an elevated BMI, higher than the values of World Health Organisation (>=30.0 kg/m^2), of overweight (BMI=25–29.9 kg/m^2) and obesity is dramatically increasing and it has been estimated that more than 1.6 thousand million people are overweight. Obviously there are striking differences among the different areas of the world, but also in Africa and Asia the obesity has increased. It must to be taken in mind that the relatively long latency period observed between the onset of obesity and a subsequent increase in cancer incidence, can explain the incidence in adult patients, particularly elderly of hematological malignancies.

As seen above, such tumours are associated to autoimmune and chronic inflammatory diseases. On the other hand, obesity alters the immune system and is related to chronic inflammatory conditions, having the capacity to constitute a risk factor especially for HL and NHL. In adulthood, and particularly in the elderly, the effect of obesity can be divided into two categories: the result of a greater mass of fat which directly affects the organ functioning and the result of an expansion of endocrine compartment, owing to the enlarged number of fat cells and the effect on target tissues. The increase of several hormones related to adiposity accounts for the cancer development [22].

A recent meta-analysis found that a 5 kg/m^2 increment in BMI was associated with a 7 % increased risk of NHL. Only few studies were performed on HL and have observed that obesity was statistically correlated with HL, especially the risk tended to be higher in the older rather than younger patients [23, 24]. A higher number of studies has observed a close association between the excess of body weight and development of MM. A very large prospective study, developed in US on 900,000 adults, has found that for lymphomas, leukaemia and MM the mortality relative risk (RR) was significantly higher and increased with aging [25].

Large cohort studies have assessed that obesity influences incidence and mortality of hematological cancers [26, 27]. However, the most investigations have not analysed the risk for each type of leukaemia or subtypes of lymphomas, presumably because of the relative small number of available cases. Notwithstanding, a meta-analysis has been carried out investigating, through cohort studies, the relationships between the excess of BMI and the incidence of leukaemia as a whole and each major subtypes [28]. They have found higher RRs for overweight in all four types of leukaemia. As regards lymphoma subtypes, the diffuse large B-cell lymphoma showed a stronger correlation, more frequent in the elderly [27].

Ionising Radiation

The close correlation between exposure to ionising radiation and the development of haematopoietic tumours has been largely assessed. Unfortunately, the atomic bomb and the nuclear weapon tests have provided enough evidence, substituting experimental essays. The radiations, after a latency of 5–7 years, cause the developing of acute leukaemia and CML. The response to the risk factor is different according to the specific cellular type and the linkage with CCL is weaker [21]. In addition to the tragic experience of war survivors, scientific evidence has been provided by those authors investigating the role played by the exposure to low dose radiation for people working or living near nuclear power stations [29]. Therefore, the leukaemia as a whole are the type of tumour most frequently induced by ionising radiation. On the contrary, lymphomas are very rarely associated to this kind of exposure and the risk is practically similar to that of general population [21].

Chemicals Compounds

A higher risk of leukaemia has been identified for occupational exposure to benzene, formaldehyde and dioxins. Also organic solvents, agriculture pesticides have been associated to an increased risk. Benzene deserves a particular attention because it is a chemical among the most studied in the last century, with a clear evidence of a negative effect of acute and chronic exposure on blood system both in animal and humans. In particular, chronic and heavy exposures are a powerful risk factor especially for acute myeloid leukaemia. Other tumours and different workplaces have been investigated, but the results have not been supported by evocal epidemiological studies. Some authors have suggested that a chronic exposure to high level of airborne benzene may cause a risk excess for lymphomas, multiple myeloma and other haematopoietic malignancies [30].

Numerous epidemiological analyses have confirmed the association of lymphomas with different chemicals such as herbicides, insecticides and fertilisers compounds. Farmers are an occupational category very exposed because agriculture chemicals could be all potentially carcinogenic and lead to a chronic immunological stimulation [31]. Some studies have demonstrated very high risks of NHL for a frequent usage of herbicides, highlighting a correlation between exposure time and lymphomas risk. However, some authors have hypothesise that the striking increase of incidence occurred in the last two decades could be due to the widespread use of herbicides, in particular 2, 4-dichlorophenoxyacetic acid [32, 33].

Finally, it is important to mention the role played by anti-tumour treatment in co-operation to the development of haematic cancers. There is the possibility that some chemotherapeutic regimens and radiotherapy can induce AML. A second AML is more frequently associated to treatment for HL and MM,

In all with a latency of 5–10 years, accounting for 10–20 % of all the leukaemia of this type [34].

Ultraviolet Radiations (UVR) and Sun Exposure

A possible association between UVR and growth of incidence of lymphomas has been carefully studied. In 1990s some analyses found a risk increase of NHL correlated with the intensity of UVR [35]. The radiations would have an immunosuppressive effect and thus they would be able to favour cancerogenesis of lymphatic system. Nevertheless, several authors have not confirmed completely this hypothesis and have found no or only a weak correlation [21, 36, 37]. A more recent study of 2004 has reported that sun exposure was linked to a decreased risk of NHL, confirming the lack of any association with UVR [38].

Socio-Economic Status (SES)

Cancer is a chronic disease whose occurrence is closely related to SES. It is possible to assess that it is a real "social disease" and that the elderly are the individuals most affected by a poor SES [39, 40]. NHL is not an exception and some studies have found that mortality and survival are correlated to the deprivation level of patients. A Danish population-based study observed that mortality was 40 % higher in patients suffering from NHL with a lower attained educational level. In addition, mortality grows in unemployed individuals, with low income and singles. This prognostic disadvantage could be due to difficulties of access to health care, with a consequent more advanced disease stage at diagnosis [41].

A recent study has found that also AML is correlated with SES. Particularly, in UK mortality was nearly 50 % higher for the most deprived group. Moreover, a gradient was observed for HD, differing in accordance of the patient's age. A protective social environment (in young adults) or an overcrowded social context (in children and in the elderly) was related to an excess of risk. The study did not found any linear association for leukaemia [42]. The same authors in a very large population-based study have found that the most deprived individual were less likely to undergo bone marrow transplant even after adjusting for confounding factors. These results are in accordance with a further investigation demonstrating an association between low survival and blue-collar workers both in AML and MM [43].

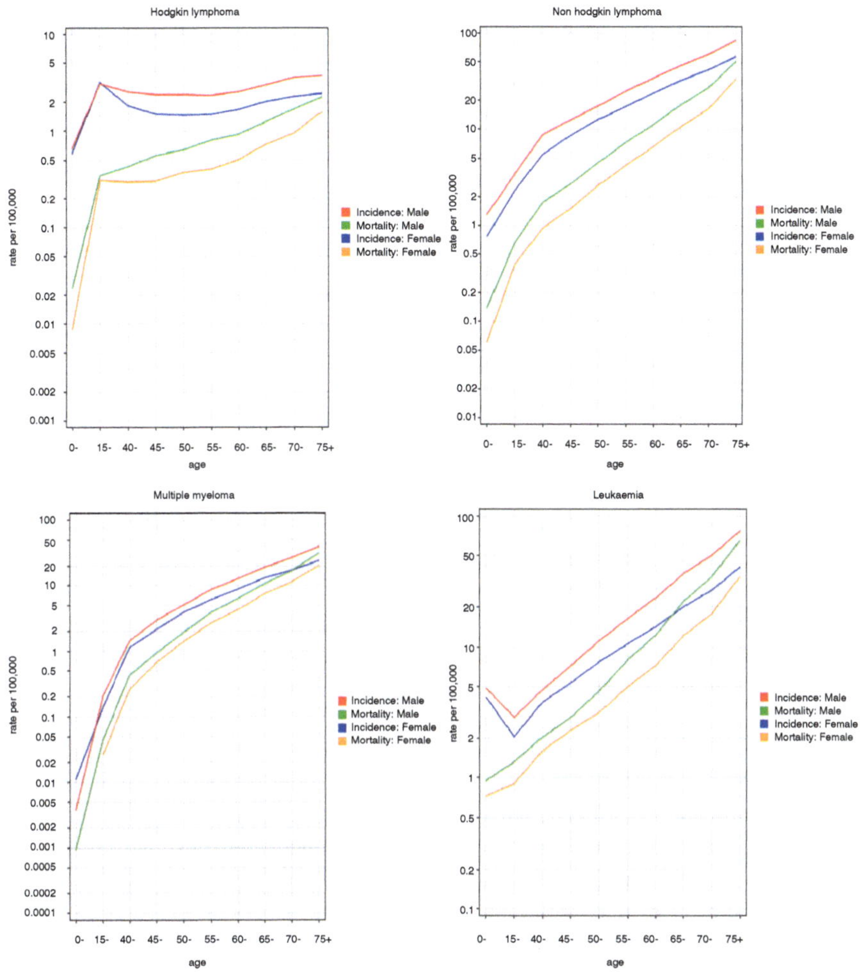

Fig. 1.2 Haematopoietic system cancers: age curves of incidence and mortality in the more developed countries by site and gender (rates per 100,000)

Descriptive Epidemiology

Age Distribution

Figure 1.2 displays age curves by sex of incidence and mortality for each hematological tumour site in more developed regions. For NHL the age curve showed an increase quite stable both in incidence and mortality up to older individuals. Rates of women were lower than those of men. Rates in both sexes did not exceed 9 cases per 100,000 and 2 per 100,000 until 40 years of age, for incidence and mortality respectively. Afterwards at 75 years incidence reached 83 cases per

100,000 in men and 56 in women, while mortality 50 in men and 33 in women. The initial gap between mortality and incidence decreased progressively with age and after 70 years the two indexes were very similar. Out of total NHL new cases, those occurring over 70 years were 42 and 51 % in men and women respectively, while deaths achieved 58 and 69 %. Practically more than half of newly diagnosed tumours and more than 2/3 of deaths were diagnosed in elderly women [1, 44].

Leukaemia showed incidence curves different from others considered haematopoietic neoplasm. In fact, there was a first incidence peak within the first year of age (5 and 4 incident cases per 100,000 in men and women respectively), followed by a successive decline up to 15 years old adolescents; finally incidence rates started to increase very quickly reaching a second peak at 75 and more years (77 and 41 cases per 100,000 in men and women respectively). As for mortality, the curve did not have the early decline, but the rates began to increase since birth in both sexes. Mortality grew up at a quicker pace than incidence and, over 75 years, the beginning gap between incidence and mortality disappeared (65 and 35 deaths per 100,000 in men and women respectively). Out of the total leukaemia, in the elderly the percentages of new cases (45 and 50 % in men and women respectively) and deaths (58 and 64 %) were very high and similar to those of NHL.

These curves were in accordance with a tumour hitting in paediatric age. For example, acute lymphoid leukaemia (ALL) is a subtype typical of children, not frequent in adulthood. Nevertheless most cases of leukaemia occurred in middle aged adults and in elderly. In particular, AML presents a median age at diagnosis of 64 years and therefore is mainly an adults' disease. Also CML arises seldom in children or adolescents, while many cases occur in older people. In a similar way, CLL is a disease of the elderly, with a median age of 70 years. For this reason it is the more common leukaemia subtype in more developed countries.

Among hematological malignancies MM was the tumour decidedly most characteristic of older age, with a median age of onset of about 65–70 years. Until 40 years incidence and mortality remained lower than 2 cases per 100,000, afterwards new cases grew exponentially, reaching values of 39 (in men) and 24 (in women) cases per 100,000 in the aged 75 or more years. Also mortality rates increased strikingly and reached 31 and 20 deaths. The new cases of MM occurring over 70 years were 52 and 58 % in men and women respectively, while deaths reached the highest values of 64 and 71 %, confirming that this is the cancer more common in the elderly among all hematological types.

HL is not a tumour of old age. It presents two peaks in childhood and adulthood, primarily hitting young adults usually between 25 and 30 years and then older adults after 50. The age curve in Figure 1.2a shows in fact a first increase of incidence and mortality rates in both sexes in children, reaching a peak at 15 years. Then rates almost levelled off and increased, only slightly, with a successive peak over 75 years. The rates were a little bit higher in men than women. Only 13 % in men and 15 % in women of newly cases was diagnosed in elderly over 70 years, while 31 % and 41 % of deaths occurred in the elderly, confirming that this tumour affects prevalently young people.

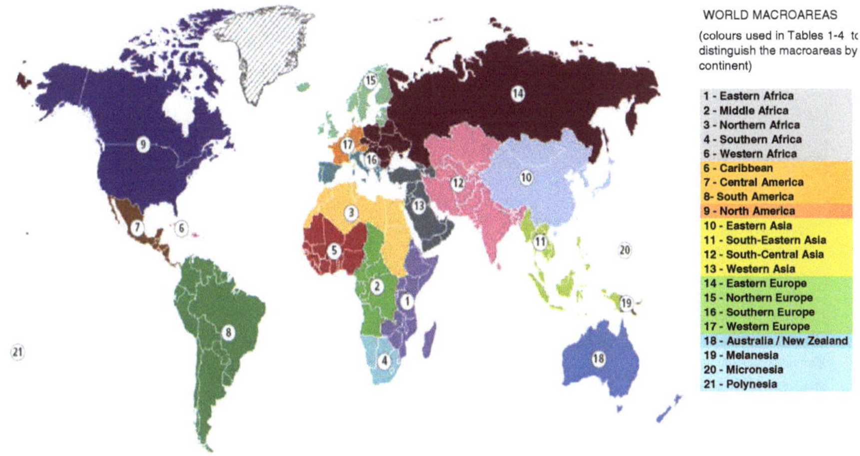

Fig. 1.3 WORLD MACROAREAS. Source: American Cancer Society – Global Cancer Facts & Figures 2007

Apart HL, these data confirmed that hematological tumours constituted a very high burden and, due to the ageing of population, they will be a major challenge which health systems must to cope with.

Geographic Distribution

Each broad hematological entity comprehends subtypes with different genetic profiles and immunophenotype. Each subtype has different histopathology, clinical procedures and epidemiological picture. These patterns correspond to different epidemiological profile which have a particular distribution across countries. Moreover, the distribution by area is partly caused by various etiological factors according to their prevalence in a specific geographical region. Notwithstanding, owing to the not clear knowledge of aetiology, it is difficult to explain exhaustively the different distribution according to the spread of determined risk factors confounded also by the huge differences in socio-economic status of people resident in the different macro-areas.

Substantial variations in incidence and mortality across the world have been observed, like shown in Figure 1.3 and Tables 1.1, 1.2, 1.3, 1.4, 1.5, 1.6, 1.7 and 1.8. Figure 1.3 shows how the macro-regions have been defined (according to sub-continental areas assessed by WHO) and on the right side of the figure the macro-regions differently coloured on the basis of the considered continent. In Tables 1.7 and 1.8 the incidence and mortality age standardised rates (ASR, world standard per 100,000), the crude rates and the yearly numbers of cancers estimated in 2008, by sex and two age groups (0–69 and 70 or more years) are listed [1].

Table 1.1 Incidence and mortality by world macro-areas, site and gender. Numbers, crude rates and ASR(W)

HODGKIN LYMPHOMA-INCIDENCE

Aged 0-69 years - MEN

MACROAREA	N°	Crude Rate	ASR (W)
Eastern Asia	3572	0.5	**0.4**
Polynesia	1	0.3	**0.4**
Melanesia	14	0.3	**0.5**
Middle Africa	229	0.4	**0.6**
Western Africa	807	0.6	**0.6**
South-Eastern Asia	1913	0.7	**0.7**
Caribbean	195	1.0	**1.0**
Central America	671	0.9	**1.0**
South-Central Asia	8008	0.9	**1.0**
Sub-Saharan Africa	3170	0.8	**1.0**
Southern Africa	300	1.1	**1.1**
World	36042	1.1	**1.1**
South America	2162	1.2	**1.2**
Micronesia	4	1.5	**1.4**
Eastern Africa	1834	1.2	**1.7**
Northern Africa	1650	1.6	**1.7**
Central & Eastern Europe	2840	2.2	**2.0**
Western Asia	2134	1.9	**2.0**
Western Europe	1911	2.3	**2.1**
Australia/New Zealand	298	2.6	**2.4**
Northern America	4293	2.7	**2.5**
Northern Europe	1217	2.8	**2.5**
Southern Europe	1988	3.0	**2.6**

Aged 70 years and more - MEN

MACROAREA	N°	Crude Rate	ASR (W)
Micronesia	0	0.0	**0.0**
Polynesia	0	0.0	**0.0**
South-Eastern Asia	116	1.3	**1.3**
Caribbean	20	2.0	**1.8**
Melanesia	1	1.6	**1.8**
Eastern Asia	840	2.0	**2.0**
Southern Africa	10	1.9	**2.0**
Western Africa	59	2.7	**2.5**
Northern Africa	74	2.8	**2.8**
Middle Africa	25	2.9	**2.9**
Central & Eastern Europe	272	2.9	**2.9**
South-Central Asia	672	3.0	**3.0**
World	4223	3.0	**3.0**
South America	247	3.4	**3.4**
Central America	91	3.5	**3.4**
Western Asia	109	3.8	**3.8**
Australia/New Zealand	40	3.9	**3.8**
Northern Europe	178	3.9	**3.9**
Western Europe	376	3.9	**3.9**
Sub-Saharan Africa	244	4.0	**4.0**
Southern Europe	343	4.3	**4.2**
Northern America	600	4.7	**4.7**
Eastern Africa	150	6.1	**6.1**

Aged 0-69 years - WOMEN

MACROAREA	N°	Crude Rate	ASR (W)
Micronesia	0	0.0	**0.0**
Polynesia	0	0.0	**0.0**
Melanesia	5	0.1	**0.1**
Eastern Asia	1758	0.2	**0.2**
Middle Africa	161	0.3	**0.4**
South-Central Asia	3812	0.5	**0.5**
South-Eastern Asia	1358	0.5	**0.5**
Western Africa	571	0.4	**0.5**
South America	1226	0.7	**0.6**
Sub-Saharan Africa	1801	0.5	**0.6**
Central America	536	0.7	**0.7**
Southern Africa	191	0.7	**0.7**
World	24111	0.8	**0.7**
Eastern Africa	878	0.6	**0.8**
Caribbean	187	0.9	**0.9**
Northern Africa	1087	1.1	**1.1**
Western Asia	1455	1.4	**1.4**
Australia/New Zealand	227	2.0	**1.9**
Central & Eastern Europe	2935	2.2	**1.9**
Western Europe	1621	2.0	**1.9**
Northern Europe	921	2.1	**2.0**
Northern America	3579	2.3	**2.1**
Southern Europe	1604	2.4	**2.3**

Aged 70 years and more - WOMEN

MACROAREA	N°	Crude Rate	ASR (W)
Melanesia	0	0.0	**0.0**
Micronesia	0	0.0	**0.0**
Polynesia	0	0.0	**0.0**
Western Africa	7	0.3	**0.3**
Southern Africa	5	0.6	**0.6**
Middle Africa	10	0.9	**0.9**
South-Central Asia	262	1.0	**1.0**
Eastern Asia	566	1.1	**1.0**
Sub-Saharan Africa	77	1.0	**1.0**
Central & Eastern Europe	291	1.5	**1.5**
World	3543	1.8	**1.8**
South-Eastern Asia	197	1.7	**1.8**
Eastern Africa	55	1.8	**1.8**
Caribbean	24	2.0	**1.9**
Western Europe	345	2.3	**2.3**
Australia/New Zealand	31	2.3	**2.3**
South America	233	2.3	**2.3**
Northern Europe	182	2.7	**2.8**
Central America	96	2.9	**2.8**
Northern Africa	88	2.7	**2.8**
Western Asia	112	3.0	**3.0**
Southern Europe	398	3.3	**3.3**
Northern America	642	3.5	**3.4**

*Age-Standardised Rates, World standard (per 100,000)
Source: GLOBOCAN 2008, IARC.

Table 1.2 Incidence and mortality by world macro-areas, site and gender. Numbers, crude rates and ASR(W)

HODGKIN LYMPHOMA - MORTALITY

Aged 0-69 years - MEN

MACROAREA	N°	Crude Rate	ASR (W)
Micronesia	0	0.0	**0.0**
Polynesia	0	0.0	**0.0**
Eastern Asia	1204	0.2	**0.1**
Australia/New Zealand	26	0.2	**0.2**
Western Europe	226	0.3	**0.2**
Northern America	497	0.3	**0.3**
Northern Europe	154	0.4	**0.3**
South America	607	0.3	**0.3**
South-Eastern Asia	1050	0.4	**0.4**
Southern Europe	345	0.5	**0.4**
Caribbean	106	0.5	**0.5**
Central America	306	0.4	**0.5**
Melanesia	13	0.3	**0.5**
Middle Africa	187	0.3	**0.5**
South-Central Asia	4053	0.5	**0.5**
Western Africa	653	0.5	**0.5**
World	14964	0.5	**0.5**
Central & Eastern Europe	1079	0.8	**0.7**
Southern Africa	229	0.8	**0.9**
Sub-Saharan Africa	2564	0.7	**0.9**
Northern Africa	1298	1.3	**1.4**
Western Asia	1436	1.3	**1.4**
Eastern Africa	1495	1.0	**1.5**

Aged 70 years and more - MEN

MACROAREA	N°	Crude Rate	ASR (W)
Polynesia	0	0.0	**0.0**
Micronesia	0	0.0	**0.0**
South-Eastern Asia	103	1.2	**1.2**
Eastern Asia	597	1.4	**1.4**
Melanesia	1	1.6	**1.8**
Northern America	261	2.0	**1.9**
Western Europe	197	2.1	**1.9**
Northern Europe	91	2.0	**1.9**
Australia/New Zealand	20	1.9	**1.9**
South America	158	2.2	**2.1**
Central & Eastern Europe	209	2.2	**2.2**
Southern Africa	11	2.1	**2.2**
World	3292	2.3	**2.3**
Caribbean	31	3.1	**2.8**
Western Africa	72	3.3	**3.0**
Southern Europe	249	3.1	**3.0**
Middle Africa	28	3.2	**3.3**
Northern Africa	88	3.4	**3.4**
South-Central Asia	779	3.5	**3.5**
Western Asia	106	3.7	**3.7**
Central America	113	4.4	**4.3**
Sub-Saharan Africa	289	4.8	**4.8**
Eastern Africa	178	7.3	**7.3**

Aged 0-69 years - WOMEN

MACROAREA	N°	Crude Rate	ASR (W)
Micronesia	0	0.0	**0.0**
Polynesia	0	0.0	**0.0**
Australia/New Zealand	18	0.2	**0.1**
Eastern Asia	671	0.1	**0.1**
Melanesia	5	0.1	**0.1**
Western Europe	132	0.2	**0.1**
Northern America	388	0.2	**0.2**
Northern Europe	119	0.3	**0.2**
South America	352	0.2	**0.2**
Caribbean	63	0.3	**0.3**
Central America	176	0.2	**0.3**
Middle Africa	140	0.2	**0.3**
South-Central Asia	2036	0.2	**0.3**
South-Eastern Asia	790	0.3	**0.3**
Southern Europe	218	0.3	**0.3**
World	9002	0.3	**0.3**
Central & Eastern Europe	754	0.6	**0.4**
Western Africa	478	0.3	**0.4**
Southern Africa	148	0.5	**0.5**
Sub-Saharan Africa	1492	0.4	**0.5**
Eastern Africa	726	0.5	**0.6**
Northern Africa	847	0.9	**0.9**
Western Asia	941	0.9	**0.9**

Aged 70 years and more - WOMEN

MACROAREA	N°	Crude Rate	ASR (W)
Polynesia	0	0.0	**0.0**
Micronesia	0	0.0	**0.0**
Melanesia	0	0.0	**0.0**
Western Africa	7	0.3	**0.3**
Southern Africa	5	0.6	**0.6**
Eastern Asia	501	1.0	**0.9**
Middle Africa	10	0.9	**0.9**
South-Central Asia	264	1.0	**1.0**
Sub-Saharan Africa	80	1.0	**1.0**
Central & Eastern Europe	245	1.2	**1.2**
Western Europe	203	1.4	**1.2**
World	2644	1.4	**1.3**
Australia/New Zealand	19	1.4	**1.3**
Northern Europe	114	1.7	**1.5**
Northern America	309	1.7	**1.5**
South America	155	1.6	**1.5**
Eastern Africa	58	1.9	**1.8**
South-Eastern Asia	200	1.7	**1.8**
Southern Europe	237	2.0	**1.9**
Western Asia	96	2.5	**2.5**
Caribbean	34	2.8	**2.6**
Central America	93	2.9	**2.7**
Northern Africa	94	2.9	**2.9**

*Age-Standardised Rates, World standard (per 100,000)
Source: GLOBOCAN 2008, IARC.

Table 1.3 Incidence and mortality by world macro-areas, site and gender. Numbers, crude rates and ASR(W)

NON HODGKIN LYMPHOMA - INCIDENCE

Aged 0-69 years - MEN

MACROAREA	N°	Crude Rate	ASR (W)
Eastern Asia	21252	2.8	2.5
Micronesia	5	1.8	2.6
South-Central Asia	20935	2.4	2.9
Caribbean	645	3.3	3.4
Central America	2491	3.5	4.0
Central & Eastern Europe	6227	4.9	4.0
Western Africa	4509	3.1	4.0
South America	7211	3.9	4.3
Middle Africa	1754	2.9	4.5
World	141282	4.3	4.6
Sub-Saharan Africa	13549	3.5	4.7
Southern Africa	1100	4.0	4.8
South-Eastern Asia	11926	4.3	5.0
Western Asia	4566	4.1	5.1
Eastern Africa	6186	4.1	5.3
Melanesia	162	3.8	5.5
Polynesia	16	4.9	5.9
Northern Africa	5841	5.8	7.1
Southern Europe	6827	10.2	7.6
Western Europe	9284	11.3	7.9
Northern Europe	5348	12.3	8.9
Australia/New Zealand	1637	14.2	10.9
Northern America	23360	14.8	11.9

Aged 70 years and more - MEN

MACROAREA	N°	Crude Rate	ASR (W)
Micronesia	0	0.0	0.0
South-Central Asia	3647	16.3	16.3
Eastern Asia	9599	22.5	22.2
Western Africa	556	25.3	24.3
Central America	646	25.1	24.8
Central & Eastern Europe	2353	25.0	24.9
Sub-Saharan Africa	1550	25.7	25.6
Eastern Africa	630	25.7	25.7
Southern Africa	132	25.7	25.9
Middle Africa	232	26.7	27.0
Caribbean	274	27.3	27.1
Western Asia	946	33.1	33.0
South-Eastern Asia	2995	34.5	34.4
South America	2706	37.8	36.7
Northern Africa	994	38.1	38.2
World	58454	41.3	40.6
Polynesia	4	41.3	41.3
Southern Europe	4678	58.1	56.6
Melanesia	38	61.5	60.8
Western Europe	7148	74.9	72.7
Northern Europe	3844	84.7	82.2
Australia/New Zealand	1114	108.2	104.2
Northern America	15918	124.0	119.5

Age 0-69 years - WOMEN

MACROAREA	N°	Crude Rate	ASR (W)
Eastern Asia	13582	1.9	1.6
South-Central Asia	12375	1.5	1.8
Caribbean	477	2.4	2.4
Central & Eastern Europe	5082	3.7	2.6
Micronesia	5	1.8	2.6
South America	4751	2.6	2.7
Central America	1816	2.5	2.8
Melanesia	92	2.3	3.0
Western Africa	3271	2.3	3.0
World	97746	3.1	3.1
South-Eastern Asia	8322	3.0	3.2
Eastern Africa	4128	2.7	3.4
Sub-Saharan Africa	10193	2.6	3.4
Southern Africa	908	3.2	3.6
Western Asia	3160	3.0	3.7
Polynesia	10	3.2	3.9
Northern Africa	3477	3.5	4.3
Middle Africa	1886	3.1	4.5
Southern Europe	5050	7.6	5.6
Western Europe	6930	8.5	5.6
Northern Europe	4024	9.3	6.3
Australia/New Zealand	1188	10.4	7.7
Northern America	17213	11.0	8.3

Aged 70 years and more - WOMEN

MACROAREA	N°	Crude Rate	ASR (W)
Western Africa	237	8.9	8.9
South-Central Asia	2684	10.5	10.5
Eastern Africa	359	11.6	11.6
Sub-Saharan Africa	932	12.0	11.9
Middle Africa	145	12.6	12.5
Eastern Asia	8815	16.7	15.9
Central & Eastern Europe	3196	16.2	16.3
Central America	671	20.6	20.4
South-Eastern Asia	2361	20.3	20.4
Micronesia	2	22.9	20.7
Caribbean	261	21.2	21.0
Southern Africa	191	21.4	21.0
Northern Africa	746	23.2	23.3
Western Asia	934	24.6	24.5
South America	2695	27.1	25.7
Melanesia	19	26.4	25.8
World	58949	30.7	29.5
Polynesia	4	32.0	32.9
Southern Europe	6013	50.6	47.8
Western Europe	7827	53.2	50.9
Northern Europe	3934	58.7	56.6
Australia/New Zealand	1061	79.3	75.6
Northern America	16795	91.4	88.1

*Age-Standardised Rates, World standard (per 100,000)
Source: GLOBOCAN 2008, IARC.

Table 1.4 Incidence and mortality by world macro-areas, site and gender. Numbers, crude rates and ASR(W)

NON HODGKIN LYMPHOMA - MORTALITY

Aged 0-69 years - MEN

MACROAREA	N°	Crude Rate	ASR (W)
Eastern Asia	10641	1.4	1.2
Western Europe	2418	2.9	1.9
Caribbean	375	1.9	2.0
Central America	1226	1.7	2.0
Central & Eastern Europe	3194	2.5	2.0
South-Central Asia	14129	1.6	2.0
South America	3640	2.0	2.2
Northern Europe	1470	3.4	2.3
Southern Europe	2168	3.2	2.3
World	71570	2.2	2.3
Northern America	4739	3.0	2.4
Australia/New Zealand	397	3.4	2.5
Micronesia	5	1.8	2.6
Polynesia	8	2.4	3.2
Western Africa	3691	2.6	3.3
Western Asia	3008	2.7	3.4
South-Eastern Asia	8383	3.0	3.6
Middle Africa	1434	2.4	3.7
Southern Africa	848	3.1	3.8
Sub-Saharan Africa	11065	2.9	3.8
Eastern Africa	5092	3.4	4.3
Melanesia	136	3.2	4.6
Northern Africa	4568	4.5	5.6

Aged 70 years and more - MEN

MACROAREA	N°	Crude Rate	ASR (W)
Micronesia	0	0.0	0.0
South-Central Asia	3357	15.0	15.0
Eastern Asia	7631	17.9	17.4
Central & Eastern Europe	1721	18.3	18.2
Caribbean	204	20.3	19.6
Central America	527	20.4	20.0
Western Africa	535	24.3	23.4
Southern Africa	125	24.3	24.5
Eastern Africa	606	24.8	24.8
Sub-Saharan Africa	1498	24.8	24.8
South America	1865	26.0	25.4
Western Asia	733	25.7	25.6
World	37914	26.8	26.1
Middle Africa	232	26.7	26.9
South-Eastern Asia	2825	32.6	32.5
Southern Europe	2998	37.2	35.1
Northern Africa	953	36.5	36.6
Western Europe	4086	42.8	40.4
Polynesia	4	41.3	41.3
Northern Europe	2221	48.9	45.7
Northern America	6639	51.7	47.8
Australia/New Zealand	616	59.8	55.1
Melanesia	36	58.2	57.6

Aged 0-69 years - WOMEN

MACROAREA	N°	Crude Rate	ASR (W)
Eastern Asia	5936	0.8	0.7
Central & Eastern Europe	2135	1.6	1.1
Western Europe	1486	1.8	1.1
Caribbean	242	1.2	1.2
South-Central Asia	8183	1.0	1.2
Micronesia	2	0.7	1.3
Southern Europe	1373	2.1	1.3
Central America	848	1.2	1.4
Northern Europe	923	2.1	1.4
South America	2480	1.3	1.4
Northern America	3209	2.1	1.5
World	46123	1.5	1.5
Australia/New Zealand	249	2.2	1.6
Polynesia	5	1.6	2.2
South-Eastern Asia	5768	2.1	2.3
Western Asia	2057	2.0	2.4
Western Africa	2711	1.9	2.5
Melanesia	78	1.9	2.6
Eastern Africa	3428	2.2	2.8
Sub-Saharan Africa	8401	2.2	2.8
Southern Africa	699	2.5	2.9
Northern Africa	2748	2.8	3.4
Middle Africa	1563	2.6	3.7

Aged 70 years and more - WOMEN

MACROAREA	N°	Crude Rate	ASR (W)
Micronesia	0	0.0	0.0
Western Africa	213	8.0	8.0
South-Central Asia	2508	9.8	9.8
Central & Eastern Europe	2135	10.8	10.6
Eastern Africa	335	10.8	10.8
Sub-Saharan Africa	858	11.0	11.0
Eastern Asia	6376	12.1	11.2
Middle Africa	141	12.2	12.2
Caribbean	172	14.0	13.6
Central America	504	15.4	15.0
Western Asia	674	17.8	17.6
World	35992	18.8	17.6
South America	1863	18.7	17.9
South-Eastern Asia	2120	18.3	18.2
Southern Africa	169	19.0	18.6
Northern Africa	658	20.5	20.6
Melanesia	18	25.0	24.5
Southern Europe	3400	28.6	25.7
Western Europe	4369	29.7	26.3
Northern Europe	2270	33.9	29.8
Polynesia	4	32.0	32.9
Northern America	7495	40.8	36.0
Australia/New Zealand	568	42.4	38.1

*Age-Standardised Rates, World standard (per 100,000)
Source: GLOBOCAN 2008, IARC.

Table 1.5 Incidence and mortality by world macro-areas, site and gender. Numbers, crude rates and ASR(W)

MULTIPLE MYELOMA - INCIDENCE

Aged 0-69 years - MEN

MACROAREA	N°	Crude Rate	ASR (W)
Micronesia	0	0.0	0.0
Melanesia	3	0.1	0.1
Western Africa	232	0.2	0.3
Eastern Asia	3523	0.5	0.4
South-Central Asia	3879	0.4	0.6
Sub-Saharan Africa	1403	0.4	0.7
South-Eastern Asia	1780	0.6	0.8
Middle Africa	265	0.4	0.9
Central America	499	0.7	0.9
Eastern Africa	701	0.5	0.9
Southern Africa	205	0.7	1.1
World	30934	0.9	1.1
Central & Eastern Europe	2076	1.6	1.2
South America	1861	1.0	1.2
Polynesia	3	0.9	1.2
Western Asia	998	0.9	1.3
Northern Africa	1018	1.0	1.4
Caribbean	274	1.4	1.5
Southern Europe	2204	3.3	2.2
Western Europe	3078	3.7	2.3
Northern Europe	1620	3.7	2.5
Australia/New Zealand	459	4.0	2.9
Northern America	6256	4.0	3.0

Aged 70 years and more - MEN

MACROAREA	N°	Crude Rate	ASR (W)
Melanesia	2	3.2	3.0
Western Africa	99	4.5	4.6
Middle Africa	50	5.8	5.6
South-Eastern Asia	545	6.3	6.3
Eastern Africa	156	6.4	6.4
Sub-Saharan Africa	385	6.4	6.4
South-Central Asia	1469	6.6	6.6
Eastern Asia	3024	7.1	7.0
Northern Africa	222	8.5	8.5
Central America	251	9.7	9.6
Central & Eastern Europe	1116	11.8	11.8
Western Asia	372	13.0	13.0
South America	1042	14.5	14.4
Southern Africa	80	15.6	15.6
World	23989	17.0	16.6
Caribbean	188	18.7	18.4
Micronesia	2	29.7	28.4
Southern Europe	2686	33.3	32.1
Northern Europe	1860	41.0	39.3
Western Europe	4063	42.6	41.0
Polynesia	4	41.3	41.3
Northern America	6191	48.2	46.6
Australia/New Zealand	567	55.1	52.0

Aged 0-69 years - WOMEN

MACROAREA	N°	Crude Rate	ASR (W)
Micronesia	0	0.0	0.0
Melanesia	3	0.1	0.1
Eastern Asia	2915	0.4	0.3
Western Africa	238	0.2	0.3
South-Central Asia	3288	0.4	0.5
Sub-Saharan Africa	1145	0.3	0.5
South-Eastern Asia	1554	0.6	0.6
Eastern Africa	482	0.3	0.6
Middle Africa	240	0.4	0.7
Southern Africa	185	0.7	0.8
World	24824	0.8	0.8
Central America	432	0.6	0.8
South America	1495	0.8	0.9
Central & Eastern Europe	2240	1.6	1.0
Northern Africa	744	0.7	1.0
Western Asia	725	0.7	1.0
Caribbean	242	1.2	1.2
Western Europe	2144	2.6	1.6
Northern Europe	1143	2.6	1.7
Australia/New Zealand	324	2.8	2.0
Northern America	4346	2.8	2.0
Southern Europe	2078	3.1	2.0
Polynesia	6	1.9	2.7

Aged 70 years and more - WOMEN

MACROAREA	N°	Crude Rate	ASR (W)
Polynesia	0	0.0	0.0
Melanesia	0	0.0	0.0
Western Africa	89	3.3	3.3
Middle Africa	42	3.6	3.6
South-Central Asia	954	3.7	3.7
South-Eastern Asia	498	4.3	4.3
Sub-Saharan Africa	358	4.6	4.6
Eastern Asia	2823	5.4	5.1
Eastern Africa	166	5.4	5.5
Northern Africa	193	6.0	6.0
Central America	210	6.4	6.5
Southern Africa	61	6.8	7.0
Central & Eastern Europe	1465	7.4	7.6
Western Asia	323	8.5	8.5
South America	1143	11.5	11.2
World	23079	12.0	11.5
Caribbean	199	16.2	15.4
Northern Europe	1732	25.8	24.1
Southern Europe	3202	26.9	25.1
Micronesia	2	22.9	25.7
Western Europe	4105	27.9	26.3
Northern America	5430	29.5	28.5
Australia/New Zealand	441	32.9	30.4

*Age-Standardised Rates, World standard (per 100,000)
Source: GLOBOCAN 2008, IARC.

Table 1.6 Incidence and mortality by world macro-areas, site and gender. Numbers, crude rates and ASR(W)

MULTIPLE MYELOMA - MORTALITY

Aged 0-69 years - MEN

MACROAREA	N°	Crude Rate	ASR (W)
Micronesia	0	0.0	**0.0**
Melanesia	3	0.1	**0.1**
Western Africa	204	0.1	**0.3**
Eastern Asia	2217	0.3	**0.3**
South-Central Asia	3043	0.4	**0.5**
Sub-Saharan Africa	1235	0.3	**0.6**
World	18566	0.6	**0.6**
Polynesia	2	0.6	**0.7**
South-Eastern Asia	1394	0.5	**0.7**
Eastern Africa	621	0.4	**0.8**
Central America	425	0.6	**0.8**
Central & Eastern Europe	1298	1.0	**0.8**
South America	1407	0.8	**0.9**
Southern Africa	173	0.6	**0.9**
Middle Africa	237	0.4	**0.9**
Western Europe	1376	1.7	**1.0**
Western Asia	732	0.7	**1.0**
Southern Europe	981	1.5	**1.0**
Australia/New Zealand	183	1.6	**1.1**
Caribbean	196	1.0	**1.1**
Northern Africa	886	0.9	**1.2**
Northern America	2419	1.5	**1.2**
Northern Europe	769	1.8	**1.2**

Aged 70 years and more - MEN

MACROAREA	N°	Crude Rate	ASR (W)
Melanesia	2	3.2	**3.0**
Western Africa	103	4.7	**4.7**
Middle Africa	54	6.2	**6.0**
Eastern Asia	2685	6.3	**6.2**
South-Central Asia	1479	6.6	**6.6**
Eastern Africa	165	6.7	**6.7**
Sub-Saharan Africa	407	6.7	**6.7**
South-Eastern Asia	595	6.9	**6.9**
Northern Africa	242	9.3	**9.3**
Central America	249	9.7	**9.5**
Central & Eastern Europe	971	10.3	**10.2**
Western Asia	340	11.9	**11.8**
South America	962	13.4	**13.2**
World	19229	13.6	**13.2**
Southern Africa	85	16.5	**16.6**
Caribbean	177	17.6	**17.2**
Southern Europe	2183	27.1	**25.3**
Micronesia	2	29.7	**28.4**
Northern America	3952	30.8	**28.7**
Western Europe	3076	32.2	**30.4**
Northern Europe	1507	33.2	**30.9**
Australia/New Zealand	396	38.5	**35.4**
Polynesia	4	41.3	**41.3**

Aged 0-69 years - WOMEN

MACROAREA	N°	Crude Rate	ASR (W)
Polynesia	0	0.0	**0.0**
Melanesia	3	0.1	**0.1**
Eastern Asia	1756	0.2	**0.2**
Western Africa	214	0.2	**0.3**
Eastern Africa	422	0.3	**0.5**
South-Eastern Asia	1246	0.4	**0.5**
World	15406	0.5	**0.5**
South-Central Asia	2978	0.4	**0.5**
Sub-Saharan Africa	1002	0.3	**0.5**
Middle Africa	209	0.3	**0.6**
Central & Eastern Europe	1334	1.0	**0.6**
Southern Europe	828	1.2	**0.7**
Southern Africa	157	0.6	**0.7**
South America	1167	0.6	**0.7**
Western Europe	954	1.2	**0.7**
Central America	370	0.5	**0.7**
Northern Europe	553	1.3	**0.8**
Northern America	1709	1.1	**0.8**
Western Asia	542	0.5	**0.8**
Australia/New Zealand	148	1.3	**0.9**
Northern Africa	643	0.6	**0.9**
Caribbean	171	0.9	**0.9**
Micronesia	2	0.7	**1.3**

Aged 70 years and more - WOMEN

MACROAREA	N°	Crude Rate	ASR (W)
Polynesia	0	0.0	**0.0**
Melanesia	0	0.0	**0.0**
Western Africa	92	3.5	**3.5**
South-Central Asia	929	3.6	**3.6**
South-Eastern Asia	487	4.2	**4.2**
Middle Africa	49	4.2	**4.2**
Eastern Asia	2513	4.8	**4.5**
Sub-Saharan Africa	366	4.7	**4.7**
Eastern Africa	161	5.2	**5.3**
Central America	204	6.3	**6.3**
Northern Africa	207	6.4	**6.5**
Central & Eastern Europe	1305	6.6	**6.6**
Western Asia	269	7.1	**7.1**
Southern Africa	64	7.2	**7.3**
World	19252	10.0	**9.5**
South America	1082	10.9	**10.6**
Caribbean	205	16.7	**15.9**
Southern Europe	2424	20.4	**18.5**
Northern America	3977	21.6	**19.8**
Western Europe	3319	22.6	**20.4**
Micronesia	2	22.9	**20.7**
Northern Europe	1599	23.8	**21.2**
Australia/New Zealand	364	27.2	**24.2**

*Age-Standardised Rates, World standard (per 100,000)
Source: GLOBOCAN 2008, IARC.

Table 1.7 Incidence and mortality by world macro-areas, site and gender. Numbers, crude rates and ASR(W)

LEUKAEMIA - INCIDENCE

Aged 0-69 years - MEN

MACROAREA	N°	Crude Rate	ASR (W)
Western Africa	2276	1.6	2.2
Eastern Africa	2653	1.7	2.4
Sub-Saharan Africa	6616	1.7	2.4
Middle Africa	1092	1.8	2.6
Southern Africa	595	2.2	2.6
Melanesia	108	2.6	3.0
Caribbean	616	3.1	3.3
South-Central Asia	26138	3.0	3.3
Northern Africa	3221	3.2	3.8
Micronesia	10	3.7	4.0
South America	7289	4.0	4.3
South-Eastern Asia	11963	4.3	4.6
World	143446	4.4	4.6
Eastern Asia	38325	5.0	4.8
Western Asia	4604	4.1	4.8
Central America	3692	5.2	5.3
Central & Eastern Europe	8115	6.3	5.6
Polynesia	17	5.2	6.0
Northern Europe	3472	8.0	6.5
Southern Europe	5251	7.8	6.6
Western Europe	7024	8.5	6.6
Northern America	15751	10.0	8.8
Australia/New Zealand	1234	10.7	9.1

Aged 70 years and more - MEN

MACROAREA	N°	Crude Rate	ASR (W)
Middle Africa	62	7.1	7.3
Western Africa	246	11.2	10.9
South-Central Asia	3235	14.5	14.4
Sub-Saharan Africa	888	14.7	14.7
Melanesia	9	14.6	15.3
Eastern Africa	408	16.7	16.7
South-Eastern Asia	1537	17.7	17.7
Northern Africa	523	20.1	20.0
Central America	555	21.5	20.7
Eastern Asia	9230	21.7	21.3
Micronesia	2	29.7	28.4
Caribbean	307	30.6	28.9
Western Asia	909	31.9	31.6
South America	2391	33.4	32.1
Southern Africa	172	33.5	34.4
World	52010	36.8	35.8
Central & Eastern Europe	4136	43.9	43.7
Polynesia	5	51.6	51.4
Southern Europe	5069	62.9	59.9
Northern Europe	3134	69.1	66.0
Western Europe	6860	71.9	68.9
Australia/New Zealand	987	95.9	90.1
Northern America	12233	95.3	90.2

Aged 0-69 years - WOMEN

MACROAREA	N°	Crude Rate	ASR (W)
Eastern Africa	2008	1.3	1.6
Sub-Saharan Africa	5001	1.3	1.7
Western Africa	1751	1.2	1.8
Southern Africa	454	1.6	1.8
Middle Africa	788	1.3	1.9
Melanesia	79	1.9	2.1
South-Central Asia	19013	2.3	2.5
Micronesia	6	2.2	2.5
Northern Africa	2330	2.3	2.6
Caribbean	530	2.7	2.7
South America	5850	3.2	3.3
World	111347	3.5	3.6
Western Asia	3467	3.3	3.7
Central & Eastern Europe	6856	5.0	4.0
South-Eastern Asia	10937	3.9	4.2
Eastern Asia	31455	4.4	4.2
Northern Europe	2305	5.3	4.4
Western Europe	4698	5.8	4.6
Central America	3269	4.5	4.7
Polynesia	14	4.5	5.3
Southern Europe	4122	6.2	5.5
Northern America	10617	6.8	6.0
Australia/New Zealand	798	7.0	6.1

Aged 70 years and more - WOMEN

MACROAREA	N°	Crude Rate	ASR (W)
Micronesia	0	0.0	0.0
Middle Africa	24	2.1	2.1
Eastern Africa	153	4.9	5.0
Melanesia	4	5.6	5.7
Sub-Saharan Africa	586	7.5	7.6
South-Central Asia	2080	8.2	8.1
Southern Africa	94	10.5	10.8
Northern Africa	361	11.2	11.4
Western Africa	315	11.8	11.6
South-Eastern Asia	1470	12.7	12.6
Eastern Asia	7099	13.5	13.1
Central America	500	15.3	14.7
Western Asia	590	15.6	15.3
Caribbean	253	20.6	18.9
South America	2258	22.7	21.3
World	43631	22.7	21.7
Central & Eastern Europe	4435	22.5	22.5
Polynesia	4	32.0	32.9
Southern Europe	4373	36.8	33.8
Northern Europe	2556	38.1	35.5
Western Europe	6010	40.8	37.6
Australia/New Zealand	731	54.6	50.2
Northern America	10322	56.2	51.8

*Age-Standardised Rates, World standard (per 100,000)
Source: GLOBOCAN 2008, IARC.

Table 1.8 Incidence and mortality by world macro-areas, site and gender. Numbers, crude rates and ASR(W)

LEUKAEMIA - MORTALITY

Aged 0-69 years - MEN

MACROAREA	N°	Crude Rate	ASR (W)
Polynesia	5	1.5	1.6
Western Africa	2159	1.5	2.0
Eastern Africa	2503	1.7	2.2
Sub-Saharan Africa	6236	1.6	2.2
Southern Africa	538	2.0	2.3
Middle Africa	1036	1.7	2.4
South-Central Asia	20566	2.4	2.6
Northern Europe	1490	3.4	2.6
Western Europe	3039	3.7	2.6
Caribbean	503	2.6	2.7
Australia/New Zealand	408	3.5	2.8
Melanesia	104	2.5	2.9
Northern America	5494	3.5	2.9
Southern Europe	2656	4.0	3.0
South America	5534	3.0	3.2
World	99297	3.0	3.2
Northern Africa	2977	3.0	3.4
Eastern Asia	28140	3.7	3.5
Central & Eastern Europe	5346	4.2	3.5
Micronesia	8	3.0	3.7
Western Asia	3791	3.4	3.9
Central America	2649	3.7	3.9
South-Eastern Asia	10351	3.7	4.0

Aged 70 years and more - MEN

MACROAREA	N°	Crude Rate	ASR (W)
Middle Africa	64	7.4	7.5
Western Africa	240	10.9	10.7
Sub-Saharan Africa	875	14.5	14.5
Melanesia	9	14.6	15.3
South-Central Asia	3451	15.4	15.4
Eastern Africa	401	16.4	16.4
South-Eastern Asia	1492	17.2	17.2
Eastern Asia	8333	19.5	19.2
Northern Africa	519	19.9	19.8
Central America	561	21.8	20.9
Caribbean	280	27.9	26.6
Micronesia	2	29.7	28.4
Western Asia	838	29.4	29.1
World	44258	31.3	30.3
South America	2296	32.0	30.7
Southern Africa	170	33.1	34.1
Central & Eastern Europe	3499	37.2	36.7
Polynesia	4	41.3	41.3
Northern Europe	2456	54.1	50.3
Southern Europe	4738	58.8	54.7
Western Europe	5888	61.7	57.8
Australia/New Zealand	668	64.9	59.5
Northern America	8349	65.0	59.9

Aged 0-69 years - WOMEN

MACROAREA	N°	Crude Rate	ASR (W)
Micronesia	0	0.0	0.0
Polynesia	4	1.3	1.4
Eastern Africa	1898	1.2	1.5
Southern Africa	419	1.5	1.6
Sub-Saharan Africa	4736	1.2	1.6
Northern Europe	980	2.3	1.7
Western Africa	1671	1.2	1.7
Western Europe	1958	2.4	1.7
Australia/New Zealand	251	2.2	1.8
Middle Africa	748	1.2	1.8
Northern America	3477	2.2	1.8
South-Central Asia	15068	1.8	2.0
Southern Europe	1773	2.7	2.0
Caribbean	425	2.1	2.1
Melanesia	76	1.9	2.1
Central & Eastern Europe	4377	3.2	2.4
Northern Africa	2164	2.2	2.4
South America	4398	2.4	2.5
World	76883	2.4	2.5
Eastern Asia	22502	3.2	3.0
Western Asia	2926	2.8	3.1
Central America	2306	3.2	3.4
South-Eastern Asia	9462	3.4	3.6

Aged 70 years and more - WOMEN

MACROAREA	N°	Crude Rate	ASR (W)
Middle Africa	23	2.0	2.0
Eastern Africa	152	4.9	4.9
Melanesia	4	5.6	5.7
Sub-Saharan Africa	557	7.1	7.2
South-Central Asia	2142	8.4	8.3
Southern Africa	87	9.8	10.0
Northern Africa	343	10.7	10.7
Western Africa	295	11.1	10.9
South-Eastern Asia	1353	11.7	11.6
Eastern Asia	6310	12.0	11.6
Western Asia	535	14.1	13.7
Central America	495	15.2	14.5
World	36723	19.1	18.0
Caribbean	251	20.4	18.8
Central & Eastern Europe	3815	19.4	18.9
South America	2127	21.4	20.1
Micronesia	2	22.9	20.7
Northern Europe	2155	32.1	28.3
Southern Europe	3996	33.6	29.9
Western Europe	5356	36.4	31.9
Northern America	6751	36.7	32.1
Polynesia	4	32.0	32.9
Australia/New Zealand	527	39.4	34.2

*Age-Standardised Rates, World standard (per 100,000)

Source: GLOBOCAN 2008, IARC.

As regards developing countries, the rates were low, but the data from Asia and Africa in particular, have to be taken with caution owing to the low percentage of population observed by cancer registries, which must afford a hard challenge to provide complete and reliable data.

Considering all hematological tumours, and comparing the incidence and mortality rates in developing and developed countries, it is possible to individuate two specific patterns; in contrast to incidence which was always higher in Europe, Australia and Northern America both in younger and older age groups and in both sexes, mortality under 70 years had a less clear worldwide distribution, with developing countries showing often the highest rates. Only in the elderly, the developed countries showed the highest mortality values.

Non Hodgkin's Lymphomas

For NHL all more developed countries have higher incidence rates than developing ones (Table 1.1): in men aged from 0 to 69 years, the values of men ranged from 2.5 in Eastern Asia to 11.9 in Northern America and those of women from 1.6 in Eastern Asia to 8.3 in Northern America. In the elderly the rank of considered countries did not change but rates strikingly higher with respect younger patients were recorded; in men rates ranged from 16.3 in South-Central Asia to 119.5 in Northern America and in women from 8.9 in Western Africa to 88.1. A very huge gap was observed between older and younger age groups: in more developed countries the elderly showed rates 10 times higher than in younger people, both in women and men.

For mortality the rank of countries was less definite than for incidence (Table 1.2). In younger age groups both in men and women the lowest rates (under the mean of the world) were registered not only in developing countries but also in some developed areas. Not surprisingly the highest values were observed in African macro-areas, probably due to a more diffuse exposure to infectious agent risks. A different situation was reported in the elderly, with higher mortality rates registered in more developed macro-areas, exception made for Central-Eastern Europe, while those lower in countries of the third world. This model was very similar to that observed for incidence, and a very wide difference between the elderly and younger people was observed also for mortality (rates were about 10 times higher in older compared to younger age group, in both sexes). Intriguing was the exception of Melanesia and Polynesia which followed the Australian rates and the very low rates of Central and Eastern Europe occurring for incidence and mortality in both sexes.

Among more developed countries, US had the tendency to show always rates higher than those reported in European areas. In these countries and in North America the most frequent histological types are nodal and follicular disease which account for 30 % of NHL in US and 20 % in Europe; such types are rare in developing world [45, 46]. Asiatic countries more frequently show intermediate-grade, high-grade diffuse aggressive [47] or peripheral T-cell NHL, extranodal disease, strongly associated with EBV and human T-cell leukaemia/lymphoma virus type 1

(HTLV-1) infection [48], whereas follicular lymphomas are rare. In Africa an excess of high-grade NHL has been observed, while the follicular subtype is rare. Burkitt's lymphoma is very common, accounting for 25–44 % of all NHL [49] and occurring more frequently in children with a peak around seven years and involving more rarely older individuals.

Leukaemia

Like for NHL, also leukaemia incidence showed a clear pattern, similar in younger and older age groups (Table 1.3). Both in young and elderly people, all developed countries had the highest rates, followed by Central America, Asian countries and lastly Africans. The mortality pattern was partially different (Table 1.4). For the young group in both sexes Asian macro-areas had the highest rates followed by Central America, Europe and Northern America and Africa ones. Considering elderly patients the pattern was again similar to that of incidence with all developed countries showing the highest rates followed by Central America, Asia and Africa. The differences between the two age groups were striking, and in the developed countries the elderly had rates 15 and 10 times higher than younger people in men and women respectively. It is interesting to underline that many of the single countries at higher incidence (data not shown) often are those were in the recent past the inhabitants could be exposed to radiations (depleted uranium bullets) or chemical agents (defoliants as the orange agent) during the conflicts that bathed in blood these for many years.

Multiple Myeloma

The country rank, reported for incidence of NHL and leukaemia, still recurred for MM (Table 1.5). In fact, both in the two age groups and in both sexes the highest rates were observed for developed countries followed by Central and South America and African macro-regions. Central and Eastern Europe represented, as already seen above, an exception within the European continent, showing much lower rates, almost at level of developing countries.

The pattern observed for leukaemia mortality recurred also for MM (Table 1.6). For the young group the highest rates were registered not only in the developed countries, but also in some unexpected developing regions of Africa, Central America and Asia. With respect to the elderly, the distribution returned to be "classic", with more affluent countries having the highest rates, followed by macro-regions with decreasing affluence. The exception of the low rates in Central and Eastern Europe still remained as well as the bizarre behaviour of insular areas of Oceania. The differences in incidence rates by age group were highest in affluent areas with rates 17 and 11 times higher in the elderly than in younger people, for men and women respectively. For mortality the same ratios increased to 34 and 19.

Hodgkin's Lymphoma

This hematological malignancy is typical of children and adolescents, representing in the elderly only a very small part of all combined cancers. The incidence rates for both sexes did not overcome 2.6 in the young group and 6.1 in the elderly, while mortality rates did not exceed 1.5 in younger people and 7.3 in the elderly (Table 1.7). In the younger group incidence pattern showed the "classic", already observed, gradient: developed countries had the highest rates followed, as usual, by the poorer populations, in both sexes and age groups. Less definite was the rank for the elderly with some African areas having rates among the highest in the world. The older individuals of Northern America and Southern Europe had rates around 2 times higher than the younger ones and in women this ratio was even lower, demonstrating that this tumour is prevalently a paediatric tumour.

This gradient was completely inverted for mortality (Table 1.8). The highest rates were observed for African and Asian areas, followed by Central and South America and, finally, by the affluent Western macro-areas. However, the rates were so low that any comment is probably unreliable and it must be taken with caution.

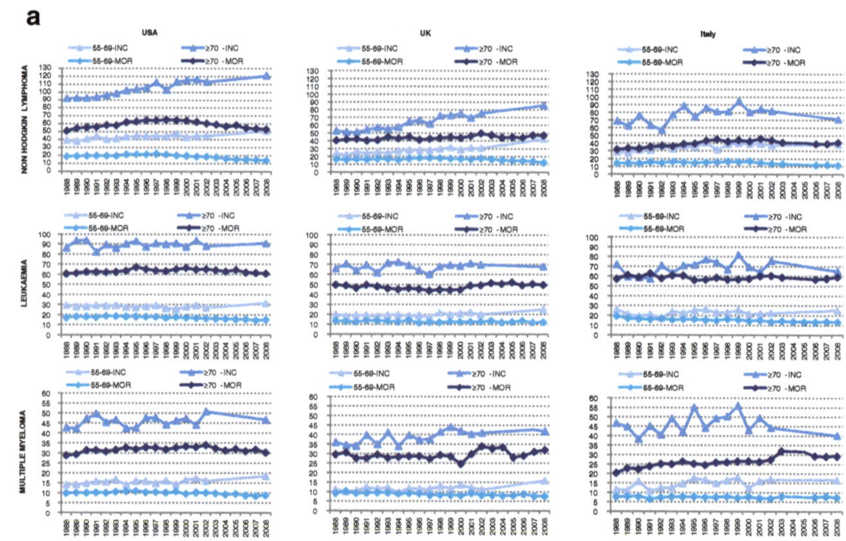

Fig. 1.4 (**a**) Incidence and mortality trend of Non-Hodgkin Lymphomas, Multiple Myeloma and Leukemia in USA, UK (England & Wales) and Italy. MEN – Aged ≥70 years vs. the 55–69 ones (ASR-W). (**b**) Incidence and mortality trend of Non-Hodgkin Lymphomas, Multiple Myeloma and Leukemia in USA, UK (England & Wales) and Italy. WOMEN – Aged ≥70 years vs. the 55–69 ones (ASR-W)

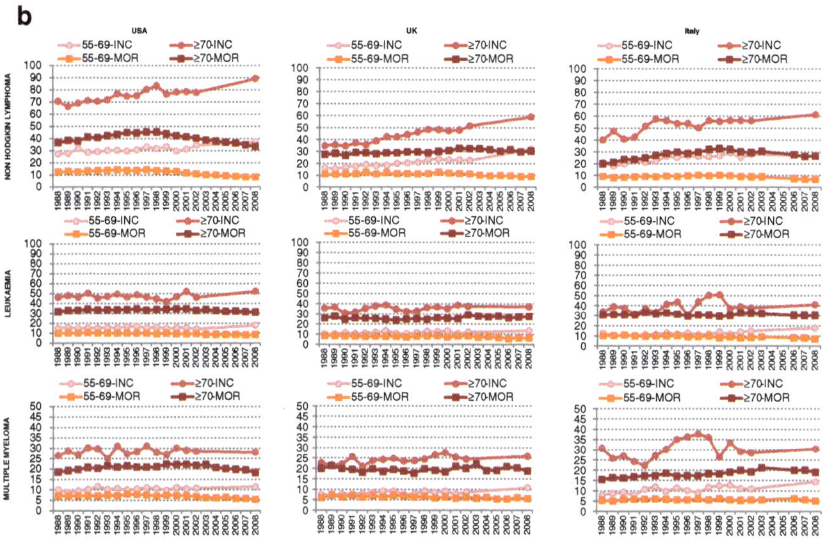

Fig. 1.4 (continued)

Time Trends

Figure 1.7 for men and Fig. 1.8 for women give incidence and mortality time trends (age standardised rates according to world standard population) from 1988 to 2008 for NHL, leukaemia and MM, comparing middle aged adults (55–69 years) with the elderly aged 70 or more years. The HL trends are not reported due to the low numbers and their instability in time.

We choose three examples of developed countries, having a high occurrence of hematological malignancies, such as Italy and UK for Southern and Northern Europe as well as US.

Incidence rates from 1988 to 2002 came from the IARC publication of Cancer Incidence in five Continents, therefore directly observed by cancer registries (9 for US, 5 for UK and 6 for Italy) [44], while the expected rates of 2008 were drawn from the database of Globocan estimates [1], that came from modelling procedures, and data for the 2003–2007 intermediate period were interpolated. For this reason the more recent estimated part of trend should be interpreted cautiously.

Death certification data derived by WHO databank [50]. Italian mortality data for 2004 and 2005 not produced by ISTAT (the Italian national institute of statistics) were interpolated [51].

Incidence and mortality trends were analysed by means of Join point regression models, using the Joinpoint Regression Program in order to obtain the Annual

Percent Changes (APCs) and the Joinpoints years (JPs). The time-trend is divided into segments and the number of segments depends on the number of JPs. The JP year is the point in time when we estimate a variation in time trend [52].

Non Hodgkin's Lymphomas

NHL incidence rates increased in all the three countries, both sexes and age groups. The largest variations were observed for UK, where all the rates grew about 3 % yearly, with younger people showing a faster pace since 2003–2004. Over the whole period in the elderly rates increased from 53 to 86 new cases per 100,000 in men and from 35 to 59 in women. The rise was marked also in US with a significant upward trend in younger individuals of both sexes (APC around 1.1–1.4), while in the elderly women showed an increase from 71 to 89 new cases and in men, after a quick rise, a levelling from 2000 (rates from 92 to 121 over the whole period). In Italy the picture was a little better. In middle aged adults of both sexes an early growth until 1994 was observed, followed by a levelling leading to an overall rise of 1.4 and 1.7 % in men and women respectively. In elderly men the rates increased quickly until 2000 thereafter decreased from 81 to 72, in women increased from 40 to 62 during the entire period.

Summarising, the epidemic growth of NHL observed during the second half of twentieth century was not finished in 2008, especially in UK and US. However, we found an encouraging levelling or a slight decline from the early 2000s in Italian elderly of both sexes and in older American men.

As regards mortality, trends were more favourable. Downward trends were noted in the three countries for almost every age or sex. After a strike increase until the end of 1990s a reversal of trend was reported, particularly in Italy and US; in contrast, in UK the rates of the elderly still increased. In younger Italian people of both sexes mortality fell since 1999 (APC about −4 %), while the corresponding value of older patients were slightly lower (about −1.5 %). A similar picture appeared in US where the APCs were equal to those reported in Italy. The rates declined since 1998 from 65 to 54 and since 1997 from 46 to 34 in men and women respectively. The trends were good also in English younger groups, with decreasing rates since the end of 1990s (−5 and −3.4 % in men and women). On the contrary the rates of the elderly continued to increase over the entire period from 41 to 47 in men and from 28 to 30 in women.

Summarising, NHL showed a very clear and definite pattern: an early rise followed by decreasing rates, very quick in younger adults and little bit slower in older ones; the older group had not encouraging trends in UK.

NHL are one of the few tumours whose incidence and mortality have been increasing in Europe and North America over the last decades. Unlike incidence, still rising, mortality rates have started to level off or even to declined during the most recent years [53]. Some authors affirm that the striking incidence growth could be related with improved diagnostic procedures over time [54]. Moreover, a role at least partial could be played by changes in classification and registration [55, 56]. However, it is probable that these two phenomena have not caused a so large and generalised increase and it is conceivable that the overall growth of newly diagnosed cases is real, although a plausible causal hypothesis has not been found.

Leukaemia

Unlike NHL, leukaemia incidence trends did not present a definite pattern. The rates were very often stable or weakly growing, without any tendency to decrease. In Italy the rates of both sexes and age groups were quite stable, exception made for an upward trend in younger women (APC 2.6 %). In UK trends were slightly poorer: rates increased steadily and significantly over the whole period for each considered group (APC ranging from 0.5 to 1.2 %), except for elderly men who had a stable trend. Also American trends were less favourable than those of Italy. In middle aged adults of both sexes after an early period of stability followed a rise from the early 2000s, while the trends of the older age groups were stable in both sexes.

At a first glance at leukaemia mortality in all the three countries, it is possible to highlight an encouraging general picture with rates often decreasing. The American trends were the most favourable; at the beginning, the rates were stable or growing, thereafter since 1990s declining in both age groups and sexes. The rates of elderly decreased since 2000 from 67 to 61 (APC −1 %) in men and from 35 to 31 (APC −1.3 %) in women. In Italy trends differed by age; in younger individuals of both sexes a continuous decline was registered (APC around −1.5 %), whilst in the elderly the rates were completely steady. In UK mortality trends had various behaviours; in the middle aged adults trends were stable in men and decreasing since 2002 in women. In the elderly we found stable rates in women and a rise since 1997 in men (from 44 to 50, APC 1.4 %).

Summarising, unlike incidence which had no tendency to decrease, mortality was often declining or at least steady also in the elderly (especially in US).

Multiple Myeloma

Incidence rates of MM were almost all increasing for both sexes and the two age groups, without any particular characteristic related to ageing. However, notwithstanding the significant APCs, the growth was weak, and differences in the number of cases from 1988 to 2008 ranged from 2 to 5 cases per 100,000 in different age groups and sexes.

Only in Italian elderly people of both sexes a tendency to level off was observed, as well as in elderly American women. Mortality trends were more favourable in younger than in older people. In Italy the rates in the younger adults of both sexes were steady, whilst in the elderly increased from 21 to 29 (APC 1.7 %) in men and from 16 to 19 (APC 1.3 %) in women. In UK the younger individuals of both sexes had downward trends (−1.5 % in men and −1 % in women), whereas trends of the elderly were stable. Also in US a similar pattern was found: decrease of rates in younger group of both sexes since 1996 and stability in elderly men and women.

Summarising, nevertheless the low rates reported especially for incidence, it was possible to note how the elderly of both sexes were slightly disadvantaged with respect the younger counterpart.

Survival

Table 1.9 illustrates the relative survival at 1 (RS-1 %) and 5 years (RS-5 %) from diagnosis, and their confidence intervals at 95 % level, in US and Italy by sex and the two age groups of elderly (70 or more years) and middle aged adults (55–69 years). Italian data came from 19 cancer registries belonging to the association of Italian cancer registry (database AIRTUM), while US data came from 18 cancer registries belonging to SEER Program.

Table 1.9 shows the differences in prognosis between the two groups, computed in order to underline the prognostic disadvantage of older people with respect to younger individuals.

RS is a net survival measure representing cancer survival in the absence of other causes of death and it is defined as the ratio of observed survivors proportion in a cohort of cancer patients to the proportion of expected survivors in a comparable set of cancer free individuals. To an easy comprehension the ratios are presented multiplied per 100.

We applied the method of period analysis for estimating RS rates; this methodology better reflects the survival experience of cancer patients diagnosed during the last available period (2005–2007) [57]. All the analyses have been performed through SEER*Stat software [58].

RS-1 % and RS-5 % in the 55–69 Age Group

RS-1 % in US ranged from 77 to 96 % in younger men and from 74 to 97 % in younger women, AML representing the tumour with the lowest figures (44 % in men and 47 % in women). In Italy the corresponding values ranged from 82 to 99 % and from 73 to 98 %, whilst AML showed the lowest rates (57 % in men and 43 % in women).

In Italian men the highest rates of RS-1 % were observed for CLL and CML (99 % and 92 %), followed by NHL, overall leukaemia, MM and HL (values higher than 82 %). The situation was very similar in women, except for HL, which had rates higher than in men (92 % vs 84 %).

In Italy the highest RS-5 % rates were registered for CLL (82 % in men and 84 % in women), whilst the rates of other tumours fell, moving the attention from 1 to 5 years from diagnosis. In men rates ranged from 54 to 69 % for NHL, overall leukaemia, MM, HL and CML, whilst AML had the lowest survival (only 14 %). In women the rates were quite similar to those of men for MM, CLL, AML and CML, whereas they differed for NHL (69 % in men and 77 % in women), overall

Table 1.9 Relative survival rates (%) at 1 and 5 years since diagnosis (RS-1 % and RS-5 %) by site and gender in United States of America and Italy (2005–2007 period)

	United States of America													
	RS-1 %	***CI 95 %***		**RS-1 %**	***CI 95 %***		**1-year differences**[a]	**RS-5 %**	***CI 95 %***		**RS-5 %**	***CI 95 %***		**5-years differences**[a]
		Inf.	*Sup.*		*Inf.*	*Sup.*			*Inf.*	*Sup.*		*Inf.*	*Sup.*	
	MEN 55–69 years			**MEN 70+ years**				**MEN 55–69 years**			**MEN 70+ yrs**			
Non Hodgkin's Lymphomas	84.3	*83.5*	*85.1*	71.0	*70.0*	*72.0*	**13.3**	68.7	*67.4*	*69.8*	53.3	*51.9*	*54.7*	**15.4**
Leukaemia	77.1	*75.8*	*78.3*	57.5	*56.2*	*58.8*	**19.6**	58.0	*56.3*	*59.5*	37.4	*35.8*	*38.9*	**20.6**
Multiple Myeloma	80.2	*78.6*	*81.7*	64.5	*62.8*	*66.2*	**15.7**	46.2	*44.1*	*48.3*	27.4	*25.4*	*29.3*	**18.8**
Hodgkin's Lymphoma	83.2	*79.9*	*86.0*	59.7	*54.8*	*64.3*	**23.5**	67.6	*63.0*	*71.8*	42.9	*36.5*	*49.1*	**24.7**
Chronic Lymphoid Leukaemia	95.6	*94.5*	*96.5*	87.5	*85.9*	*88.9*	**8.1**	82.8	*80.7*	*84.7*	65.1	*62.5*	*67.6*	**17.7**
Acute Myeloid Leukaemia	44.1	*41.1*	*47.0*	17.8	*16.1*	*19.5*	**26.3**	15.7	*13.4*	*18.1*	3.7	*2.8*	*4.8*	**12.0**
Chronic Myeloid Leukaemia	83.8	*80.2*	*86.8*	66.4	*62.8*	*69.8*	**17.4**	57.4	*52.5*	*61.9*	32.0	*27.9*	*36.2*	**25.4**
	WOMEN 55–69 years			**WOMEN 70+**				**WOMEN 55–69 years**			**WOMEN 70+**			
Non Hodgkin's Lymphomas	87.2	*86.4*	*88.1*	71.6	*70.7*	*72.6*	**15.6**	75.9	*74.7*	*77.1*	56.3	*54.9*	*57.6*	**19.6**
Leukaemia	73.5	*71.9*	*75.1*	56.0	*54.6*	*57.4*	**17.5**	55.9	*53.9*	*57.8*	39.3	*37.7*	*41.0*	**16.6**
Multiple Myeloma	82.1	*80.3*	*83.8*	64.6	*62.8*	*66.4*	**17.5**	48.3	*45.8*	*50.7*	26.9	*25.1*	*28.8*	**21.4**
Hodgkin's Lymphoma	83.4	*79.2*	*86.8*	59.1	*54.1*	*63.7*	**24.3**	72.6	*67.3*	*77.3*	40.7	*35.0*	*46.3*	**31.9**
Chronic Lymphoid Leukaemia	97.3	*96.0*	*98.2*	88.9	*87.3*	*90.4*	**8.4**	87.8	*85.3*	*89.9*	72.4	*69.5*	*75.0*	**15.4**

(continued)

Table 1.9 (continued)

Acute Myeloid Leukaemia	46.5	*43.2*	*49.8*	17.3	*15.5*	*19.2*	**29.2**	21.6	*18.8*	*24.5*	4.5	*3.4*	*5.9*	**17.1**
Chronic Myeloid Leukaemia	85.5	*81.3*	*88.8*	63.6	*59.5*	*67.4*	**21.9**	63.7	*57.8*	*68.9*	31.5	*27.3*	*35.8*	**32.2**
	Italy													
	RS-1 %	***CI 95 %***		**RS-5 %**	***CI 95 %***		**1-year differences[a]**	**RS-1 %**	***CI 95 %***		**RS-5 %**	***CI 95 %***		**5-years differences[a]**
		Inf.	*Sup.*		*Inf.*	*Sup.*			*Inf.*	*Sup.*		*Inf.*	*Sup.*	
	MEN 55–69 years			**MEN 70+ years**				**MEN 55–69 years**			**MEN 70+ yrs**			
Non Hodgkin's Lymphomas	85.5	*83.2*	*87.5*	70.8	*68.1*	*73.4*	**14.7**	69.3	*66.4*	*72.1*	52.6	*49.2*	*55.9*	**16.7**
Leukaemia	82.3	*78.3*	*85.7*	53.3	*48.9*	*57.5*	**29.0**	57.0	*52.4*	*61.4*	30.0	*26.0*	*34.1*	**27.0**
Multiple Myeloma	86.3	*82.1*	*89.5*	73.3	*69.0*	*77.1*	**13.0**	53.8	*49.0*	*58.4*	34.7	*30.0*	*39.4*	**19.1**
Hodgkin's Lymphoma	83.7	*73.7*	*90.1*	60.0	*47.2*	*70.7*	**23.7**	66.0	*55.2*	*74.7*	35.1	*23.5*	*46.9*	**30.9**
Chronic Lymphoid Leukaemia	99.0	*92.4*	*99.9*	87.6	*80.1*	*92.4*	**11.4**	81.9	*75.5*	*86.8*	58.9	*50.0*	*66.8*	**23.0**
Acute Myeloid Leukaemia	56.9	*47.4*	*65.4*	21.3	*15.8*	*27.3*	**35.6**	13.7	*8.4*	*20.4*	5.2	*2.7*	*8.9*	**8.5**
Chronic Myeloid Leukaemia	92.2	*80.2*	*97.1*	75.7	*64.2*	*84.0*	**16.5**	59.4	*45.7*	*70.7*	37.3	*26.0*	*48.5*	**22.1**
	WOMEN 55–69 years			**WOMEN 70+**				**WOMEN 55–69 years**			**WOMEN 70+**			
Non Hodgkin's Lymphomas	89.1	*86.8*	*91.0*	66.9	*64.2*	*69.4*	**22.2**	76.9	*73.9*	*79.5*	50.7	*47.6*	*53.7*	**26.2**
Leukaemia	73.3	*67.2*	*78.5*	52.9	*48.0*	*57.7*	**20.4**	50.5	*44.8*	*56.0*	31.0	*26.6*	*35.5*	**19.5**
Multiple Myeloma	85.7	*81.2*	*89.2*	73.2	*68.9*	*76.9*	**12.5**	52.1	*46.9*	*57.1*	34.7	*30.4*	*39.1*	**17.4**
Hodgkin's Lymphoma	91.5	*80.3*	*96.5*	73.8	*60.2*	*83.4*	**17.7**	81.3	*68.8*	*89.1*	51.7	*37.3*	*64.4*	**29.6**

Chronic Lymphoid Leukaemia	97.7	*88.9*	*99.5*	81.2	*72.2*	*87.5*	**16.5**	84.1	*75.7*	*89.8*	59.8	*50.0*	*68.3*	**24.3**
Acute Myeloid Leukaemia	43.3	*32.6*	*53.5*	24.1	*17.4*	*31.4*	**19.2**	17.6	*11.2*	*25.2*	3.8	*1.5*	*7.6*	**13.8**
Chronic Myeloid Leukaemia	94.9	*78.8*	*98.9*	69.2	*54.9*	*79.7*	**25.7**	60.7	*45.9*	*72.6*	31.4	*20.5*	*42.8*	**29.3**

[a]Differences between relative survival of the elderly aged 70 years or more and that of middle aged adults (55–69 years)

leukaemia (57 % in men and 51 % in women) and HL (66 % in men and 81 % in women).

In American men the highest RS-1 % was observed for CLL (96 %), like in Italy, followed by NHL, CML, HL, MM and overall leukaemia (values over 77 %); AML only had rates lower than 45 %. For women the tumour rank and the absolute values were similar. As regards RS-5 % in men, CLL showed the best prognosis (83 %) followed by NHL, HL, overall leukaemia, CML, which maintained a fairly good prognosis (ranging from 58 to 69 %). MM showed lower values (46 %), while AML had a very poor prognosis (16 %). Women showed values similar to those of men for overall leukaemia and MM, while the rates of NHL, HL, CLL, AML and CML where higher in women.

RS-1 % and RS-5 % in Patients Aged 70 or More Years

As expected, RS-1 % showed values higher than RS-5 % for all hematological tumours in both sexes, as already noted for younger patients. The fact that the elderly had always rates lower than those of middle aged adults, both for RS-1 % and RS-5 %, was noteworthy.

In Italian men RS-1 % remained fairly good, over 53 % for all considered tumours, except AML showing much lower rates (around 21 %). Survival declined largely at 5 years after diagnosis for all tumours whose rates were always under 53 %, except CLL (59 %), reaching the poorest prognosis for AML (5 %). In women RS-1 % was lower than in men, except HL and AML. RS-5 % of women was very similar to men, except HL (35 % in men and 52 % in women) and CML (37 % in men and 31 % in women).

In US, elderly men and women showed almost identical RS-1 % rates for every considered tumour.

The prognoses were quite good ranging in both sexes from about 57 % for overall leukaemia to 88–89 % for CLL, exception made for AML with very low rates (around 17 %). Also RS-5 % was almost identical by gender, except CLL. Survival rates were always under 56 %, with the exception of CLL, which had the best prognosis (65 % and 72 % in men and women respectively) like in Italy. AML, as usually, was the subtype of leukaemia with the poorest prognosis (under 5 %).

Differences by Age

In the last decade some articles dealing with the differences in prognosis between elderly and middle aged adults have been published [59, 60]. All these works have found a very high mortality excess in the elderly, with a particular disadvantage in women for gynaecological cancers and NHL, even if also men presented death risks very high. The excess of deaths was greater at 1 compared to 5 years from diagnosis because an elderly patient, who survives the first period of diagnostic and therapeutic procedures, experiences a prognosis similar to that of a younger one.

In the present study a clear difference by gender was not noted: elderly women showed survival sometimes higher, sometimes lower than men. Second, the disadvantage of the elderly, usually more marked at 1 year since diagnosis, now is similar to that at 5 years. Third, there was no systematic difference in survival between the two countries, although some minor variations existed.

The most relevant result is the confirmation of a really great difference in prognosis between the elderly and middle aged adults, depending neither by sex nor by time after diagnosis or by country, but exclusively by the type of considered hematological malignancy.

For RS-1 % in both countries, CLL, NHL and MM showed the lowest differences between the two age groups, that is the smallest prognostic disadvantage of the elderly compared to younger adults: for CLL in US about 8 units in both sexes, in Italy 11 and 17 units in men and women; for NHL in US about 14 units in both sexes, in Italy 15 and 22 in men and women; for MM in US about 16 in men and 18 in women, in Italy 13 in both sexes. On the contrary the largest elderly disadvantage was reported for AML (in US 26 in men and 29 in women, in Italy 36 in men and 19 in women) and HL (in US 24 in both sexes, in Italy 24 in men and 18 in women). At a first glance differences by countries did not exist.

Also for RS-5 % the lowest disadvantage of elderly was reported in US for CLL (around 16 in both sexes), NHL (15 in men and 20 in women) and AML (12 in men and 17 in women). An intermediate difference by age was observed for MM and overall leukaemia. The elderly experienced a very large prognostic disadvantage for CML and HL (25 in men and 32 in women). In Italy the smallest gap was observed for NHL in women (17), overall leukaemia in women (20), MM (19 in men and 17 in women) and AML (9 in men and 14 in women). Very large differences were noted for overall leukaemia in man (27), HL (31 in men and 30 in women), CLL (23 in men and 24 in women) and CML (22 in men and 29 in women).

Summarising, elderly patients experienced a marked disadvantage in survival with respect middle aged adults. This gap did not depend on gender, country or time of follow up, but was correlated strongly to the type of hematological neoplasm.

The causes of these differences can be various; first of all, a difficult health care access linked to clinical problems. The impaired physiological status of old patients, along with different comorbid conditions, can mask the real symptoms of a tumour, influencing a not timely diagnosis and, as a consequence, an advanced stage [61]. A delayed access to health care, particularly for the elderly, can be related to socio-economic status: a low income, a low educational level attained, an insufficient social support (elderly women are often widow) may lead to a delay in seeking medical advice [59].

Treatment procedures represent the second main cause of prognostic gap. Elderly patient can be treated only on the basis of chronological age"per se", without a comprehensive geriatric assessment, which could evaluated the whole condition of an old individual. In this case undertreatment, without a curative intent may represent one of the main reasons of the survival differences [62–64].

References

1. Ferlay J, Shin HR, Bray F, Forman D, Mathers C, Parkin DM. GLOBOCAN 2008 v2.0, Cancer Incidence and Mortality Worldwide: IARC CancerBase No. 10 [Internet]. Lyon: International Agency for Research on Cancer; 2010. Available from: http://globocan.iarc.fr.
2. Berg SL, Steuber P, Poplack DG. Clinical manifestations of acute lymphoblastic leukemia. In: Hoffman R, Benz Jr EJ, Shattil SJ, Furie B, Cohen HJ, Silberstein LE, McGlave P, editors. Hematology, basic principles and practice. New York: Churchill Livingstone; 2000. p. 1070–8.
3. Rubnitz JE, Look AT. Pathobiology of acute lymphoblastic leukemia. In: Hoffman R, Benz Jr EJ, Shattil SJ, Furie B, Cohen HJ, Silberstein LE, McGlave P, editors. Hematology, basic principles and practice. New York: Churchill Livingstone; 2000. p. 1052–69.
4. Allman D, Miller JP. The aging of early B-cell precursors. Immunol Rev. 2005;205:18–29.
5. Min H, Montecino-Rodriguez E, Dorshkind K. Effects of aging on early B- and T-cell development. Immunol Rev. 2005;205:7–17.
6. Woolthuis CM, de Haan G, Huls G. Aging of hematopoietic stem cells: intrinsic changes or micro-environmental effects? Curr Opin Immunol. 2011;23(4):512–7.
7. Johnson KM, Owen K, Witte PL. Aging and developmental transitions in the B cell lineage. Int Immunol. 2002;14:1313–23.
8. Heng TS, Goldberg GL, Gray DH, Sutherland JS, Chidgey AP, Boyd RL. Effects of castration on thymocyte development in two different models of thymic involution. J Immunol. 2005;175:2982–93.
9. Stephan RP, Reilly CR, Witte PL. Impaired ability of bone marrow stromal cells to support Blymphopoiesis with age. Blood. 1998;91:75–88.
10. Solana R, Pawelec G, Tarazona R. Aging and innate immunity. Immunity. 2006;24:491–4.
11. Weng NP. Aging of the immune system: how much can the adaptive immune system adapt? Immunity. 2006;24:495–9.
12. Müller AM, Ihorst G, Mertelsmann R, Engelhardt M. Epidemiology of non-Hodgkin's lymphoma (NHL): trends, geographic distribution, and etiology. Ann Hematol. 2005;84:1–12.
13. Gale RP, Opelz G. Commentary: does immune suppression increase risk of developing acute myeloid leukemia? Leukemia. 2012;26(3):422–3.
14. van de Schans SAM, van Spronsen DJ, Hooijkaas H, Janssen-Heijnen MLG, Coebergh JWW. Excess of autoimmune and chronic inflammatory disorders in patients with lymphoma compared with all cancer patients: a cancer registry-based analysis in the south of the Netherlands. Autoimmun Rev. 2011;10:228–34.
15. Seaberg EC, Wiley D, Martínez-Maza O, Chmiel JS, Kingsley L, Tang Y, Margolick JB, Jacobson LP, Multicenter AIDS Cohort Study (MACS). Cancer incidence in the multicenter AIDS Cohort Study before and during the HAART era: 1984 to 2007. Cancer. 2010;116(23):5507–16.
16. Marcucci F, Mele A. Hepatitis viruses and non-Hodgkin lymphoma: epidemiology, mechanisms of tumorigenesis, and therapeutic opportunities. Blood. 2011;117:1792–8.
17. Engels EA, Cho ER, Jee SH. Hepatitis B virus infection and risk of non-Hodgkin lymphoma in South Korea: a cohort study. Lancet Oncol. 2010;11(9):827–34.
18. Kuppers RB. Cells under influence: transformation of B cells by Epstein-Barr virus. Nat Rev Immunol. 2003;3:801–12.
19. Deschler B, Lübbert M. Acute myeloid leukemia: epidemiology and etiology. Cancer. 2006;107:2099–107.
20. Franchini G, Fukumoto R, Fullen JR. T-cell control by human T-cell leukemia/lymphoma virus type 1. Int J Hematol. 2003;78:280–96.
21. Rodriguez-Abreu D, Bordoni A, Zucca E. Epidemiology of hematological malignancies. Ann Oncol. 2003;18(Supplement 1):i3–8.
22. Tilg H, Moschen AR. Adipocytokines: mediators linking adipose tissue, inflammation and immunity. Nat Rev Immunol. 2006;6:772–83.

23. Larsson SC, Wolk A. Body mass index and risk of non-Hodgkin's and Hodgkin's lymphoma: a meta-analysis of prospective studies. Eur J Cancer. 2011;47:2422–30.
24. Willett EV, Roman E. Obesity and the risk of Hodgkin lymphoma (United Kingdom). Cancer Causes Control. 2006;17:1103–6.
25. Calle EE, Rodriguez C, Walker-Thurmond K, et al. Overweight, obesity, and mortality from cancer in a prospectively studied cohort of U.S. adults. N Engl J Med. 2003;348:1625–38.
26. Samanic C, Gridley G, Chow WH, et al. Obesity and cancer risk among white and black United States veterans. Cancer Causes Control. 2004;15:35–43.
27. Lichtman MA. Obesity and the risk for a hematological malignancy: leukemia, lymphoma, or myeloma. Oncologist. 2010;15:1083–101.
28. Larsson SC, Wolk A. Overweight and obesity and incidence of leukemia: a meta-analysis of cohort studies. Int J Cancer. 2008;122:1418–21.
29. Krestinina L, Preston DL, Davis FG, Epifanova S, Ostroumova E, Ron E, Akleyev A. Leukemia incidence among people exposed to chronic radiation from the contaminated Techa River, 1953–2005. Radiat Environ Biophys. 2010;49(2):195–201.
30. Galbraith D, Gross SA, Paustenbach D. Benzene and human health: a historical review and appraisal of associations with various diseases. Crit Rev Toxicol. 2010;40(S2):1–46.
31. Pearce N, Bethwaite P. Increasing incidence of non-Hodgkin's lymphoma: occupational and environmental factors. Cancer Res. 1992;52:5496s–500.
32. Palackdharry CS. The epidemiology of non-Hodgkin's lymphoma: why the increased incidence? Oncology. 1994;8:67–73.
33. Zahm SH, Blair A. Pesticides and non-Hodgkin's lymphoma. Cancer Res. 1992;52:5485s–8.
34. Gojo I, Karp JE. The impact of biology on the treatment of secondary AML. Cancer Treat Res. 2001;108:231–55.
35. Bentham G. Association between incidence of non-Hodgkin's lymphoma and solar ultraviolet radiation in England and Wales. Br Med J. 1996;312:1128–31.
36. Freedman DM, Zahm SH, Dosemeci M. Residential and occupational exposure to sunlight and mortality from non-Hodgkin's lymphoma: composite (threefold) case–control study. Br Med J. 1997;314:1451–5.
37. Sasieni P, Bataille V. Non-Hodgkin's lymphoma and skin cancer. Ultraviolet light is unlikely explanation for association. Br Med J. 1995;311:749.
38. Hu S, Ma F, Collado-Mesa F, Kirsner RS. Ultraviolet radiation and incidence of non-Hodgkin's lymphoma among. Hispanics in the United States. Cancer Epidemiol Biomarkers Prev. 2004;13:59–64.
39. Quaglia A, Lillini R, Mamo C, Ivaldi E, Vercelli M, SEIH (Socio-Economic Indicators, Health) Working Group. Socio-economic inequalities: a review of methodological issues and the relationships with cancer survival. Crit Rev Oncol Hematol. 2013;85:266–77.
40. Vercelli M, Villini R, Capocaccia R, Micheli A, Coebergh JWW, Quinn M, Martinez-Garcia C, Quaglia A, The ELDCARE Working Group. Cancer survival in the elderly: Effects of socio-economic factors and health care system features (ELDCARE project). Eur J Cancer. 2006;42:234–42.
41. Frederiksen BL, Dalton SO, Osler M, Steding-Jessen M, de Nully Brown P. Socioeconomic position, treatment, and survival of non-Hodgkin lymphoma in Denmar - - nationwide study. Br J Cancer. 2012;106(5):988–95 [Epub 2012 Feb 7].
42. Bhayat F, Das-Gupta E, Smith C, McKeever T, Hubbard R. The incidence of and mortality from leukaemias in the UK: a general population-based study. BMC Cancer. 2009;9:252–8.
43. Kristinsson SY, Derolf AR, Edgren G, Dickman PW, Bjo¨rkholm M. Socioeconomic differences in patient survival Are increasing for acute myeloid leukemia and multiple myeloma in Sweden. J Clin Oncol. 2009;27:2073–80.
44. Ferlay J, Parkin DM, Curado MP, Bray F, Edwards B, Shin HR, Forman D. Cancer Incidence in Five Continents, Volumes I to IX: IARC CancerBase No. 9 [Internet]. Lyon: International Agency for Research on Cancer; 2010. Available from: http://ci5.iarc.fr.
45. Newton R, Ferlay J, Beral V, Devesa SS. The epidemiology of non-Hodgkin's lymphoma: comparison of nodal and extra-nodal sites. Int J Cancer. 1997;72:923–30.

46. Anderson JR, Armitage JO, Weisenburger DD. Epidemiology of the non-Hodgkin's lymphomas: distributions of the major subtypes differ by geographic locations. Non-Hodgkin's lymphoma classification project. Ann Oncol. 1998;9:717–20.
47. Sukpanichnant S, Sonakul D, Piankijagum A, Wanachiwanawin W, Veerakul G, Mahasandana C, Tanphaichitr VS, Suvatte V. Malignant lymphoma in Thailand: changes in the frequency of malignant lymphoma determined from a histopathologic and immunophenotypic analysis of 425 cases at Siriraj Hospital. Cancer. 1998;83:1197–204.
48. Lymphoma Study Group of Japanese Pathologists. The World Health Organization classification of malignant lymphomas in Japan: incidence of recently recognized entities. Pathol Int. 2000;50:696–702.
49. Echimane AK, Ahnoux AA, Adoubi I, Hien S, M'Bra K, D'Horpock A, Diomande M, Anongba D, Mensah-Adoh I, Parkin DM. Cancer incidence in Abidjan, Ivory Coast: first results from the cancer registry, 1995–1997. Cancer. 2000;89:653–63.
50. World Health Organization, mortality database http://www.who.int/whosis/mort/download/en/index.html.
51. ISTAT. Geo-Demo. Demography in figures, http://demo.istat.it/.
52. Joinpoint Regression Program, Version 3.3.1. April 2008; Statistical Research and Applications Branch, National Cancer Institute. U.S.A.
53. McKean-Cowdin R, Feigelson HS, Ross RK, Pike MC, Henderson BE. Declining cancer rates in the 1990s. J Clin Oncol. 2000;18:2258–68.
54. Armitage JO, Bierman PJ, Bociek RG, Vose JM. Lymphoma 2006: classification and treatment. Oncology (Williston Park). 2006;20:231–9.
55. Harris NL, Jaffe ES, Diebold J, Flandrin G, Muller-Hermelink HK, Vardiman J. Lymphoma classification—from controversy to consensus: the R.E.A.L. and WHO Classification of lymphoid neoplasms. Ann Oncol. 2000;11:3–10.
56. Jaffe E, Harris NL, Stein H, Vardiman J. World Health Organization classification of tumours: pathology and genetics of tumours of hematopoietic and lymphoid tissue. Lyon: IARC; 2001.
57. Brenner H, Gefeller O. An alternative approach to monitoring 591 cancer patient survival. Cancer. 1996;78:2004–10.
58. Surveillance Research Program, National Cancer Institute SEER*Stat software (www.seer.cancer.gov/seerstat) version 7.1.0.
59. Quaglia A, Tavilla A, Shack L, Brenner H, Janssen-Heijnenf M, Allemani C, Colonna M, Grande E, Grosclaude P, Vercellia M and the EUROCARE Working Group. The cancer survival gap between elderly and middle-aged patients in Europe is widening. Eur J Cancer. 2009;45:1006–16.
60. Quaglia A, Capocaccia R, Micheli A, Carrani E, Vercelli M and the EUROCARE-3 Working Group. A wide difference in cancer survival between middle aged and elderly patients in Europe. Int J Cancer. 2007;120:2196–201
61. Janssen-Heijnen ML, Maas HA, Houterman S, Lemmens VE, Rutten HJ, Coebergh JW. Comorbidity in older surgical cancer patients: influence on patient care and outcome. Eur J Cancer. 2007;43:2179–93.
62. Repetto L, Fratino L, Audisio RA, et al. Comprehensive geriatric assessment adds information to ECOG performance status in elderly cancer patients: an Italian group for geriatric oncology study. J Clin Oncol. 2002;20:494–502.
63. Bouchardy C, Rapiti E, Fioretta G, et al. Undertreatment strongly decreases prognosis of breast cancer in elderly women. J Clin Oncol. 2003;21:3580–7.
64. Fentiman IS. Are the elderly receiving appropriate therapy for cancer? Ann Oncol. 1996;7:657–8.

Chapter 2
Anemia, Fatigue and Aging

Lodovico Balducci

Keywords Anemia • Aging • Elderly • Cancer • Inflammation

Introduction

The incidence and prevalence of anemia increase with age [1–8] The prevalence of this condition a is higher among institutionalized than among home-dwelling elderly [9–12]. Cancer and anemia are commonly associated [13, 14]. In younger individuals this association is related to cancer itself or cancer treatment. In the older ones this association may also reflect the increasing prevalence of comorbidity with age, as many comorbid conditions may cause anemia. Irrespective of the causes, anemia in older individuals has been associated with unfavourable outcomes [1–8]. Thus the practitioner managing cancer in the older aged person needs to be aware of the causes, the potential complications and the treatment of anemia.

In this chapter we will explore:

- The definition of anemia in the older aged person;
- The causes of anemia.
- The medical consequences of anemia
- The treatment of anemia and the reversal of its medical consequences.

L. Balducci, MD
H. Lee Moffitt Cancer Center and Research Institute,
University of South Florida College of Medicine,
12902 Magnolia Dr., Tampa, FL 33612, USA
e-mail: balducci@moffitt.usf.edu

U. Wedding, R.A. Audisio (eds.), *Management of Hematological Cancer in Older People*, DOI 10.1007/978-1-4471-2837-3_2

Definition of Anemia

According to the WHO anemia is defined as hemoglobin concentrations lower than 13.5 g/dl for men and 12.0 g/dl for women [15]. This definition is controversial, as it is obtained by averaging the values of hemoglobin in a large population of apparently normal individuals. A more meaningful approach, utilized in recent studies, defined normal hemoglobin levels as those at which the lowest risk of medical events was seen The medical events of interest in an older population include death, loss of independence and reduction of active life expectancy. Among the studies that took this approach was the Woman Health and Aging Study (WHAS). A longitudinal study of 1,003 women 65 and older living in the Baltimore area, the WHAS showed that hemoglobin levels lower than 13.4 g/dl represented a risk factor for mortality and values lower than 13.0 g/dl a risk factor of disability and functional dependence [16, 17]. Likewise, the cardiovascular health study found that hemoglobin levels below 12.6 g/dl were an independent risk factor for mortality in women 65 and older [18]. Based on these findings it would appear reasonable to consider the lowest normal hemoglobin levels in older women between 12.5 and 13.0 g/dl. When these levels are adopted, the difference in incidence and prevalence of anemia between older men and women disappears.

According to the WHO definition the prevalence of anemia is higher in men than in women after age 65 and is higher in black than in white people for any age group. If one uses a hemoglobin level of 12.5 g/dl as the lower threshold for anemia in women, the prevalence of anemia after age 65 is similar in both genders.

The issue whether African Americans should be considered anemic at lower hemoglobin levels than individuals of other ethnic origin is still controversial. A recent study of the population aged 70–79 in Memphis, TN, revealed that the risk of mortality and functional disability for older blacks increased only for hemoglobin levels 2 g lower than the WHO standard, over a 2 year observation time [7]. In the meantime, a longitudinal study of older African Americans at Duke's University showed that the risk of mortality and disability was increased for levels of hemoglobin below the WHO standards [19]. Similar finding were reported in a longitudinal study of individuals 65 and older in Chicago, over 13 years [20]. For the present time it appears prudent to consider anemic aging African Americans with hemoglobin levels lower than the WHO standards.

Causes of Anemia

The causes of anemia in aged individuals in the outpatient setting are shown in Table 2.1 [1, 4–6]. The variation between different studies may be partly explained by the fact that they were conducted at different times and in different populations and that the extent of the diagnostic investigations was different. The Biella [5] and the Chicago [6] studies were conducted in specialized anemia clinics, where patients

Table 2.1 Causes of anemia in older individuals

	NHANES III [1]	Olmsted county [4]	Biella [5]	Chicago [6]
Iron deficiency	16 %	15 %	16 %	25 %
Anemia of Chronic Inflammation (ACI)	33.6 %	36 %	17 %	10 %
B12 and/or folate deficiency	14.3 %	NA	10 %	3.4 %
Renal Failure	12 %	8 %	15 %	3.5 %
Hematology malignancies	NA	NA	7.4 %	NA
Thalassemia	NA	NA	4.5	7.5 %
Unknown cause	24 %	33 %	26 %	44 %

underwent a thorough evaluation of the causes of anemia. Neither in the NHANES [1] or the Olmstead county studies [4] the causes of anemia were consistently investigated. In all studies one may recognize some common trends:

- In more than 50 % cases the cause of anemia is treatable. This findings supports a thorough investigation of the causes of anemia, even of mild anemia in older individuals.
- In at least a third of cases the cause of anemia remains unexplained, even after an intensive work up. Approximately one fourth of the patients with anemia of unknown causes developed myelodysplasia during the follow up period in the Biella study. This finding begs the question whether early diagnosis of myelodysplasia is feasible and may improve the prognosis of this condition.
- Anemia of multiple causes is common and in the Biella study anemia of multiple causes accounted for more than half of all cases.

In older age the main cause of iron deficiency is blood loss, especially from the gastro-intestinal tract [21–24]. Even in the absence of symptoms, and in the face of negative hemoccult stool test the gastrointestinal tract should be evaluated with colonoscopy and gastroduedonoscopy [21]. If these exams fail to reveal a bleeding lesion a camera endoscopy of the small bowel is indicated. In 30–50 % of adult individuals a cause of blood loss may not identifiable. In these situations iron malabsorption from atrophic gastritis, H. Pylori infections, celiac disease or medications may be responsible for iron deficiency.

Incidence and prevalence of cobalamin deficiency increase with age [25, 26]. Inability to digest food B12 from decreased gastric production of hydrochloric acid and of pepsin, is the most common cause. As the production of intrinsic factor is not compromised cobalamin deficiency may be ameliorated with oral crystalline B12 [25, 26]. Drug induced B12 deficiency is becoming increasingly common [27], especially with the use of proton pump inhibitors and metformin In addition to anemia, B12 deficiency may be a cause of neurologic disorders including dementia, and posterior column lesions.

Some cases of anemia of unknown causes may be accounted for by early myelodysplasia or chronic renal insufficiency that become more prevalent with age. For a glomerular filtration rate (GFR) lower than 60 ml/min as many as 75 % of patients develop anemia [28, 29]. These GFR values are common at age 65 and older and are almost universal after age 80. Hypogonadism may account for some anemia of unknown causes [30]. In the INCHIANTI study Ferrucci et al. found low levels of circulating testosterone in three fourth of older men and women with anemia. Low testosterone levels in non-anemic subjects were predictive of anemia during the following 3 years. The role of testosterone in promoting erythropoiesis is well documented by a number of clinical observations. In men testosterone replacement therapy and in women testosterone –producing ovarian tumors are associated with erythocytosis [31, 32]. After aromatization to estrogen androgens stimulate the proliferation of hemopoietic stem cells through estrogen receptor alpha that activates the TET gene and leads to increased telomerase synthesis [33]. Consistent with these findings, androgen deprivation therapy of prostate cancer and aromatase inhibition therapy of breast cancer may be associated with anemia.

Nutrition may play an important role in anemia of unknown causes [34] In addition to protein/calorie malnutrition that becomes more common with aging, the lack of specific nutrients may be important. Recent studies identified deficiency of Vitamin D [35] and copper [36] as potential causes of anemia in older individuals.

Relative erythropoietin deficiency may represent an important mechanism of anemia of unknown causes in the elderly. Whereas in the presence of iron deficiency an inverse relation exists between the hemoglobin and erythropoietin levels, older individuals with anemia of unknown origin lose the ability to raise the levels of circulating erythropoietin when the hemoglobin levels decline [6]. Ferrucci et al. found that the levels of erythropoietin were more elevated in the presence of normal hemoglobin levels, but failed to increase appropriately when the hemoglobin levels dropped, in patients with increased concentrations of inflammatory cytokines in the circulation [37]. Inflammatory cytokines may both reduce the sensitivity of erythropoietic precursors to erythropoietin and inhibit erythropoietin secretion. In other words, most cases of anemia of unknown origin would represent a form of anemia of inflammation. This is reasonable as aging is seen as a form of chronic and progressive inflammation [38]. A recent study showing that no relation exists between the excretion of hepcidin in the urines of older individuals and their hemoglobin levels questions this hypothesis, however [39]. Another group of investigators also found decreased erythropoietin sensitivity in the absence of increased hepcidin levels in elderly individuals with anemia of unknown causes [40]. Hepcidin is an enzyme that shuts down the transport of iron from the gastrointestinal tract and from the storages to the bone marrow by destroying the iron transporting protein ferroportin [41]. The production of hepcidin occurs in the liver and is stimulated by inflammatory cytokines, and in particular interleukin 6. Increased levels of hepcidin are considered essential to anemia of inflammation. While it is clear that the sensitivity to and the production of erythropoietin decline with the concentration of inflammatory cytokines in the circulation, it may not be concluded that this form of anemia is a classical anemia of inflammation. In this, elevated levels of hepcidin play a critical role.

Table 2.2

	Anemia of inflammation	Iron deficiency anemia
Serum Iron	Low	Low
Total iron binding capacity	Decreased	Increased
Ferritin levels	Increased	Decreased
Soluble transferrin receptor	Decreased	Increased
Hepcidin levels	Increased	Decreased

An area of controversy is whether anemia may develop in older individuals in absence of a specific disease from an exhaustion of hemopoietic reserves, which may include numeric as well as functional abnormalities of the hemopoietic stem cells and failure of the hemopoietic microenvironment to support the viability of these elements. In older mammals, including humans, the stem cells are primed to differentiate into the myeloid rather than the erythroid series [42]. Also, the accumulation of oxidative damage may reduce the ability of human stem cell self renewal [43]. It is not clear whether these changes are sufficient to cause anemia in the aged. In some cross-sectional studies the average hemoglobin levels appeared consistent in all age groups at least up to age 85, though the prevalence of anemia increased with age [3, 44–46] suggesting that anemia is not a necessary consequence of age. Two longitudinal studies, one from Japan [47] and the other from Sweden [48] revealed a small but progressive decline in hemoglobin concentration with age. Such findings suggest that a progressive erythropoietic exhaustion, of low degree may occur with aging. It may become significant in condition of erythropoietic stress, such as blood loss with a delayed and incomplete correction of anemia.

As anemia may have multiple causes in as many as 50 % of anemic elderly [5] the diagnosis of the causes of anemia in the older person involves some unique problems. Perhaps the most important diagnostic issue is the recognition of iron deficiency in the presence of anemia of inflammation (table 2.2). A foolproof diagnostic test does not exist, but elevated levels of soluble transferrin receptors and low circulating levels of hepcidin suggest some degree of iron deficiency. In this situation an improvement of anemia following iron treatment may confirm the diagnosis of iron deficiency [49–52]. The distinction is important not only for therapeutic reasons. A diagnosis of iron deficiency should trigger investigations for occult bleeding especially from the gastrointestinal tract [20].

Figure 2.1 illustrates a reasonable approach to the evaluation of anemia in the older aged person. High reticulocyte count indicates loss of read blood cells though acute hemorrhage or hemolysis, while low count reveals anemia due to decreased production, that is the most common form of chronic anemia in the elderly. The size of the red blood cells (Mean Cellular Volume of MCV) may suggest to the cause of anemia:

- Microcytosis indicates decreased production of hemoglobin. The main causes of this in older people are iron deficiency or chronic inflammation. Hemoglobinopathy such as thalassemia may contribute to microcytosis as well.

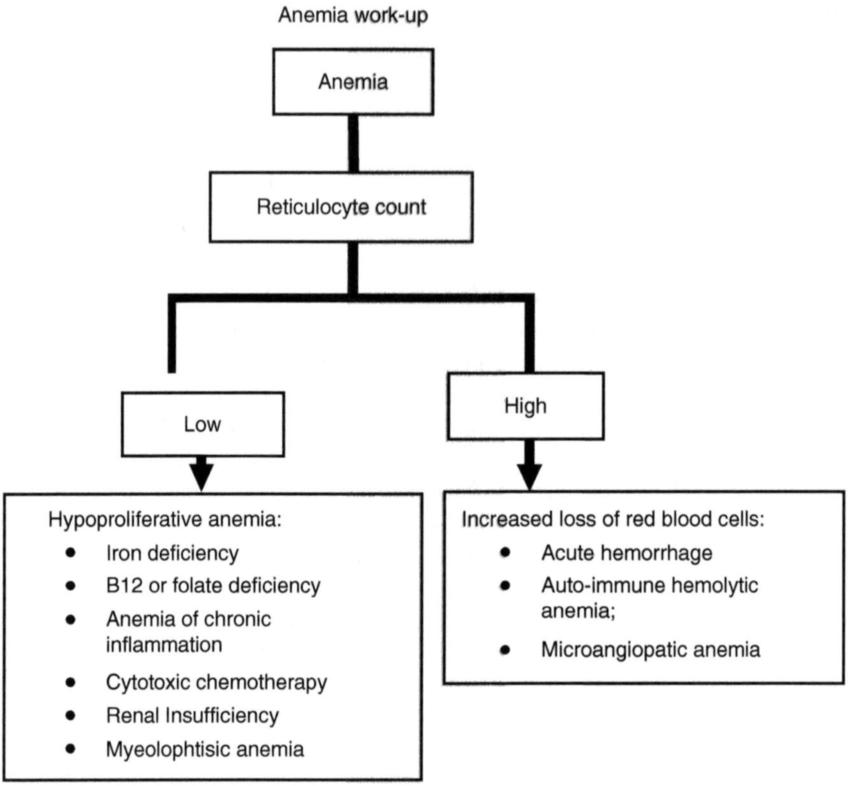

Fig. 2.1 Suggested basic work-up of anemia

- Macrocytosis or enlarged red blood cells is generally due to reduced synthesis of DNA. The cells are overgrown because they cannot divide. The most common cause is cytotoxic chemotherapy of cancer or of autoimmune diseases. Other causes include B12 and folate deficiency. Hypothyroidism, copper deficiency, and myelodysplasia may also lead to macrocytosis. Macrocytosis may rarely be seen in conditions where the red blood cell membrane is over-expanded due to accumulation of cholesterol as in liver failure with L-CAT (lysolicetin-cholesterol acetyl transferase).
- Normocytosis suggests erythropoietin deficiency (renal failure, chronic inflammation) or decreased production of RBC due to exhaustion of red blood cell precursors (aplastic anemia).

The MCV may not be very reliable in older individuals because multiple causes of anemia may have different effects on MCV. For example the combination of iron and B12 deficiency may lead to normocytosis [5, 50]. When the B12 levels are borderline (that is lower than 300 ug/dl), one should also check the methymalonic acid levels. An increased concentration of this substance suggest functional B12 deficiency.

Table 2.3 Consequences of anemia in older individuals

Decreased survival
Fatigue and functional dependence
Increased risk of therapeutic complications, including chemotherapy-related toxicity
Increased risk of coronary death
Increased risk of congestive heart failure
Increased risk of dementia

Bone marrow examination is required when one suspects the diagnosis of myelodysplasia or of marrow occupying diseases (myelofibrosis, cancer, infections). If myelodysplasia or a neoplastic disorder of the marrow is suspected, cytogenetics and flow cytometry of the marrow should be obtained

Consequences of Anemia

The clinical consequences of anemia are listed in Table 2.3 [3].

A number of studies demonstrated that anemia is an independent risk factor for mortality in older individuals [11, 16–18, 53–56]. In the Women Health and Aging Study (WHAS) the risk of mortality for home dwelling women aged 65+ was increased for hemoglobin levels <13.4 g/dl [53].

Functional dependence that is the inability to live alone [57–60] is a common and devastating complication of anemia in the aged. The WHAS [56], the EPESE [57], and the Chianti study [60] all demonstrated that anemia after age 65 was associated with some degree of dependence in the instrumental activities of daily livings (IADLs) and with mobility limitations. There was an inverse linear relation between risk of functional dependence, mobility impairment and hemoglobin levels <13.5 g/dl, indicating that even mild anemia may have serious health and social consequences.

As for therapeutic complications, four studies showed anemia as an independent risk factor for the complications of cytotoxic chemotherapy [61–64]. As the majority of antineoplastic agents are bound to red blood cells, one may expect that the concentration of free drug in the circulation, and the risk of toxicity may increase with anemia [61]. At the meantime, the condition of chronic hypoxia caused by anemia may enhance the vulnerability of normal tissues to treatment complications. Cerebral hypoxia is a likely explanation for the increased risk of post-operative delirium associated with anemia [65].

The association of chronic anemia and congestive heart failure is well known. A review of Medicare records showed that individuals 65 and older with myocardial infarction and hematocrit lower than 30 % were more likely to die if they did not receive any blood transfusions [66].

Anemia has been associated with cognitive impairment in older individuals. Cognitive decline was more common among chronic renal failure patients whose anemia had not been corrected with erythropoietin. [67]. In breast cancer patients receiving chemotherapy a correlation was found between hemoglobin levels and performance of three cognitive tests [68]. A systematic review of three longitudinal studies showed that anemia was an independent risk factors for dementia [69].

The prevalence of other geriatric syndromes was increased in the presence of anemia. In particular anemia was frequently identified as an independent risk factor for falls [10, 70]

Anemia, Cancer and Aging: A Crossroad

Anemia may represent a crossroad of cancer and aging. The roads that are crossing include:

- Age-related hemopoietic exhaustion: aging is associated with functional abnormalities of hemopoietic stem cells. These include increased heterogeneity of stem cells, with overexpression of micro RNA as it is found in myelodysplasia [41, 71], oxidative damage of these elements that compromise their viability [43], preferential commitment of the stem cells to the myeloid series [72]. Studies in rodents revealed that the concentration of stem cells decline with age [73] but this finding was never conclusively demonstrated in humans.
- Cancer and its treatment may enhance and aggravate the effects of hemopoietic exhaustion: both chemotherapy and radiotherapy are myelosuppressive [72]. In addition cancer itself may associated with chronic inflammation and anemia of inflammation [41, 73–75].
- Aging too is associated with chronic and progressive inflammation [6, 37, 38]: as already mentioned this inflammation is associated with relative erythropoietin deficiency (that is decreased sensitivity to and decreased production of erythropoietin) [37]. For some unexplained reason the inflammation of aging is not associated with increased production of hepcidin.
- A reduction in GFR is universal with age, and is associated with reduced erythropoietin production [26, 27].
- The incidence and prevalence of geriatric syndromes and the risk of mortality are increased in older individuals with anemia. This findings suggests that anemia may enhance the unfavourable effects of aging.
- Anemia is associated with fatigue, which is also a complication of cancer and of chemotherapy [74]. Likewise, comorbidity of aging is associated with fatigue [75]. In older individuals fatigue is associated both with functional dependence [59, 76] and death [77].
- Anemia is associated with unfavourable outcome in cancer patients as well including increased risk of mortality, functional dependence, and fatigue [2, 78]. While it is clear that anemia is associated with a number of serious adverse events, it is not been established as yet that reversal of anemia may prevent the poor outcome of aging and of cancer. An ongoing multicenter study explores the benefit of managing mild anemia in older individuals

Treatment of Anemia

The treatment must be based on the specific causes of anemia (Fig. 2.1).

Correction of nutritional deficiencies including iron, cobalamin and copper, and treatment of underlying metabolic conditions such as hypothyroidism is indicated. Intravenous iron may be preferable to oral iron in older individuals as the ability to absorb iron may be compromised both by medications and by gastric hypochloridria [79]. Several intravenous iron preparations are available [79]. In the USA low molecular weight iron dextran is the preparation of most common use. The advantage of this preparation includes the ability to administer the full amount of iron over a single session. The disadvantages include the risk of anaphylactoid reaction and the need for administration over several hours. Ferumoxytol (FeraHeme) is approved in the USA for the treatment of iron deficiency in patients with chronic renal insufficiency. The advantages include the administration over few minutes and the absence of immediate adverse reactions. Disadvantages include the high cost and the fact that only 510 mg can be administered during a single session. Other preparation of irons available in Europe include Ferric Carboxymaltorse and Ferumoxytol. Both appear free of immediate reaction and may be administered over few minutes [80].

Vitamin B12 (cobalamin) is effective orally at high doses in patients with pernicious anemia [81]. It is reasonable, albeit unproven, to assume that oral preparation may be effective also in older individuals without pernicious anemia, whose major problem appear inadequate digestion of food B12. Indefinite B12 replacement was considered desirable until recently. This assumption was questioned in a recent study showing a direct relationship between vitamin B12 levels and mortality among older hospitalized patients [82]. Until the meaning of this association is clarified if is reasonable to limit the replacement treatment until normal blood levels of B12, methylmalonic acid and cystein (that are markers of B12 deficiency) are achieved.

The biggest controversy concerns the management of anemia of inflammation, that is the most common form of anemia in older individuals, with erythropoietic stimulating agents (ESA) such as epoetin α or β and darbepoetin α [83–86]. These compounds were effective in improving the fatigue and the quality of life of cancer patients, but a number of recent studies suggested that they may cause deep vein thrombosis and may stimulate the growth of some tumors, especially cancer of the breast and of the head and neck. It should be underlined that these complications were observed mainly in patients not receiving chemotherapy for their cancer and almost exclusively when hemoglobin levels were raised about 12 g/dl. Also, a meta-analysis of studies using exclusively darbepoetin in patients receiving chemotherapy failed to show any increase in tumor growth [85].

These findings led to a halt of all attempts to treat anemia of inflammation in older individuals with ESA. Hopefully these studies may be resumed in the future, once that the risks of ESAs are clarified. If erythropoietin is used for the management of anemia of inflammation addition of iron intravenously may improve the efficacy of the compounds [83].

The treatment of anemia involves the use of blood transfusions, but the indications of this treatment are controversial at present [87]. General agreement exists on transfusing patients who are symptomatic with dyspnea at mild exercise or severe fatigue. Recent studies indicating that blood transfusions were associated with increased mortality in patients treated in intensive care units [88] as well as in cancer patients [89] suggest that allogeneic red blood cells may have some serious unfavourable effects, whose mechanism is poorly understood. In the USA it is common practice among oncologists to transfuse red blood cells in patients receiving chemotherapy whose hemoglobin is lower than 8.0 g/dl even if they are asymptomatic. This is based on the observation that symptoms become more common for hemoglobin levels lower that 8 g/dl and that the hemoglobin levels are likely to drop after cytotoxic chemotherapy.

Conclusions

Anemia, even mild anemia has a negative influence on survival, function and health of older individuals. Anemia should be considered present in older women for hemoglobin levels lower than 13 g/dl. There are no good reasons at present to use different standards for the definition of anemia in African American and Caucasian patients.

Anemia is associated with increased mortality, increased risk of functional dependence, geriatric syndromes, and therapeutic complications in older individuals, but it is not clear whether the reversal of anemia will reverse these risks.

Frequently, anemia in older individuals has more than one cause; in approximately 50 % of cases these causes of anemia are treatable.

The major area of controversy concerns the treatment of anemia of inflammation with ESA. More studies are urgently needed in this area.

References

1. Guralnick JM, Eisenstaedt RS, Ferrucci L, et al. Prevalence of anemia in persons 65 year and older in the United States: evidence for a high rate of unexplained anemia. Blood. 2004;104: 2063–8.
2. Ferrucci L, Balducci L. Anemia of aging: role of chronic inflammation and cancer. Semin Hematol. 2008;45:242–9.
3. Beghe C, Wilson A, Ershler WB. Prevalence and outcomes of anemia in geriatrics: a systematic review of the literature. Am J Med. 2004;116(Suppl 7A):3S–10.
4. Anía BJ, Suman VJ, Fairbanks VF, Rademacher DM, Melton 3rd LJ. Incidence of anemia in older people: an epidemiologic study in a well defined population. J Am Geriatr Soc. 1997;45: 825–31.
5. Tettamanti M, Lucca U, Gandini F, et al. Prevalence, incidence and types of "mild anemia" in the elderly: the "Health and Anemia" population bases study. Hematologica. 2010;95:1849–56.

6. Artz AS, Thirman MJ. Unexplained anemia predominates despite an intensive evaluation in a racially diverse cohort of older adults from a Referral Anemia Clinic. J Gerontol A Biol Sci Med Sci. 2011;66A:925–32.
7. Patel KV, Harris TB, Faulhaber M. Racial Variation in relationship of anemia with mortality and morbidity disability among older adults. Blood. 2007;109:4663–70.
8. Pang W, Schrier SL. Anemia in the elderly. Curr Opin Hematol. 2012;19:133–40.
9. Robinson B, Artz AS, Culleton B, et al. Prevalence of anemia in the nursing home: contribution of chronic renal disease. J Am Geriatr Soc. 2007;55:1566–70.
10. Pandya N, Bookhart B, Mody SH, et al. Study of Anemia in Long term Care (SALT): prevalence of anemia and itsrelationship with the risk fo falls in nursing home residents. Curr Med Res Opin. 2008;24:2139–49.
11. Landi F, Russo A, Danese P, et al. Anemia status, hemoglobin concentration, and mortality in nursing home residents. J Am Med Dir Assoc. 2007;8:322–7.
12. Sabol VK, Resnick B, Galik E, et al. Anemia and its impact in function in nursing home residentd. What do we know? J Am Acad Nurse Pract. 2010;22:3–16.
13. Rodgers GM, Becker PS, Blinder M, et al. Cancer and chemotherapy-induced anemia. J Natl Compr Canc Netw. 2012;10:628–53.
14. Spivak JL, Gascon P, Ludwig H. Anemia management in oncology and hematology. Oncologist. 2009;14 Suppl 1:43–56.
15. World health organization definition of anemia: report of a WHO scientific group. Geneva; 1968
16. Semba RD, Ricks MO, Ferrucci L, et al. Types of anemia and mortality among elderly disabled women living in the community: the women's health and Aging Study 1. Aging Clin Exp Res. 2007;19:259–64.
17. Chaves PH. Functional outcome of anemia in older adults. Semin Hematol. 2008;45:255–60.
18. Zakai NH, Katz R, Hirsch C, et al. A prospective study of anemia status, hemoglobin concentration, and mortality in an elderly cohort: the Cardiovascular health Study. Arch Intern Med. 2005;165:2214–20.
19. Denny SD, Kuchibhatla MN, Cohen HJ. Impact of anemia on mortality, cognition, and function in community-dwelling elderly. Am J Med. 2006;119(4):327–34.
20. Dong X, Mendes de Leon C, Artz A, et al. A population-based study of hemoglobin, race, and mortality in elderly persons. J Gerontol A Biol Sci Med Sci. 2008;63:873–8.
21. Vannella L, Aloe Spiriti MA, DoGiulio E. Upper and lower gastrointestinal causes of iron deficient anemia in elderly compared with adult outpatients. Minerva Gastroenterol Dietol. 2010;56:397–404.
22. Karlsson T. Comparative evaluation of the reticulocyte hemoglobin content assay when screening for iron deficiency in elderly anemic patients. Anemia. 2011. Epub 2011.
23. Jolobe OM. Does this elderly patients have iron deficiency anemia and what is the underlying cause. Postgrad Med. 2000;76:195–8.
24. Annibale B, Capurso G, Chistolini A, et al. Gastrointestinal causes of refractory iron deficient anemia in patients without gastrointestinal symptoms. Am J Med. 2001;111:439–45.
25. Selhub J, Morris MS, Jacques PF, et al. Folate-Vitamin B12 interaction in relation to cognitive impairment, anemia, and biochemical indicators of Vitamin B-12 deficiency. Am J Clin Nutr. 2009;89(2):702S–6.
26. Stabler SP. Prevalence and mechanisms of B12 deficiency. In: Balducci L, Ershler WH, DeGaetano G, editors. Blood disorders in the elderly. Cambridge: Cambridge University Press; 2008. p. 181–91.
27. Langan RC, Zawistosky KJ. Update on vitamin B12 deficiency. Am Fam Physician. 2011;83:1425–30.
28. McClellan W, Aronoff SL, Bolton WK, et al. The prevalence of anemia in patients with chronic kidney diseases. Curr Med Res Opin. 2004;20:1501–10.
29. Robinson BE. Epidemiology of chronic kidney disease and anemia. J Am Med Dir Assoc. 2006;7(9 suppl):S3–6.

30. Ferrucci L, Maggio M, Bandinelli S, et al. Low testosterone levels and the risk of anemia in older men and women. Arch Intern Med. 2006;166(13):1380–8.
31. Alagarsamy F, Khanna G, Emerson G, et al. Testosterone-induced erythrocytosis affecting hematocrit prediction of fluid responsiveness. Br J Hosp Med. 2012;73:234.
32. Muechler EK. Testosterone-producing ovarian tumor associated with erythrocytosis, hyperuricemia, and recurrent deep vein thrombosis. Am J Obstet Gynecol. 1977;129:467–9.
33. Calado RT, Yewdell WT, Wilkerson KL, et al. Sex Hormone acting on TERT gene increase telomerase activity in human primary hematopoietic cells. Blood. 2009;114:2236–43.
34. Thomson CA, Stanaway J, Neuhouser ML, et al. Nutrient Intake and anemia risk in the WHi observational study. J Am Diet Assoc. 2011;111:532–41.
35. Peristein TS, Pande R, Berliner N, et al. Prevalence of 25-hydroxyvitaminD deficiency in subgroups of elderly persons with anemia: association with anemia of inflammation. Blood. 2011;117:2800–6.
36. Halfdanarson TR, Kumar N, Li CY, et al. Hematological manifestations of copper deficiency. A retrospective review. Eur J Haematol. 2008;80:523–32.
37. Ferrucci L, Guralnik JM, Woodman RC, et al. Proinflammatory state and circulating erythropoietin in persons with and without anemia. Am J Med. 2005;118(11):1288.
38. Ferrucci L, Corsi A, Lauretani F, et al. The origin of age-related pro-inflammatory state. Blood. 2005;105:2294–9.
39. Ferrucci L, Semba RD, Guralnik JM. Pro-inflammatory status, aging, and anemia in older persons. Blood. 2010;115(18):3810–6.
40. Waalen J, von Lohenisen K, Lee P, et al. Erythropoietin, GDF-15; IL6, Hepcidine and testosterone levels in a large cohort of elderly individuals with anaemia of known and unknown cause. Eur J Haematol. 2011;87:107–16.
41. Ganz T, Nemeth E. Iron metabolism interactions with normal and disordered erythopoiesis. Cold Spring Harb Perspect Med. 2012;2:a011668.
42. Muller-Sieburg CE, Sieburg HB, Bernitz JM, et al. Stem cell heterogeneity: implications ofr aging and regenerative medicine. Blood. 2012;119:3900–7.
43. Yahata T, Takanashi T, Muguruma Y, et al. Accumulation of oxidative DNA damage restricts the self renewal capacity of human hematopoietic stem cells. Blood. 2011;118:2941–50.
44. Imelmen EM, Alessio MD, Gatto MRA, et al. Descriptive analysis of the prevalence of anemia in a randomly selected sample of elderly people at home: some results of an Italian Multicentric Study. Aging Clin Exper Res. 1994;6:81–9.
45. Izaks GJ, Westendorp RGJ, Knook DL. The definition of anemia in older persons. JAMA. 1999;281(18):1714–7.
46. Kikuchi M, Inagaki T, Shinagawa N. Five-year survival of older people with anemia: variation with hemoglobin concentration. J Am Geriatr Soc. 2001;49:1226–8.
47. Yamada M, Wong FL, Suzuki G. RERF's (Radiation Effects Research Foundation) Adult Health Study. Longitudinal trends of hemoglobin levels in a Japanese population–RERF's Adult Health Study subjects. Eur J Haematol. 2003;70(3):129–35.
48. Nilsson-Ehle H, Jagenburg R, Landahl S, Svanborg A. Blood haemoglobin declines in the elderly: implications for reference intervals from age 70 to 88. Eur J Haematol. 2000;65(5):297–305.
49. Jolobe OM. Criteria for iron deficiency anemia of unknown cause shoula allow for confounding effects of inflammation. Eur J Int Med. 2012. Epub ahead of publication.
50. Petrsovan I, Blaison G, Andres E, et al. Anemia in the elderly: an aetiologic profile of a prospective cohort of 95mhospitalised patients. Eur J Intern Med. 2012;23:524–8.
51. Rimon E, Levy S, Sapir A, et al. Diagnosis of iron deficiency anemia in elderly patients by transferrin receptor/ferritin index. Arch Intern Med. 2002;162:445–9.
52. Thuerl I, Aigner E, Theurl M, et al. Regulation of iron homeostasis in anemia of chronic disease and iron deficient anemia: diagnostic and therapeutic implications. Blood. 2009;113:5277–86.
53. Chaves PH, Xue QL, Guralnik JM, et al. What constitutes normal hemoglobin concentration in community-dwelling disabled older women? J Am Geriatr Soc. 2004;52:1811–6.

54. den Elzen WP, Willems JM, Westendorp RG. Effect of anemia and comorbidity on functional status and mortality in old age: results from the Leiden 85-plus Study. CMAJ. 2009;181(3–4): 151–7.
55. Anía BJ, Suman VJ, Fairbanks VF, Rademacher DM, Melton JL. Incidence of anemia in older people: an epidemiologic study in a well defined population. J Am Geriatr Soc. 1997;45: 825–83.
56. Culleton BF, Manns BJ, Zhang J, et al. Impact of anemia on hospitalization and mortality in older adults. Blood. 2006;107(10):3841–6.
57. Chaves PH, Ashar B, Guralnik JM, et al. Looking at the relationship between hemoglobin concentration and prevalent mobility difficulty in older women > Should the criteria currently used to define anemia in older people be reevaluated? J Am Geriatr Soc. 2002;1527–1564.
58. Penninx BW, Pahor M, Cesari M, et al. Anemia is associated with disability and decreased physical perdormance and muscle strength in the elderly. J Am Geriatr Soc. 2004;52:719–24.
59. Luciani A, Ascione G, Bertuzzi C. Detecting disabilities in older patients with cancer: comparison between comprehensive geriatric assessment and vulnerable elders survey-13. J Clin Oncol. 2010;28(12):2046–50.
60. Penninx BW, Guralnik JM, Onder G, et al. Anemia and decline in physical performance among older persons. Am J Med. 2003;115:104–10.
61. Ratain MJ, Schilsky RL, Choi KE, et al. Adaptive control of etoposide administration: impact of interpatient pharmacodynamic variability. Clin Pharmacol Ther. 1989;45:226–33.
62. Silber JH, Fridman M, Di Paola RS, et al. First-cycle Blood counts and subsequent neutropenia, dose reduction or delay in early stage breast cancer therapy. J Clin Oncol. 1998;16: 2392–400.
63. Extermann M, Boler I, Reich R. Predicting the risk of chemotherapy toxicity in older patients. The Chemotherapy Risk Assessment Scale for High Age Patient (CRASH). Cancer. 2012;118: 3377–86.
64. Schijvers D, Highley M, DeBruyn E, et al. Role of red blood cell in pharmakinetics of chemotherapeutic agents. Anticancer Drugs. 1999;10:147–53.
65. Marcantonio ER, Flacker JM, Michaels M, et al. Delirium is independently associated with poor functional recovery after hip fracture. J Am Geriatr Soc. 2000;48:618–24.
66. Wen-Chih WC, Rathore SS, Wang Y, et al. Blood transfusions in elderly patients with acute myocardial infarction. N Engl J Med. 2001;345:1230–6.
67. Pickett JL, Theberge DC, Brown WS, Schweitzer SU, Nissenson AR. Normalizing hematocrit in dialysis patients improves brain function. Am J Kidney Dis. 1999;33(6):1122–30.
68. Jacobsen PB, Garland LL, Booth-Jones M, et al. Relationship of hemoglobin levels to fatigue and cognitive functioning among cancer patients receiving chemotherapy. J Pain Symptom Manage. 2004;28:7–18.
69. Peters R, Burch L, Warner J, Beckett N, et al. Haemoglobin, anaemia, dementia and cognitive decline in the elderly, a systematic review. BMC Geriatr. 2008;8:18.
70. Dharmarajan TS, Avula S, Norkus EP. Anemia increases risk for falls in hospitalized older adults: an evaluation of falls in 362 hospitalized, ambulatory, long-term care, and community patients. J Am Med Dir Assoc. 2007;8(3 Suppl 2):e9–15.
71. Laurencet F. Qualitative changes of hemopoiesis. In: Balducci L, Ershler WB, DeGaetano G, editors. Blood disorders in the elderly. Cambridge: Cambridge University Press; 2008. p. 95–119.
72. Pang WW, Price CA, Sahoo D, et al. Human bone marrow hematopoietic stem cells are increased in frequency and myeloid-biased with age. Proc Natl Acad Sci U S A. 2011;108: 2012–7.
73. Yates J, Van Zant G. Stem cell exhaustion and aging. In: Balducci L, Ershler WB, DeGaetano G, editors. Blood disorders in the elderly. Cambridge: Cambridge University Press; 2008. p. 57–70.
74. Glaspy J. Anemia and fatigue in cancer patients. Cancer. 2001;96(6 suppl):1719–24.
75. Hardy SE, Studenski SA. Qualities of fatigue and associated chronic conditions among older adults. J Pain Symptom Manage. 2010;39:1033–42.

76. Hardy SE, Studenski SA. Fatigue and function over 3 years in older adults. J Gerontol A Biol Sci Med Sci. 2008;63:1389–92.
77. Hardy SE, Studenski SA. Fatigue predicts mortality in older adults. J Amer Geriatr Soc. 2008;56:1910–4.
78. Hoffe S, Balducci L. Cancer and age: general considerations. Clin Geriatr Med. 2012; 28:1–18.
79. Baillie GR. Adverse events associated with intravenous iron preparations. A comparison of reported rates. Clin Adv Hematol Oncol. 2012;10:600–2.
80. Wilson PD, Hutchings A, Jeans A, et al. An analysis of the health service efficiency and patient experience with two different iron preparation in a UK anemia clinics. J Med Econ. 2013;16:108–14.
81. Kuzminski AM, Del Giacco EJ, Allen RH, et al. Effective treatment of cobalamin deficiency with oral cobalamin. Blood. 1998;92:1191–8.
82. Tal S, Shavit Y, Stern F, et al. Association between vitamin B12 levels and mortality in hospitalized older adults. J Am Geriatr Soc. 2010;58:523–6.
83. Auerbach M, Ballard H, Glaspy J. Clinical update: intravenous iron for anemia. Lancet. 2007;369:1502–4.
84. Bennett CL, Silver SM, Djulbegovic B, et al. Venous thromboembolism and mortality associated with recombinant erythropoietin and darbepoetin administration for the treatment of cancer-associated anemia. JAMA. 2008;299(8):914–24.
85. Bohlius J, Schmidlin K, Brillant C et al. Erythropoietin or Darbepoetin for patients with cance--eta-analysis based on individual patient data. Cochrane Database Syst Rev. 2009;8(3): CD007303. Review.
86. Ludwig H, Crawford J, Österborg A, et al. Pooled analysis of individual patient-level data from all randomized, double-blind, placebo-controlled trials of darbepoetin Alfa in the treatment of patients with chemotherapy-induced anemia. J Clin Oncol. 2009;27:2838–47.
87. Vincent JL. Indications for blood transfusions: too complex to base on a single number? Ann Intern Med. 2012;157:71–2.
88. Lelubre C, Vincent JL. Red blood cell transfusions in the critically ill patients. Ann Intensive Care. 2011;1:1–43.
89. Acheson AG, Brookes MJ, Spahn DR. Effects of allogenei red blood cell transfusions on clinical outcomes in patients undergoing colorectal cancer surgery. A systematic review and meta-analysis. Ann Surg. 2012;256:235–44.

Chapter 3
Myelodysplastic Syndromes in Older Patients

Reinhard Stauder

Abstract Myelodysplastic syndromes (MDS) represent typical diseases of the elderly. MDS cover a broad spectrum of clonal hematopoietic stem cell diseases characterized by a dysplastic hematopoiesis and cytopenias in the peripheral blood. Clinical manifestations of MDS are variable and range from mild symptoms related to anemia, thrombocytopenia or granulocytopenia to the transformation to acute myeloid leukemia. The availability of promising treatment options including disease-modifying agents and supportive therapy, imposes the need to develop strategies and algorithms for individualized risk assessment and treatment algorithms in elderly MDS-patients.

Keywords Myelodysplastic Syndromes • MDS • Elderly • Individualised

Myelodysplastic syndromes (MDS) represent one of the most frequent hematologic diseases of the elderly. MDS cover a broad spectrum of clonal hematopoietic stem cell diseases characterized by a dysplastic hematopoiesis and cytopenias in the peripheral blood. Clinical manifestations of MDS are variable and range from mild symptoms related to anemia, thrombocytopenia or granulocytopenia to the transformation to acute myeloid leukemia (AML). MDS represent a typical disease of the elderly as the median age at diagnosis is 70+ years in most registries: 72 years in the Düsseldorf registry; 76 in the Tyrol registry and 74 in the European Leukemia Net registry [1, 2]. The incidence of MDS increases significantly at higher age displaying age specific incidences of 9, 25, and 31/100,000/year for the age groups 60–70, 71–80, and 80+, respectively. Actually MDS might be the underlying disease in a relevant proportion of elderly with unexplained

R. Stauder, MD, MSc
Department of Internal Medicine V (Haematology and Oncology),
Innsbruck Medical University, Anichstraße 35, Innsbruck 6020, Austria
e-mail: reinhard.stauder@i-med.ac.at

U. Wedding, R.A. Audisio (eds.), *Management of Hematological Cancer in Older People*, DOI 10.1007/978-1-4471-2837-3_3

anemia. The number of elderly MDS-patients will increase within the next years based on the increasing proportion of elderly and the occurrence of secondary, therapy-related MDS following radio- or chemotherapy for a primary tumor [3–6]. The availability of promising treatment options including disease-modifying agents and supportive therapeutic options, imposes the need to develop strategies and algorithms for individualized management and treatment of elderly MDS-patients [7].

Differences in Tumor Biology Between Older and Younger Patients

An adverse outcome in MDS is often related to an unfavourable karyotype as assessed by conventional karyotyping or FISH-analysis. Thus, the karyotype represents the most relevant prognostic factor in MDS. Whereas the distribution of distinct aberrations is different in younger and in elderly patients, the distribution of the prognostic relevant normal and abnormal karyotypes is not different [8]. However, detailed analyses of the age distribution of different karyotypes and their impact in different age groups are still missing and are analyzed in ongoing projects.

Age per se has a significant negative impact on overall survival in most analyses performed in MDS so far. In contrast, age does not represent a risk factor for leukemia transformation [8–11]. In general, the relevance of age in prognostication of survival is more relevant in good-risk MDS than in high-risk disease. As shorter survival in elderly persons is logical, prognostication should include age-adjusted parameters like the standardized mortality rate (SMR) or age-adjusted survival. Thus the survival in a given MDS patient is compared with an age- and sex-matched population [12]. Based on this analyses it was demonstrated, that even in elderly patients, MDS represent a relevant disease with a greater than threefold risk of disease-related death, resulting in a significant loss of life years in the majority of prognostic subgroups. However, in prognostic excellent subgroups, life expectancy is not different from the general population [13], pointing out the importance of integrating age-matched prognostic scoring systems in individualized treatment algorithms.

Current Diagnostic Standards

Based on a working conference in Vienna, minimal diagnostic criteria in MDS were proposed by Valent et al. [14] and updated recently [15]: two prerequisite criteria for the diagnosis of MDS are: (i) Constant cytopenia (≥6 months) and marked cytopenia in one or more of the following cell lineages: erythroid (hemoglobin <11 g/dL); neutrophilic (ANC < 1,500/μL) or megakaryocytic (platelets <100,000/μL) and (ii) exclusion of another clonal or non-clonal hematopoietic disease or non-hematopoietic disease including toxins or viral infections as the primary reason for

Table 3.1 The classification of Myelodysplastic Syndromes based on WHO 2008 [35]

Refractory cytopenias with unilineage dysplasia (RCUD) Refractory anemia (RA) Refractory neutropenia (RN) Refractory thrombocytopenia (RT)
Refractory anemia with ring sideroblasts (RARS, ≥15 % BM ringed sideroblasts)
Refractory cytopenia with multilineage dysplasia (RCMD)
Myelodysplastic syndrome unclassified (MDS-U)
MDS associated with isolated del(5q)
Refractory anemia with excess of blasts-1 (RAEB-1, 5–9 % bone marrow blasts)
Refractory anemia with excess of blasts-2 (RAEB-2, 10–19 % bone marrow blasts)

WHO world health organization

cytopenia/dysplasia. At least one out of three additional MDS-related criteria is required: (i) dysplasia in ≥10 % of erythroid cells (or >15 % ringed sideroblasts in iron stain), neutrophils and their precursors or megakaryocytes in bone marrow (BM) smears; (ii) typical cytogenetic abnormality as assessed by conventional karyotyping or FISH-analysis or (iii) a constant BM-blast count of 5–19 %. Co-criteria are suggested in patients who fulfill both prerequisite criteria and show typical clinical features of MDS, but do not demonstrate any of the three additional criteria. Co-criteria include: (i) an abnormal phenotype of bone marrow cells as determined by flow cytometry according to European Leukemia Network criteria and (ii) clear molecular signs of a monoclonal cell population based on a human androgen receptor assay, gene chip analysis, or mutation analysis (e.g. EZH2 mutations). The guidelines recommend that a complete blood count, a peripheral blood (PB) smear with differential leukocyte count, a BM aspiration for cytogenetic and morphologic evaluation, as well as a BM biopsy to assess marrow architecture, cellularity, fibrosis, blast percentage and dysmegakaryopoiesis should be performed.

Current Treatment Concepts

Classification and Risk Scoring in MDS

The most widely used classification is based on the World Health Organization (WHO) [16] (Table 3.1). To refine prognostication and risk scoring, much attention has focused on the identification of additional prognostic parameters. The International Prognostic Scoring System (IPSS) was developed based on the FAB-classification and has become the gold standard for clinical risk assessment in patients with primary MDS at initial diagnosis. IPSS-scoring divides patients into low-risk and high-risk MDS [9]. A revised version of the IPSS (IPSS-R) has been developed recently [17] (Tables 3.2 and 3.3). The IPSS-R integrates the severity of cytopenias and includes a detailed list of cytogenetic aberrations. An advantage of IPSS-R is the integration of age as an optional variable in risk scoring. An electronic

Table 3.2 The revised International Prognostic Scoring System (IPSS-R) [17]

	Score values						
Characteristics	0	0.5	1	1.5	2	3	4
Cytogenetics	Very good	–	Good	–	Intermediate	Poor	Very poor
Blasts BM, %	≤2	–	>2– <5	–	5–10	>10	–
Hb	≥10	–	8– <10	<8	–	–	–
Platelets	≥100	50– <100	<50	–	–	–	–
Neutrophils	≥0.8	<0.8	–	–	–	–	–

Total score	
Risk group	Score
Very low	≤1.5
Low	>1.5–3
Intermediate	>3–4.5
High	>4.5–6
Very high	>6

Cytogenetic risk groups			
Prognostic subgroup	Cytogenetic Aberration	Median survival; yrs	Median AML-evolution 25 %; yrs
Very good	-Y, del(11q)	5.4	NR
Good	Normal, del (5q), del (12p), del (20q), double including del (5q)	4.8	9.4
Intermediate	del (7q), +8, +19, i(17q), any other single or double independent clones	2.7	2.5
Poor	−7, inv(3)/t(3q)/del(3q), double including −7/del(7q), complex: 3 abnormalities	1.5	1.7
Very poor	Complex: >3 abnormalities	0.7	0.7

AML acute myeloid leukemia, *BM* bone marrow, *Hb* hemoglobin, *yrs* years

Table 3.3 Age-related survival rates based on the International Prognostic Scoring System (IPSS-R) [17]

	IPSS-risk categories (median survival, years)				
Age groups (years)	Very low	Low	Inter-mediate	High	Very high
All	8.8	5.3	3.0	1.6	0.8
≤60	NR	8.8	5.2	2.1	0.9
>60–70	10.2	6.1	3.3	1.6	0.8
>70–80	7.0	4.7	2.7	1.5	0.7
>80	5.2	3.2	1.8	1.5	0.7

calculator is available **[International working group for the prognosis of MDS;** www.ipss-r.com/]. The MD Anderson Cancer Center (MDACC) prognostic score for MDS was established both in de-novo and in therapy-related MDS. Beside classical parameters like cytogenetics, bone marrow blasts, anemia, thrombopenia or white blood cell counts, the items age and performance status are included, which are very relevant in the evaluation of elderly patients [10] (Table 3.4.).

Table 3.4 The MDACC global MDS risk scoring [10]

Characteristics	Score values
Performance status ≥2	2
Age, year	
60–64	1
≥65	2
Platelets, ×10*9/L	
<30	3
30–49	2
50–199	1
Hemoglobin <12 g/dL	2
Bone marrow blasts, %	
5–10	1
11–29	2
White blood cells >20×10*9/L	2
Karyotype: 7 abnormality or complex ≥3 abnormalities	3
Prior transfusion, yes	1

Survival by risk group			
Score	Survival (median, months)	% at 3 years	% at 6 years
0–4	54	63	38
5–6	25	34	13
7–8	14	16	6
≥9	6	4	0.4

MDACC MD Anderson Cancer Center, *MDS* myelodysplastic syndromes

Treatment Options in Elderly MDS Patients

Transfusion Therapy, Growth Factors and Iron Chelation

An essential goal in the treatment of senior MDS patients is to maintain or achieve red blood cell transfusion independence (RBC-TI), to counteract the consequences of cytopenias and to maintain and improve the health-related quality of life (QoL).

Anemia often represents the first symptom in MDS. Anemia is detected in 80–90 % of MDS patients and results in an impaired QoL and in a decreased overall survival. In addition a high red blood cell (RBC) transfusion frequency represents an unfavorable risk factor for survival [18]. Moreover anemia reduces functional, cognitive, and social capacities in elderly. Targeted transfusion therapy using RBC aims to reach a range of 80–100 G/L in cardio-respiratory healthy persons and >100–120 G/L in elderly and in persons displaying co-morbidities. Erythropoiesis-stimulating agents (ESAs) with or without granulocyte-colony stimulating factor (G-CSF) represent the standard of treatment for transfusion-dependent anemia in low-risk MDS (Fig. 3.1) [7, 14]. ESA-treatment aims to increase hemoglobin levels,

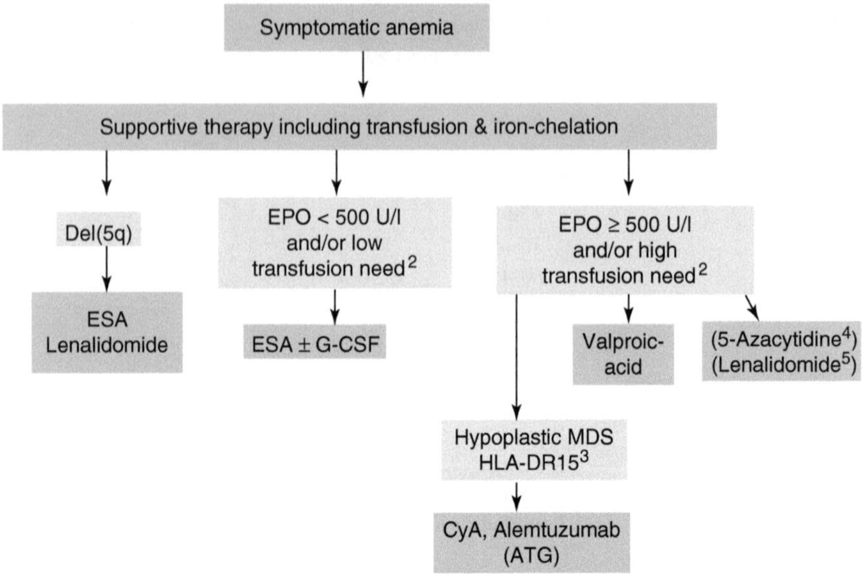

Fig. 3.1 Treatment options in anemic low-risk MDS (IPSS Low-grade und Intermediate 1). *ATG* anti-thymocyte globulin, *CMML* Chronic myelomonocytic leukemia, *ESA* erythropoiesis-stimulating agent, *CyA* Cyclosporin-A. *1* In MDS 5q – licensed by FDA and EMA. *2* Based on predictive model (Nordic score) for ESA treatment described in table 5. G-CSF might increase the erythroid response to ESAs particularly in MDS with an increase of ring sideroblasts (RARS). *3* Response more frequent in younger patients, in hypoplastic MDS and in HLADR-15. *4* 5-Azacytidine might be effective in low risk MDS. However, EMA approval so far only for high-risk MDS and CMML. In contrast FDA-approval in low-risk MDS. Role in low-risk MDS is analysed in clinical studies. *5* Clinical studies in Non-5q- low-risk MDS are ongoing

to reduce transfusion need and to improve QoL. Predictive models for ESA treatment have been developed. Low endogenous erythropoietin (EPO) levels as well as a low transfusion need result in an increased response rate. The Nordic Score thus identifies patients with low, intermediate and high probability of response (Table 3.5) [19]. In addition G-CSF might augment the erythroid response to ESAs, particularly in patients with an increase of ring sideroblasts (RARS). ESAs have been used safely in larger numbers of MDS patients with no evidence for negative impact on survival or AML evolution [20–22]. However, the increased risk of thromboembolic complications in ESA-treated patients should be considered.

In neutropenic MDS patients suffering from infections the interventional use of G-CSF is recommended [7, 14].

Platelet transfusions are applied in thrombopenic MDS patients to prevent or treat bleeding episodes. However, due to immunization frequent transfusions might cause a poor response. Thrombopoietic agents like Romiplostim or Eltrombopag, which are approved for the treatment of immune thrombocytopenic purpura (ITP), have been introduced in MDS and are currently evaluated in clinical trials. A clinical study using Romiplostim in MDS has been closed recently due to a suspected increase of disease progressions. However, in-depth analyses of this trial are pending [7, 11].

Table 3.5 The predictive Nordic Score to assess response to erythropoiesis-stimulating agents (ESAs) in MDS [19]

	Score
Transfusion requirement (RBC)	
<2 U/month	0
≥2 U/month	1
Serum Epo[a]	
<500 U/L	0
≥500 U/L	1
Total score	**Probability of response (%)**
0	74
1	23
2	7

EPO erythropoietin, *MDS* myelodysplastic syndromes
[a]Serum erythropoietin level before treatment

Due to alteration in iron hemostasis and frequent blood transfusions, many MDS-patients are characterized by an iron overload. Iron overload may cause a transfusion-related hemochromatosis, which primarily affects the heart and the liver. As the risk of events becomes apparent when RBC transfusions exceed 20 and serum ferritin levels exceed 1,500–2,000 ng/mL, the treatment with iron-chelating agents such as desferoxamine (applied either subcutaneously or intravenously) or deferasirox (orally), should be considered. In most guidelines a reasonable expected survival (at least more than 1 year) is recommended. In elderly patients treated with deferasirox renal function has to be monitored carefully [23].

Immunomodulating Agents

The immunomodulating drug (IMiD) Lenalidomide is highly active in MDS with 5q-. Lenalidomide induces major clinical and even cytogenetic responses thus forming the basis for Food and Drug Agency (FDA) and EMA approval. Lenalidomide reveals also activity in non-del5q- low risk MDS; studies to evaluate the relevance of lenalidomide in low-risk MDS are ongoing. Relevant side effects of Lenalidomide are neutropenias and thrombocytopenias. TP53 alterations in MDS represent a predictor for increased leukemia transformation and reduced lenalidomide response [24]. Immunosupressive strategies using combinations of anti-thymocyte globulin (ATG) and Cyclosporin-A (CyA) are effective in subgroups of younger patients in hypoplastic MDS and with a HLADR15 phenotype. As ATG is poorly tolerated in elderly patients, a CyA or corticoid monotherapy is generally preferred. Due to nephrotoxicity of CyA renal function has to be monitored closely. Promising data have been reported for the use of alemtuzumab [25] but application in clinical practice will depend on more data reported and the availability of the drug.

Epigenetic Therapies

The hypomethylating agents 5-azacytidine and decitabine reveal encouraging results in high-risk MDS patients. Based on the large number of studies reported, 5-azacytidine represents the standard of care in high-risk MDS patients, who are not eligible for intensive therapies like AML-induction or hematopoietic stem cell transplantation (HSCT). AZA has received an EMA approval in MDS in this indication. In low risk patients, these drugs are analyzed in clinical studies and might so far only be considered when signs of progression occur. AZA significantly extended overall survival in IPSS int-2 and high-risk MDS in comparison with conventional care regimens (CCR) including BSC only, low-dose cytarabine (LDAC), or anthracycline plus cytarabine-based intensive chemotherapy in a phase III study. Moreover AZA-treated patients required less transfusion and spent fewer days in the hospital [26]. Effectiveness of AZA in response and survival prolongation was demonstrated in a subgroup analysis even in elderly MDS patients (75 years) and in patients with an unfavourable cytogenetic profile (−7/del 7q) [27]. As the median number of cycles to achieve a response is three, evaluation of response should not be performed too early. In the absence of unacceptable toxicity or disease progression, continued AZA treatment might further improve responses in MDS. A score for AZA therapy has been identified recently, which identifies three risk groups with median OS of >24, 15 or 6.1 months [28]. The efficacy of decitabine (DAC) in high-risk MDS, including unfavourable cytogenetics, was demonstrated in several clinical studies. Whereas DAC is characterised by its favourable side-effects, so far no clear benefit in terms of survival has been demonstrated [29, 30].

Valproic acid (VPA) was used as an anticonvulsant for decades and might be effective in myeloid neoplasms by the inhibition of histone deacetylase. As VPA causes an erythroid response in about 50 % of patients in low-risk MDS, treatment with valproic acid might represent a useful alternative in low-risk MDS patients with a low probability of erythropoiesis-stimulating factors (ESF) response (Fig. 3.1). In senior patients monitoring of VPA serum concentrations is essential.

Intensive Therapies in Elderly MDS: Current Standards

The only curative treatment approach in MDS represents an allogeneic HSCT. This therapy however is associated with a relatively high risk of transplant-related morbidity and mortality. In elderly, a HSCT with reduced intensity conditioning (RIC-HSCT) can only be offered to a small cohort of patients, who are characterized by an excellent performance status and the lack of relevant co-morbidities. Intensive AML-like chemotherapy has the capacity to restore normal polyclonal hematopoiesis in subgroups of patients. However, a long-term complete remission is induced only in a minority of patients. The decision to apply intensive therapies should be based on the integration of multiple parameters including risk scoring based on

Table 3.6 Individualized therapy of high-risk MDS (IPSS Int-2 and high) in elderly patients ($\geq$70 years)

Patient category	Therapy recommended	Aim of therapy
Go-go/fit	Best supportive care[a]	Improved QoL, hematologic improvement
	Allo-HSCT[b]	Curation, prolonged OS and PFS
	Azanucleosides[c]	Prolonged OS and PFS, hematologic improvement, reduction of transfusion need, relief of symptoms, improved QoL
	Investigational agents[d,e]	
Slow-go / vulnerable	Best supportive care[a]	Improved QoL, hematologic improvement
	Azanucleosides[d]	Prolonged OS and PFS, hematologic improvement, reduction of transfusion need, relief of symptoms, improved QoL
	Investigational agents[d,e]	
No-go / frail	Best supportive care[a]	Improved QoL, hematologic improvement
	(Azanucleosides)[f]	Improved QoL, hematologic improvement, relief of symptoms
	Investigational agents[d,e]	

Allo-HSCT allogeneic hematologic stem cell transplantation, *OS* overall survival, *PFS* progression-free survival, *QoL* quality of life

[a]Supportive care represents the basis of all treatment concepts

[b]Might be feasible in a minority of selected cases with an excellent health status. Decision should be made on an individual basis, possibly after pretreatment with azanucleosides

[c]Vidaza® is approved in this indication in Europe and in the United States, Dacogen® in the United States. A predictive score for response to Vidaza® has been developed recently [28]

[d]The inclusion in clinical studies is recommended

[e]Investigational agents include an oral formulation of azacitidine, histone deacetylase inhibitors, lenalidomide and combinations thereof

[f]Even a minor portion of no-go patients might benefit from azacitidine

established scores, functional capacities, co-morbidities and preferences of patients and relatives (Fig. 3.1).

The need for Geriatric Assessment

Aspects of multidimensional geriatric assessment have just started to be integrated in the care of MDS patients. Whereas the scoring systems established so far are based on disease-specific prognostic factors like bone marrow blasts or karyotype, patient-related factors like functional capacities or co-morbidities including cardiac insufficiency or tolerance to chemotherapy are less well defined. The integration of structured co-morbidity scores to classify and quantify co-morbid conditions in clinical studies has just started. The hematopoietic stem-cell transplantation-specific co-morbidity index (HCT-CI), was found to be a significant prognostic factor for overall survival, for event-free survival as well as for non-leukemic deaths in MDS patients [31]. Several studies have proven the relevance of comorbidity scoring in the prognostication in MDS [32, 33, 34]. The systematic evaluation and integration of scores of the geriatric assessment like nutritional status, social support or cognitive function has just started [36, 37]. These parameters will be evaluated for their prognostic impact, their capacity to predict response and toxicities and will turn out to represent parameters of clinical outcome. Their integration will improve the individualized therapy-planning both in clinical studies and in medical practice in MDS.

Future Perspectives

Based on the development of innovative therapeutic options including epigenetically active drugs, immune modulating agents, thrombopoietic agents and effective iron chelators, treatment algorithms in elderly MDS have become more complex. To achieve an individualized therapy-planning and to optimize clinical outcome, not only chronological age but also aspects of age-adjusted life expectancy and assessment parameters including functional capacities, co-morbidities, quality of life and nutritional status have to be integrated in clinical studies and in daily practice.

Acknowledgement Supported by Senioren-Krebshilfe, www.senioren-krebshilfe.at.

References

1. Germing U, Strupp C, Kundgen A, Bowen D, Aul C, Haas R, Gattermann N. No increase in age-specific incidence of myelodysplastic syndromes. Haematologica. 2004;89(8):905–10.
2. de Swart L, Smith A, Fenaux P, Symenonidis A, Hellström-Lindberg E, Sanz G, Cermak J, Georgescu O, Germing U, MacKenzie M, Beyne-Rauzy O, Malcovati L, Stauder R, Droste J, Bowen D, de Witte T. Management of 1000 patients with low- and intermediate-1 risk myelodysplastic syndromes in the European LeukemiaNet MDS Registry. Leuk Res. 2011; S3(7):Supplement 1.
3. Pfeilstöcker M, Karlic H, Nösslinger T, Sperr W, Stauder R, Krieger O, Valent P. Myelodysplasia and aging: differences and common features in biology and clinic. Leukemia and Lymphoma. 2007;48(10):1900–9.
4. Stauder R, Noesslinger T, Pfeilstöcker M, Sperr WR, Wimazal F, Krieger O, Valent P. Impact of age and comorbidity in myelodysplastic syndromes. J Natl Compr Canc Netw. 2008;6(9): 927–34.
5. Stauder R. The challenge of personalized risk assessment and therapy planning in elderly high-risk myelodysplastic syndromes (MDS) patients. Ann Hematol. 2012;91(9):1333–43.
6. Neukirchen J, Schoonen WM, Strupp C, Gattermann N, Aul C, Haas R, Germing U. Incidence and prevalence of myelodysplastic syndromes: data from the Düsseldorf MDS-registry. Leuk Res. 2011;35(12):1591–6.
7. Stauder R, Wimazal F, Nösslinger T, Krieger O, Sperr WR, Sill H, Pfeilstöcker M, Valent P. Individualized management and therapy of myelodysplastic syndromes. Wien Klin Wochenschr. 2008;120:523–37.
8. Schanz J, Tüchler H, Solé F, Mallo M, Luño E, Cervera J, Granada I, Hildebrandt B, Slovak ML, Ohyashiki K, Steidl C, Fonatsch C, Pfeilstöcker M, Nösslinger T, Valent P, Giagounidis A, Aul C, Lübbert M, Stauder R, Krieger O, Garcia-Manero G, Faderl S, Pierce S, Le Beau MM, Bennett JM, Greenberg P, Germing U, Haase D. New comprehensive cytogenetic scoring system for primary myelodysplastic syndromes (MDS) and oligoblastic acute myeloid leukemia after MDS derived from an international database merge. J Clin Oncol. 2012;30(8):820–9.

9. Greenberg P, Cox C, LeBeau MM, Fenaux P, Morel P, Sanz G, Sanz M, Vallespi T, Hamblin T, Oscier D, Ohyashiki K, Toyama K, Aul C, Mufti G, Bennett J. International scoring system for evaluating prognosis in myelodysplastic syndromes. Blood. 1997;89(6):2079–88.
10. Kantarjian H, O'Brien S, Ravandi F, Cortes J, Shan J, Bennett JM, List A, Fenaux P, Sanz G, Issa JP, Freireich EJ, Garcia-Manero G. Proposal for a new risk model in myelodysplastic syndrome that accounts for events not considered in the original International Prognostic Scoring System. Cancer. 2008;113(6):1351.
11. Garcia-Manero G. Myelodysplastic syndromes: 2014 update on diagnosis, risk-stratification, and management. Am J Hematol. 2014;89(1):97–108.
12. Nösslinger T, Tüchler H, Germing U, Sperr WR, Krieger O, Haase D, Lübbert M, Stauder R, Giagounidis A, Valent P, Pfeilstöcker M. Prognostic impact of age and gender in 897 untreated patients with primary myelodysplastic syndromes. Ann Oncol. 2010;21(1):120–5.
13. Malcovati L, Porta MG, Pascutto C, Invernizzi R, Boni M, Travaglino E, Passamonti F, Arcaini L, Maffioli M, Bernasconi P, Lazzarino M, Cazzola M. Prognostic factors and life expectancy in myelodysplastic syndromes classified according to WHO criteria, a basis for clinical decision making. J Clin Oncol. 2005;23(30):7594–603.
14. Valent P, Horny HP, Bennett JM, Fonatsch C, Germing U, Greenberg P, Haferlach T, Haase D, Kolb HJ, Krieger O, Loken M, van de Loosdrecht A, Ogata K, Orfao A, Pfeilstöcker M, Rüter B, Sperr WR, Stauder R, Wells DA. Definitions and standards in the diagnosis and treatment of myelodysplastic syndromes: consensus statements and report from a working conference. Leukemia Research. 2007;31(6):727–36.
15. Platzbecker U, Santini V, Mufti GJ, Haferlach C, Maciejewski JP, Park S, Solé F, van de Loosdrecht AA, Haase D. Update on developments in the diagnosis and prognostic evaluation of patients with myelodysplastic syndromes (MDS): consensus statements and report from an expert workshop. Leuk Res. 2012;36(3):264–70.
16. Bruning RD, Orazi A, Germing U, Le Beau MM, Porwit A, Baumann I, et al. Myelodysplastic syndromes. In: Swerdlow SH, Campo E, Harris NL, Jaffe ES, Pileri SA, Stein H, Thiele J, Vardiman JW, editors. World Health Organization classification of tumours of the hematopoietic and lymphoid tissues. 4th ed. Lyon: International Agency for Research on Cancer; 2008.
17. Greenberg PL, Tuechler H, Schanz J, Sanz G, Garcia-Manero G, Solé F, Bennett JM, Bowen D, Fenaux P, Dreyfus F, Kantarjian H, Kuendgen A, Levis A, Malcovati L, Cazzola M, Cermak J, Fonatsch C, Le Beau MM, Slovak ML, Krieger O, Luebbert M, Maciejewski J, Magalhaes SM, Miyazaki Y, Pfeilstöcker M, Sekeres M, Sperr WR, Stauder R, Tauro S, Valent P, Vallespi T, van de Loosdrecht AA, Germing U, Haase D. Revised international prognostic scoring system for myelodysplastic syndromes. Blood. 2012;120(12):2454–65.
18. Malcovati L, Della Porta MG, Cazzola M. Predicting survival and leukemic evolution in patients with myelodysplastic syndrome. Haematologica. 2006;91(12):1588–90.
19. Hellström-Lindberg E, Gulbrandsen N, Lindberg G, Ahlgren T, Dahl IM, Dybedal I, Grimfors G, Hesse-Sundin E, Hjorth M, Kanter-Lewensohn L, Linder O, Luthman M, Löfvenberg E, Oberg G, Porwit-MacDonald A, Rådlund A, Samuelsson J, Tangen JM, Winquist I, Wisloff F, Scandinavian MDS Group. A validated decision model for treating the anaemia of myelodysplastic syndromes with erythropoietin+G-CSF: significant effects on quality of life. Br J Haematol. 2003;120(6):1037–46.
20. Greenberg PL, Sun Z, Miller KB, Bennett JM, Tallman MS, Dewald G, Paietta E, van der Jagt R, Houston J, Thomas ML, Cella D, Rowe JM. Treatment of MDS patients with erythropoietin with or without G-CSF: results of a prospective randomized phase 3 trial by the Eastern Cooperative Oncology Group (E1996). Blood. 2009;114:2393.
21. Jädersten M, Malcovati L, Dybedal I, Della Porta MG, Invernizzi R, Montgomery SM, Pascutto C, Porwit A, Cazzola M, Hellström-Lindberg E. Erythropoietin and G-CSF treatment associated with improved survival in MDS. J Clin Oncol. 2008;26(21):3607–13.
22. Park S, Grabar S, Kelaidi C, Beyne-Rauzy O, Picard F, Bardet V, Coiteux V, Leroux G, Lepelley P, Daniel MT, Cheze S, Mahé B, Ferrant A, Ravoet C, Escoffre-Barbe M, Adès L, Vey N, Aljassem L, Stamatoullas A, Mannone L, Dombret H, Bourgeois K, Greenberg P,

Fenaux P, Dreyfus F, GFM group (Groupe Francophone des Myélodysplasies). Predictive factors of response and survival in myelodysplastic syndrome treated with erythropoietin and G-CSF: the GFM experience. Blood. 2008;111(2):574–82.
23. Valent P, Krieger O, Stauder R, Wimazal F, Nösslinger T, Sperr WR, Sill H, Bettelheim P, Pfeilstöcker M. Iron overload in myelodysplastic syndromes (MDS) – diagnosis, treatment, and response criteria: a proposal of the Austrian MDS platform. Eur J Clin Invest. 2008;38(3):143–9.
24. Jädersten M, Saft L, Smith A, Kulasekararaj A, Pomplun S, Göhring G, Hedlund A, Hast R, Schlegelberger B, Porwit A, Hellström-Lindberg E, Mufti GJ. TP53 mutations in low-risk myelodysplastic syndromes with del(5q) predict disease progression. J Clin Oncol. 2011;29(15):1971–9.
25. Sloand EM, Olnes MJ, Shenoy A, Weinstein B, Boss C, Loeliger K, Wu CO, More K, Barrett AJ, Scheinberg P, Young NS. Alemtuzumab treatment of intermediate-1 myelodysplasia patients is associated with sustained improvement in blood counts and cytogenetic remissions. J Clin Oncol. 2010;28(35):5166–73. Epub 2010 Nov 1.
26. Fenaux P, Mufti GJ, Hellstrom-Lindberg E, Santini V, Finelli C, Giagounidis A, Schoch R, Gattermann N, Sanz G, List A, Gore SD, Seymour JF, Bennett JM, Byrd J, Backstrom J, Zimmerman L, McKenzie D, Beach C, Silverman LR, International Vidaza High-Risk MDS Survival Study Group. Efficacy of azacitidine compared with that of conventional care regimens in the treatment of higher risk myelodysplastic syndromes: a randomised, open-label, phase III study. Lancet Oncol. 2009;10(3):223–32.
27. Seymour JF, Fenaux P, Silverman LR, Mufti GJ, Hellström-Lindberg E, Santini V, List AF, Gore SD, Backstrom J, McKenzie D, Beach CL. Effects of azacitidine compared with conventional care regimens in elderly (≥75 years) patients with higher-risk myelodysplastic syndromes. Crit Rev Oncol Hematol. 2010;76(3):218–27.
28. Itzykson R, Thépot S, Quesnel B, Dreyfus F, Beyne-Rauzy O, Turlure P, Vey N, Recher C, Dartigeas C, Legros L, Delaunay J, Salanoubat C, Visanica S, Stamatoullas A, Isnard F, Marfaing-Koka A, de Botton S, Chelghoum Y, Taksin AL, Plantier I, Ame S, Boehrer S, Gardin C, Beach CL, Adès L, Fenaux P, Groupe Francophone des Myelodysplasies(GFM). Prognostic factors for response and overall survival in 282 patients with higher-risk myelodysplastic syndromes treated with azacitidine. Blood. 2011;117(2):403–11.
29. Kantarjian H, Issa JP, Rosenfeld CS, Bennett JM, Albitar M, DiPersio J, et al. Decitabine improves patient outcomes in myelodysplastic syndromes: results of a phase III randomized study. Cancer. 2006;106(8):1794–803.
30. Lübbert M, Suciu S, Baila L, Rüter BH, Platzbecker U, Giagounidis A, et al. Low-dose decitabine versus best supportive care in elderly patients with intermediate- or high-risk myelodysplastic syndrome (MDS) ineligible for intensive chemotherapy: final results of the randomized phase III study of the European Organisation for Research and Treatment of Cancer Leukemia Group and the German MDS Study Group. J Clin Oncol. 2011;29(15): 1987–96.
31. Sperr WR, Wimazal F, Kundi M, Baumgartner C, Nösslinger T, Makrai A, Stauder R, Krieger O, Pfeilstöcker M, Valent P. Comorbidity as prognostic variable in MDS: comparative evaluation of the HCT-CI and CCI in a core data Set of 582 patients of the Austrian MDS platform. Ann Oncol. 2010;21(1):114–9.
32. Naqvi K, Garcia-Manero G, Sardesai S, Oh J, Vigil CE, Pierce S, Lei X, Shan J, Kantarjian HM, Suarez-Almazor ME. Association of comorbidities with overall survival in myelodysplastic syndrome: development of a prognostic model. J Clin Oncol. 2011;29(16):2240–6. Epub 2011 May 2.
33. Wang R, Gross CP, Halene S, Ma X, et al. Comorbidities and survival in a large cohort of patients with newly diagnosed myelodysplastic syndromes. Leuk Res. 2009;33(12):1594–8.
34. Bammer C, Sperr WR, Kemmler G, Wimazal F, Nösslinger T, Schönmetzler A, Krieger O, Pfeilstöcker M, Valent P, Stauder R. Clustering of comorbidities is related to age and sex and impacts clinical outcome in myelodysplastic syndromes. J Geriatr Oncol. 2014;5(3):299–306.

35. Vardiman JW, Thiele J, Arber DA, Brunning RD, Borowitz MJ, Porwit A, et al. The 2008 revision of the World Health Organization (WHO) classification of myeloid neoplasms and acute leukemia: rationale and important changes. Blood. 2009;114(5):937–51.
36. Hamaker ME, Mitrovic M, Stauder R. The G8 screening tool detects relevant geriatric impairments and predicts survival in elderly patients with a haematological malignancy. Ann Hematol. 2014;93(6):1031–40.
37. Hamaker ME, Prins MC, Stauder R. The relevance of a geriatric assessment for elderly patients with a haematological malignancy – a systematic review. Leuk Res. 2014;38(3):275–83.

Chapter 4
Acute Myeloid Leukemia

Heidi D. Klepin and Timothy S. Pardee

Abstract The incidence of acute myelogenous leukemia (AML) increases with age. Older AML patients, often defined by age 60 years and above, have worse treatment outcomes than younger patients. Selected older patients can benefit from curative therapies, but as a group they experience increased treatment-related toxicity, are more likely to relapse, and have decreased overall survival. Age-related outcome disparity is in part explained by differences in tumor biology. Older patients are more likely to present with unfavorable cytogenetic abnormalities, multidrug resistance phenotypes, and secondary AML. However, even among older adults with favorable tumor biology, prognosis differs by age in clinical trials. Patient-specific factors such as impaired physical function and comorbidity independently predict increased treatment toxicity and decreased survival. Improved patient assessment strategies are needed to identify those patients most likely to benefit from standard induction and post-remission therapies. In addition, research is ongoing to identify more effective and tolerable induction and post-remission treatments for this population. Finally, enhanced supportive care strategies designed to minimize the negative effects of treatment on function and quality of life are needed to maximize short and longer term benefits of therapy.

Keywords Acute myeloid leukemia • Elderly • Induction chemotherapy • Treatment

Introduction

More than half of all newly diagnosed patients with AML are ≥65 years of age. Despite this, optimal therapy for older adults remains controversial. Clinical trial and registry data demonstrate a survival advantage for intensive therapy among

H.D. Klepin, MD, MS (✉) • T.S. Pardee, MD, PhD
Department of Internal Medicine,
Section on Hematology and Oncology,
Wake Forest School of Medicine, Medical Center Blvd,
Winston-Salem, NC 27157, USA
e-mail: hklepin@wakehealth.edu; tspardee@wakehealth.edu

U. Wedding, R.A. Audisio (eds.), *Management of Hematological Cancer in Older People*, DOI 10.1007/978-1-4471-2837-3_4

older adults compared to low intensity or supportive care, but outcomes remain poor. Older age (particularly >70 years) is associated with decreased overall survival (OS) and increased treatment-associated morbidity. Many older adults are therefore not offered curative therapy for AML. Age, however, is a surrogate measure for both changes in tumor biology (conferring treatment resistance) and patient characteristics (decreasing treatment tolerance). For patients with the same chronologic age, there is significant heterogeneity of tumor biology and physiologic reserve making strictly age-related treatment decisions suboptimal. Individualized treatment decision-making based on evolving stratification of tumor and patient characteristics can help inform the tailoring of treatment and supportive care interventions.

Epidemiology

In 2012, an estimated 13,780 men and women (7,350 men and 6,430 women) were diagnosed with and 10,200 men and women died of AML in the United States of America (US) [1]. The incidence of AML increases dramatically with age (Fig. 4.1). The median age of diagnosis in the US remains 66 years with approximately one-third of newly diagnosed patients ≥75 years of age. Survival for AML is age dependent with significantly lower survival rates reported for older adults [1, 2] (Fig. 4.2). Population-based statistics from the US (Surveillance End Epidemiologic Results, SEER) reporting on 5-year survival rate differences between 1975 and 2004 indicate improvement over time for adults, however the magnitude of the improvement declines with age; 50–64 (4.7–23.9 %) 65–74 (6.2–13 %) and ≥75 years (1.4–1.7 %).

The primary risk factors for developing AML are older age and a history of prior myelodysplastic syndrome (MDS). Less common risk factors which have been reported include: previous myeloproliferative neoplasm (MPN), chemotherapy drugs (alkylators, topoisomerase 2 inhibitors, and nitrosoureas), radiation or petrochemical exposure.

Current Diagnostic Standards

The clinical signs and symptoms of AML are varied and non-specific but acute in onset. Symptoms are typically related to cytopenias, often pancytopenia due to leukemic infiltration of the bone marrow. As such, patients commonly present with infections, fatigue, or bleeding. Less commonly, older adults with AML may present with severe leukocytosis, producing symptoms of leukostasis which can result in altered mental status (i.e., delirium), shortness of breath, or chest pain. Occasionally presentations related to symptoms of leukemic infiltration of tissues

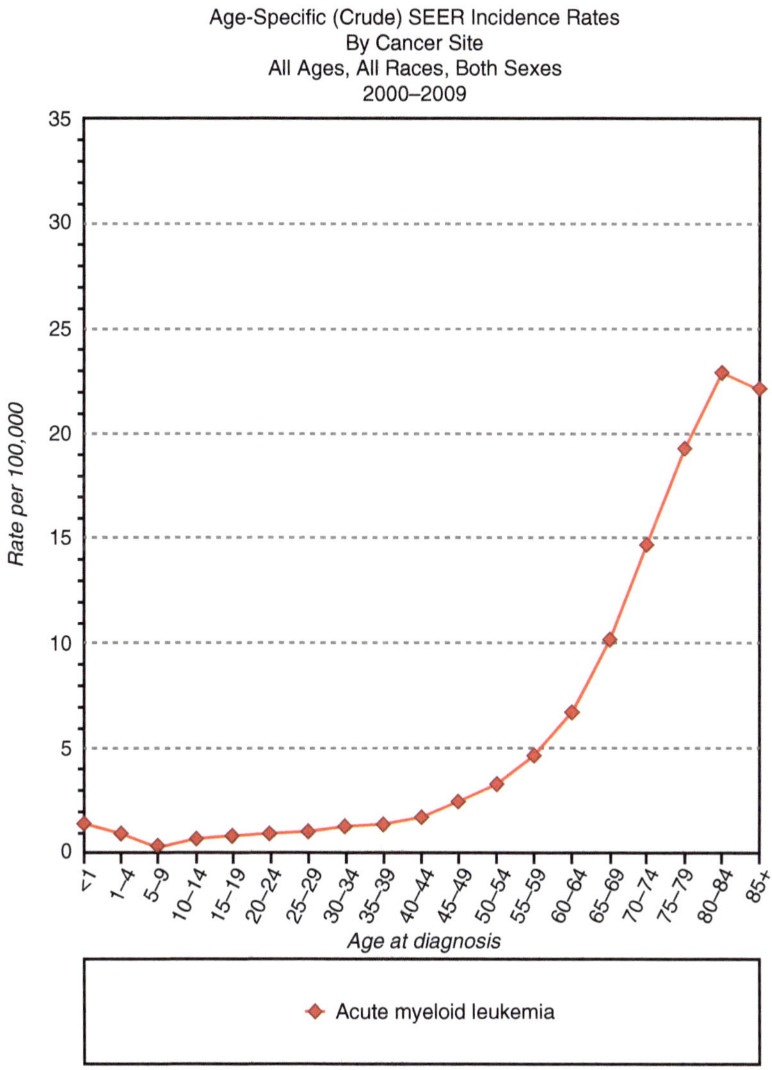

Cancer sites include invasive cases only unless otherwise noted.
Rates are per 100,000.
Incidence source: SEER 18 areas (San Francisco, Connecticut, Detroit, Hawaii, Iowa, New Mexico, Seattle, Utah, Atlanta, San Jose-Monterey, Los Angeles, Alaska Native Registry, Rural Georgia, California excluding SF/SJM/LA, Kentucky, Louisiana, New Jersey and Georgia excluding ATL/RG).

Fig. 4.1 SEER relative survival rates for AML by age group, 1988–2008. *SEER* surveillance end epidemiology and end results. http://seer.cancer.gov

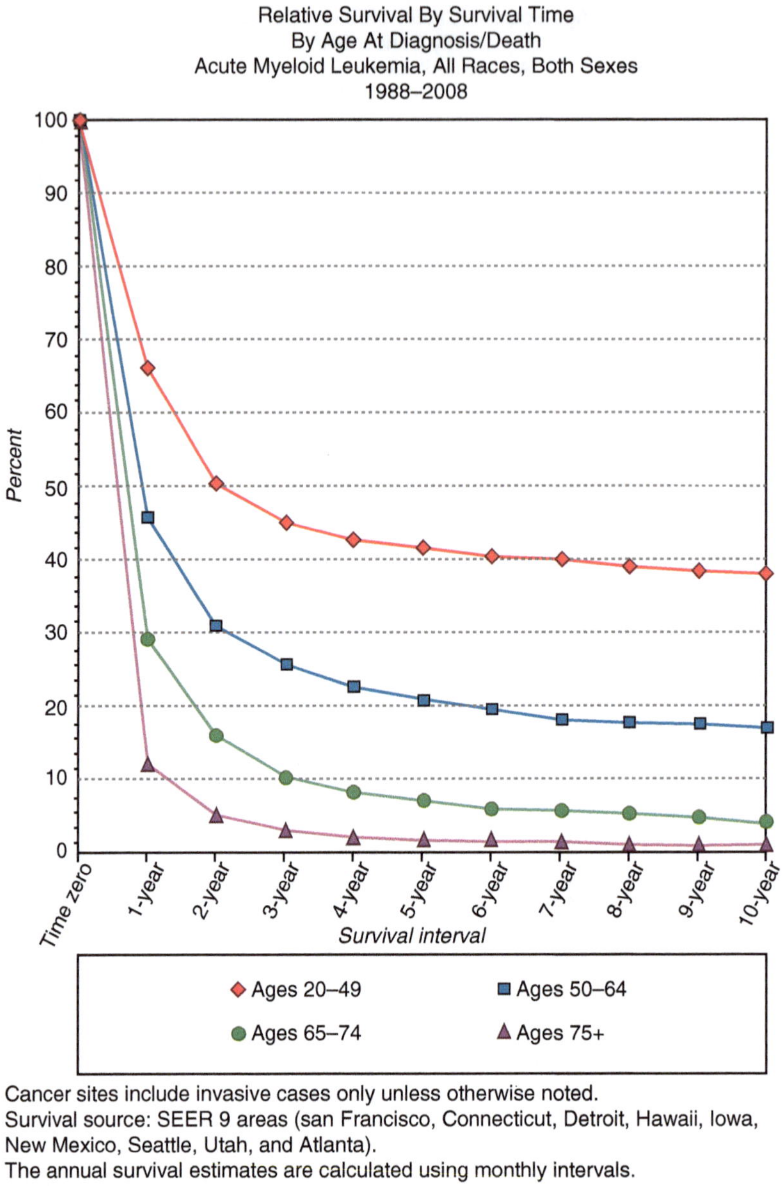

Fig. 4.2 SEER relative survival rates for AML by age group, 1988–2008. *SEER* surveillance end epidemiology and end results. http://seer.cancer.gov

outside the marrow (i.e., liver, spleen, gums, lymph nodes, skin, or central nervous system) are seen.

The diagnosis of AML requires documentation of an abnormal accumulation of leukemic blasts of myeloid origin [3]. The presence of ≥20 % blasts in the marrow or peripheral blood is diagnostic. Exceptions are made for certain genetic

Table 4.1 WHO (2008) classification of acute myeloid leukemias and related precursor neoplasms

Acute myeloid leukemia with recurrent genetic abnormalities
AML with t(8;21)(q22;q22); RUNX1-RUNX1T1
AML with inv(16)(p13.1q22) or t(16;16)(p13.1;q22); CBFB-MYH11
APL with t(15;17)(q22;q12); PML-RARA
AML with t(9;11)(p22;q23); MLLT3-MLL
AML with t(6;9)(p23;q34); DEK-NUP214
AML with inv(3)(q21q26.2) or t(3;3)(q21;q26.2); RPN1-EVI1
AML (megakaryoblastic) with t(1;22)(p13;q13); RBM15-MKL1
Provisional entity: AML with mutated NPM1
Provisional entity: AML with mutated CEBPA
Acute myeloid leukemia with myelodysplasia-related changes
Therapy-related myeloid neoplasms
Acute myeloid leukemia not otherwise specified
AML with minimal differentiation
AML without maturation
AML with maturation
Acute myelomonocytic leukaemia
Acute monoblastic/monocytic leukaemia

Acute erythroid leukaemias
  Pure erythroid leukaemia
  Erythroleukaemia, erythroid/myeloid

Acute megakaryoblastic leukaemia
Acute basophilic leukaemia
Acute panmyelosis with myelofibrosis
Myeloid sarcoma
Myeloid proliferation related to Down syndrome
Transient abnormal myelopoiesis
Myeloid leukaemia associated with Down syndrome
Blastoid plasmacytoid dendritic neoplasms

Adapted from Gilliland et al. [73]

abnormalities such as t(8;21), inv(16), t (15;17), t(16;16) and some cases of erythroleukemia. Immunohistochemical and flow cytometry techniques aid morphologic evaluation to confirm myeloid versus lymphoid origin. Conventional cytogenetics is a required component in the diagnostic evaluation of patients suspected of AML with >50 % of patients presenting with a detectable cytogenetic abnormality. Fluorescence in situ hybridization (FISH) for common prognostic chromosomal alterations should be performed if cytogenetic analysis fails. Molecular testing for mutations in *NPM1*, *CEBPA* and *FLT3* should be considered in cytogenetically normal patients. The role of molecular testing in clinical practice is rapidly evolving. The WHO classification of AML (Table 4.1) highlights the importance of cytogenetic and molecular studies for prognosis and treatment. It has become increasingly clear over recent years that AML comprises a group of distinct diseases with a broad range of tumor biology.

Tumor Biology

Age-related changes in tumor biology are a major contributor to outcomes for older adults (Table 4.2). Older patients are more likely to have unfavorable cytogenetic abnormalities (i.e., chromosome 5 and 7 abnormalities, and/or complex karyotypes) and less likely to have favorable cytogenetic abnormalities [i.e., t(8;21),t(15;17) and inv(16)] compared to younger patients at the time of presentation [2, 4, 5]. Unfavorable cytogenetic abnormalities are associated with decreased remission rates and shortened overall survival (OS) [2, 4, 6–8]. The expression of a multi-drug resistance phenotype (MDR1) is also more common in older AML patients [9]. This membrane-associated glycoprotein actively pumps out many conventional chemotherapies such as anthracyclines thereby reducing intracellular concentrations and promoting leukemia cell survival. Finally, older adults are more likely to develop AML in the setting previous hematologic disorders (MDS/MPN), which is more resistant to standard therapies [10].

While each of these risk factors independently influences remission rates, the presence of multiple poor risk features dramatically reduces the odds of achieving a complete remission (CR) with standard induction therapies. In a Southwestern Oncology Group (SWOG) study of older adults with newly diagnosed AML treated with intensive induction therapy, patients with none of these adverse risk factors (de novo AML, MDR1 negative phenotype, favorable/intermediate cytogenetics) had a CR rate of 81 % compared to 12 % of those with multiple risk factors (secondary AML, MDR1 positive phenotype, unfavorable cytogenetics) [9]. In another study focused on the small percentage of older patients with favorable cytogenetics [t(8;21), inv(16)], remission rates of 80 % with 30 % 5-year survival were reported [11] resulting in some consensus that this subgroup should be offered intensive therapy if their Eastern Cooperative Oncology Group (ECOG) performance status is <3.

The majority of older adults, however, have cytogenetically normal AML. This group remains molecularly diverse with an ever evolving understanding of the prognostic implications of gene mutations (i.e., *FLT3-ITD*, *NPM1*, *CEBPA*, *DNMT3*, *IDH1 and IDH2*, *WT1*) and overexpression (i.e., *ERG*, *BAALC*) [12–18]. The most well defined molecular risk factors are *FLT3-ITD* mutation (poor prognosis), and *NPM1* or isolated *CEBPA* mutation in absence of *FLT3-ITD* (good prognosis). The prognostic implications of these mutations are consistent between younger and older AML patients. There are molecular changes that have been observed between older and younger patients. Analysis of gene expression data comparing patients <45 years with those ≥55 years has demonstrated age-specific dysregulation of oncogenic pathways [19]. Current strategies to improve outcomes for older adults include the design of trials using novel agents to target specific molecular AML subtypes. For example, several completed and ongoing trials utilizing FLT3 inhibitors (i.e., midosaurin, sorafenib) in novel combinations were designed to investigate the efficacy of this approach for patients with FLT3 mutations. These trails have so far yielded disappointing results underscoring the genetic complexity of AML in

Table 4.2 Selected randomized trials of induction chemotherapy for adults ≥60 years of age with AML

Author	Year	Age (years)	N	Treatment Arms	CR (%)	Median OS (months)	P value for OS	Induction death rate (%)
Standard dose induction								
Lowenberg et al. [32]	1989	>65	31	Ara-C, daunorubicin, vincristine	58	5.3	<0.05	9.7
			29	Supportive care	0	2.8		N/A
Lowenberg et al. [37]	1998	>60	242	Ara-C, daunomycin	38	9.0	0.23	6.0
			247	Ara-C, mitoxantrone	47	9.7		6.0
Dose attenuated induction								
Tilly et al. [35]	1990	>65	46	Rubidazone, Ara-C	52	12.8	0.12	31
			41	Low dose Ara-C	32	8.8		10
Growth factor support								
Lowenberg et al. [41]	1997	>60	157	Daunomycin, Ara-C, GM-CSF	56	No difference	0.55	14
			161	Daunomycin, Ara-C	55			10
Stone et al. [39]	1995	>60	195	Ara-C, daunorubicin	54	9.4	0.10	16
			193	Ara-C, daunorubicin, GM-CSF	51	9.4		20
MDR1 modulation								
Baer et al. [42]	2002	≥60	61	Ara-C, daunorubicin, etoposide	46	No difference	0.48	20
			59	Ara-C, daunorubicin, etoposide, PSC-833	39			44
Van der Holt et al. [43]	2005	≥60	211	Daunorubicin, Ara-C	48	No difference	0.52	Not reported
			208	Daunorubicin, Ara-C, PSC-833	54			

(continued)

Table 4.2 (continued)

Author	Year	Age (years)	N	Treatment Arms	CR (%)	Median OS (months)	P value for OS	Induction death rate (%)
Dose Intensification								
Lowenberg et al. [44]	2009	≥60	411	Ara-C, daunorubicin 45 mg/m^2	54	No difference	0.16	11
Addition of gemtuzumab ozogamicin			402	Ara-C, daunorubicin 90 mg/m^2	64			12
Castainge et al. [45]	2012	≥50	139	Ara-C, daunorubicin, gemtuzumab ozogamicin	75[a]	11	<0.05	4
			139		81[a]	28		6
Lower intensity therapy								
Kantarjian et al. [48]	2012	≥65	243	Supportive care or low dose Ara-C	8	5	0.2	8
			242	Decitabine	18	8		9
Burnett, et al [49]	2007	≥60[b]	103	Low dose Ara-C ± ATRA	18	Improved with low dose Ara-C	<0.05	26
			99	Hydroxyurea ± ATRA	1			26

Abbreviations: *AML* acute myelogenous leukemia, *N* number of patients enrolled, *CR* complete remission, *OS* overall survival, *Ara-C* cytarabine, *N/A* not applicable, *GM-CSF* granulocyte macrophage colony stimulating growth factor

[a]Rates represent CR with incomplete platelet count recovery

[b]2 % <60 with comorbidity

older patients. It is expected that tolerable treatment options will increase for older adults with successful targeting of molecular subtypes of AML and incorporation of genetic signatures into risk stratification schema in clinical trials.

Overview of Treatment Trials for Older Adults with AML

There is ongoing debate regarding the optimal treatment strategy for older adults with AML ranging from supportive care alone to standard aggressive therapies [20–24]. This debate is fueled by low survival rates with substantial risk of treatment toxicity among elders undergoing curative therapies. These concerns translate into low rates of receipt of therapy; less than 40 % of older adults receive chemotherapy after AML diagnosis in the US [25].

Clinical trials have consistently shown worse survival outcomes among older adults with AML compared to younger patients using age cutoffs of 55, 60, and 65 years [2, 26, 27]. Older adults are less likely to achieve a CR and to remain relapse free if they have achieved a CR. For example, in an analysis of SWOG treatment trials, including 968 AML patients, treated with standard induction and consolidation therapy, CR rates were 64, 46, 39, and 33 % in age groups <56, 56–65, 66–75, and older than 75 years, respectively. Among patients with responsive disease the median disease free survival was 21.6, 7.4, 8.3 and 8.9 months, respectively; the OS for the whole population was 18.8, 9.0, 6.9, and 3.5 months, respectively [2]. Older adults are also more likely to experience treatment-related death (typically defined as death within 30 days of initiation of therapy), ranging from 15 to 30 % in clinical trials [2, 21, 22, 28]. These results likely underestimate actual treatment mortality in clinical practice as only patients fit enough to enroll on clinical trial were studied. Due to concerns regarding inferior outcomes with treatment and increased toxicity, a large proportion of older adults in the US are not considered for chemotherapy treatment for this disease [29, 30].

Induction Therapy

Standard induction chemotherapy for non-acute promyelocytic (APL) AML typically involves a treatment regimen that includes cytarabine (Ara-C) and an anthracycline given for 7 and 3 days respectively (7+3) [31]. Lowenberg et al. performed a landmark study demonstrating survival improvement for patients ≥65 years of age treated with intensive induction therapy versus supportive care alone [32] with no difference in time spent hospitalized between the two groups. This study provided supporting evidence to offer curative chemotherapy to selected older adults with AML. Population-based data from Sweden and the US similarly show a survival advantage for treatment [25, 33].

In the decades since publication of the landmark Lowenberg trial, many subsequent elderly- specific studies have been conducted. Unfortunately, most have failed to improve upon the suboptimal treatment outcomes seen in the older population (Table 4.2). In most elderly-specific trials, CR rates range from 40 to 60 %, but median survival remains less than a year [22]. Several variations of induction therapy regimens designed to improve the balance of efficacy versus toxicity have been investigated. Dose-attenuation, to minimize toxicity, has not resulted in substantial improvement in outcomes [34, 35]. Investigation of various anthracyclines, such as mitoxantrone and idarubicin, and the addition of etoposide have not improved survival for older adults [28, 36–38]. Use of growth factors including granulocyte colony stimulating factor (G-CSF) and granulocyte macrophage colony stimulating factor (GM-CSF) to decrease duration of neutropenia has not consistently been shown to improve response rates or survival; likewise they do not clearly decrease costs [28, 36, 39–41]. Modulation of the multi-drug resistant efflux pump (MDR1) was pursued using a cyclosporine analog PSC-833 with standard induction chemotherapy in two randomized trials [42, 43]. There was no benefit in response rates or survival and an increased toxic death rate on the experimental arm of the Cancer and Leukemia Group B trial [42].

Investigation of high anthracycline dose intensity has led to a positive outcome in a subset of older adults. Specifically, 90 mg/m^2 of daunorubicin improved CR rates compared to 45 mg/m^2 (64 % versus 54 % respectively) for untreated older adults receiving a 7+3 regimen [44]. While there was no significant increase in toxicity with higher dosing, the improved CR rate did not translate into better OS. In subset analyses, benefits appeared limited to adults aged 60–65 years. In this subset of "young-old" patients, a survival benefit was noted. No randomized trial data is available regarding comparison of the commonly used 60 mg/m^2 dosing with 90 mg/m^2. Two studies have shown positive outcomes when adding gemtuzumab ozogamicin to induction therapy for AML. Gemtuzumab ozogamicin is a humanized anti-CD33 monoclonal antibody linked to calicheamicin which has demonstrated efficacy in the relapsed setting but its use in older adults was after it was voluntarily withdrawn from the US market following a negative trial in younger AML patients. Recent investigations, however, testing a lower dose schedule in combination with intensive induction, suggest that the combination may be efficacious and tolerable. A phase 3 study of 280 adults aged 50–70 with untreated AML showed improvement in relapse-free (23 % versus 50 %) and overall survival (42 % versus 53 %) with the addition of gemtuzumab [45]. Benefit was most evident among patients with favorable cytogenetics. A larger study of patients >50 years old with AML or high risk MDS similarly showed a survival advantage to the addition of gemtuzumab to two different induction regimens without significant increased toxicity [46]. These studies have renewed interest in use of this agent in the curative setting, particularly among those with good risk cytogenetics, although data remains limited for adults >70 years of age. At present, gemtuzumab remains unavailable in many healthcare systems.

Lower intensity regimens have been tested for older adults, particularly for those considered "unfit" for intensive chemotherapy or presenting with more indolent disease. Use of DNA hypomethylating agents (azacitidine and decitabine) has increased significantly in recent years [25]. These agents have demonstrated activity in MDS and subset analyses of patients with low blast count AML (20–30 %) included on MDS treatment trials show evidence of increased response and survival compared to standard care (a mix of low dose Ara-C, best supportive care or 7+3) [47]. A multi-center trial of decitabine versus supportive care or low dose Ara-C for adults ≥65 years with intermediate or poor risk cytogenetics reported a CR rate of 18 % for decitabine and, in an unplanned post-hoc analysis, a small survival benefit (median 7.7 versus 6.2 months) [48]. At present, neither drug is approved for treatment of AML by the US Food and Drug Administration but both have an indication approved by the European Medicines Agency. Another low intensity option is low dose Ara-C which has limited activity and can improve survival among patients not fit for intensive chemotherapy compared to supportive care [49]. Low intensity regimens have not been compared in a randomized fashion to intensive therapy for older adults nor have rigorous definitions of fit or unfit been used in clinical trials to optimize extrapolation of data in clinical practice.

Post-remission Therapy

Optimal post-remission strategies for older adults are also undefined [31, 50]. It is generally accepted that post-remission therapy or consolidation is needed to translate a complete remission into cure [31]. Typical post-remission treatment includes high dose cytarabine or hematopoietic stem cell transplantation. For older adults with favorable or intermediate risk AML in first CR, consolidation chemotherapy without transplant is typically pursued. In a randomized study of low, intermediate and high dose cytarabine for consolidation in patients who had achieved CR, younger patients benefited from dose escalation while older patients experienced more cerebellar toxicity and no benefit in disease free survival [27]. For younger patients, high dose cytarabine (3 g/m^2) is a standard post-remission treatment option for good risk cytogenetics [31]. This treatment is too toxic for older adults and likely contributes to suboptimal outcomes seen in older adults with good risk cytogenetics. In elderly specific trials, lower dose Ara-C regimens as a single agent or in combination with an anthracycline have been tested [36, 51]. In this population, there is no clear evidence to date that multiple courses of consolidation or maintenance therapy improve outcomes when compared to a single course of consolidation therapy [34, 36, 51].

Allogeneic stem cell transplantation remains a standard post-remission treatment option with potential for long-term survival in younger adults with poor risk AML [31]. Traditional allogeneic hematopoietic cell transplantation (allo-HCT) is associated with very high treatment-related mortality in older adults and is therefore not recommended as post-remission therapy for most patients >60 years of age [52]. Advances in supportive care and use of reduced-intensity conditioning (RIC) allogeneic transplantation regimens ("non-myeloablative regimens") have resulted in a trend towards increased use of allogeneic transplantation in adults over age 50 [53]. This type of transplantation utilizes the graft versus leukemia effect and reduces acute toxicities associated with use of myeloablative therapies [54–56]. Chronologic age alone (at least up to 75 years) should not be considered a contraindication to RIC transplant. In an analysis of over 1,000 patients aged 40–79 (11 % ≥65) who received RIC for AML consolidation or MDS therapy there was no association between age and the following outcomes in multivariate analysis: non-relapse mortality, relapse, disease free and OS [57]. While this therapy may be feasible in highly selected older adults, it is yet unclear if this treatment strategy is superior to conventional approaches.

Post-remission therapy for older adults is further complicated by a higher likelihood that patients will no longer be candidates for additional treatment due to functional impairment or end organ damage resulting from induction therapy. In many cases a curative treatment approach must be aborted due to poor performance status that precludes post-remission treatment. In randomized trials, up to 20 % of older adults may not go on to receive any consolidation therapy after achieving CR [51]. Attrition is much higher for older adults considered for post-remission transplantation [54]. Outside of clinical trials even fewer older adults are likely to receive post-remission therapy since these patients are often less fit than those enrolled on clinical trials [58].

Acute Promyelocytic Leukemia

Treatment recommendations differ for patients with acute promyelocytic leukemia (APL). APL is characterized by a translocation between chromosomes 15 and 17 leading to the fusion of the promyelocytic leukemia (*PML*) gene with the retinoic acid receptor α (*RARα*) gene, resulting in disruption of normal cell differentiation [59]. While less common among older adults, response and cure rates are higher than in most AML subtypes with induction regimens that include use of all-*trans* retinoic acid (ATRA) which overcomes the differentiation block. A unique clinical feature of APL is presentation with bleeding secondary to disseminated intravascular coagulation. Hemorrhage is a frequent cause of early death. When suspected, treatment with ATRA should begin immediately. Curative treatment regimens often include induction with anthracycline and ATRA therapy followed by consolidation and maintenance therapy. Therapy may span 1–2 years with remission rates as high as 75–90 % on clinical trials. In addition, relapsed patients may respond to arsenic trioxide (ATO), with a high proportion achieving a second remission. This subtype of AML should be treated aggressively in older adults given the high probability of response. However, even among this favorable subgroup, age is a negative prognostic factor. Early death (30-day mortality) is high for all ages in population-based data (29 %) but significantly worse among those diagnosed at an older age, with poor performance status or comorbidity [60]. Despite availability of effective therapy, many older adults are not considered eligible for curative approaches [61]. Less toxic treatment approaches remain under investigation including use of ATRA and ATO during induction to minimize cytotoxic therapy.

Improving Patient Assessment Strategies

Risk stratification for older adults with AML has primarily focused on chronologic age, tumor biology, and oncology performance status (ECOG or Karnofsky). Several prognostic models for older adults (>60 years) have been developed. One model predicting induction (8-week) mortality among patients ≥70 years receiving intensive therapy includes patients age >80, complex karyotype, poor ECOG performance status (>1), and elevated creatinine (>1.3 mg/dl) [62]. Patients with none (28 %), 1 (40 %), 2 (23 %), or ≥3 (9 %) of these risk factors had early mortality rates of 16, 31, 55 and 71 %, respectively. Another model used to predict OS after induction highlights the importance of chronologic age, karyotype, NPM1 mutational status, white blood cell count, lactate dehydrogenase (LDH) levels, and CD4 expression [63]. Using this model four prognostic risk groups were illustrated: favorable, good intermediate, adverse intermediate, and high with corresponding 3-year OS rates of 39.5, 30, 10.6 and 3.3 %, respectively. A validated web-based application for prediction of CR and early death using clinical and laboratory variables (body temperature, age, secondary leukemia or antecedent hematological disease, hemoglobin, platelet count, fibrinogen and LDH) predicted CR rates ranging from 12 to 91 % if cytogenetic information was available [64]. These models demonstrate that outcomes for older adults vary widely and provide a foundation for improving risk-stratification at the time of diagnosis. Each model, however, relies on chronologic age as a surrogate for measureable underlying impairments (i.e., comorbidity, physical function, cognition) that may further improve estimates of reserve capacity during or after treatment.

Similar to the heterogeneity seen in AML biology, patient-specific factors differ substantially among older adults and translate into varied abilities to withstand the stress of treatment despite the same chronologic age. Geriatric assessment (GA) refers to the evaluation of multiple patient characteristics (physical function, comorbid disease, cognitive function, psychological state, and nutritional status) in an effort to discriminate between fit, vulnerable, and frail patients. How each of these patient characteristics influences treatment outcomes is an active field of study with AML-specific data summarized below.

Physical Function

Characterization of functional status can improve risk stratification for older adults with AML. The relationship between ECOG performance score at diagnosis, age, and 30-day mortality during induction chemotherapy is dramatic. Clinical trial data demonstrated similar 30-day mortality (11–15 %) for patients aged 56–65, 66–75, >75 with ECOG 0, contrasted with rates of 29, 47 and 82 %, respectively for baseline ECOG 3 [2]. Fit older adults, even those >75 years, may tolerate induction chemotherapy similar to those in middle age but the negative prognostic implications of poor performance status increases with age.

ECOG scores appear most useful in identifying frail patients (ECOG >2). Physiologic reserve capacity may vary widely among older adults with ECOG 0-2. Assessment of task-specific physical function or objectively measured physical performance (i.e., walking speed) may add information to oncology performance scales. In a prospective cohort of older adults considered to have "good" performance status (ECOG ≤1) treated with intensive induction therapy almost half had significant physical limitations at the time of treatment (48.2 % activities of daily living (ADL), 53.7 % objectively tested physical performance) [65]. Impairment in instrumental activities of daily living (IADLs) and physical performance (Short Physical Performance Battery [SPPB] score <9; includes walking speed, chair stands and balance testing) are independently associated with decreased survival [66, 67]. These data suggest that utilizing standardized measures to assess functional status can enhance treatment decision-making for the older adult.

Comorbidity

The presence of major comorbidity is a negative prognostic factor among older adults with AML, particularly among patients 60–80 years. In a retrospective study, 133 patients aged ≥70 years who received induction chemotherapy were evaluated using an adapted Charlson Comorbidity Index (CCI) to assess comorbidity burden [68]. Approximately one-third had major comorbidity (CCI score >1) which was an independent adverse prognostic factor for CR ($p=0.05$). The Hematopoietic Cell Transplantation Comorbidity Index (HCT-CI) developed to improve the sensitivity of the CCI in the transplant setting has been evaluated in AML. Giles et al. used this measure to assess comorbidity among 177 patients ≥60 years who received induction chemotherapy. The HCT-CI score was 0 in 22 %, 1–2 in 30 %, and ≥3 in 48 % corresponding with early death rates (3, 11, and 29 %) and OS (45, 31, and 19 weeks, respectively) [69]. While larger prospective studies are lacking, current evidence supports the use of pretreatment comorbidity assessment using the CCI or HCT-CI. The prognostic implications of individual comorbid conditions are not well-studied.

Cognitive Function

Cognitive dysfunction is prevalent among older adults. Pretreatment cognitive impairment may increase risks of complications during intensive therapy but research in this area is limited. Small studies suggest cognitive impairment may be prevalent and unrecognized among older adults undergoing therapy for AML

[66, 70]. For example, in prospective study of 74 older adults receiving intensive induction chemotherapy, pretreatment cognitive impairment was detected in 29 % of patients (median age 69) [66]. In multivariate analysis, cognitive impairment (defined by score <77 on the modified Mini Mental State Exam [3MS]) was associated with worse OS. These data support the need for more research on the prognostic value of cognitive screening in the setting of AML therapy.

Geriatric Assessment-Putting It All Together

Pretreatment assessment of older adults needs to take into account the complexity of variables that may differ from patient to patient. The additive effects of multiple impairments may be more important than individual conditions. Single institution data suggests pretreatment GA to assess multiple patient characteristics is feasible and can detect impairments among patients scheduled to receive intensive therapy: cognitive impairment, 31.5 %; depression, 38.9 %; distress, 53.7 %; impairment in ADLs, 48.2 %; impaired physical performance, 53.7 %; and comorbidity, 46.3 %. Importantly, most patients were impaired in one (92.6 %) or more (63 %) functional domains [65]. Feasibility of primarily self-administered GA is being tested in cooperative group treatment trials for older adults with AML and the prognostic significance of these impairments is under investigation. Ultimately, understanding specific patient vulnerabilities may help to: (1) predict tolerance and response to standard therapies; (2) inform adaptive clinical trial design for specific patient subgroups; and (3) identify targets for intervention to improve treatment tolerance such as exercise for physical impairment.

Recommendations for Treatment of Older Adults—Fit, Vulnerable, and Frail

Treatment recommendations for older adults with AML need to be individualized based on the complexity of tumor biology and patient characteristics. While optimal therapy for older adults as a group remains debated, there is some evidence to guide decision-making for individual patients. Older adults with newly diagnosed AML who present with an ECOG score >2 or significant comorbidity (CCI score >1, HCT-CI score >2) are more likely to experience toxicity and less likely to benefit from standard intensive induction chemotherapy. For these frail patients who are at highest risk for toxicity it would be reasonable to consider best supportive care, low intensity therapy or a clinical trial investigating novel agents. Options for less intensive therapy include low dose Ara-C or hypomethylating agents. Alternatively, older adults with good functional status (ECOG <2), minimal comorbidity, and good risk cytogenetics are likely to benefit from curative therapies regardless of chronologic age. A reasonable treatment regimen for these patients is 7 days of continuous infusion cytarabine at 100 mg/m²/day with 3 days of an anthracycline (daunorubicin at 60–90 mg/m²/day, idarubicin 12 mg/m², mitoxantrone 12 mg/m²). Consideration should be given to regimens including low dose gemtuzumab if available.

Optimal treatment for the large population of older adults who fall between these two extremes is unclear. While there is no clear evidence-based recommendation for patients with intermediate or poor risk cytogenetics those who are deemed to have good physiologic reserve capacity may benefit from intensive therapies on (preferred) or off clinical trials. One algorithm to define fit based on current evidence includes the following criteria: ECOG <2, no impairment in IADLs, no impairment in physical performance (SPPB >9), no cognitive impairment (3MS >77), and no significant comorbidity (CCI or HCT-CI ≤1). Prospective multi-site studies are needed to validate new refined criteria for fitness in this setting.

Finally, informed decision-making requires careful communication of individualized treatment options and potential outcomes. Limited evidence has suggested that older AML patients may over-estimate treatment benefit and often report not being offered treatment options [71, 72]. Careful evaluation of tumor and patient characteristics can help guide communication of treatment options for older adults.

Conclusions

Treatment decision-making for older adults with AML should be individualized taking into account both the heterogeneity of tumor biology and patient characteristics which can identify patients most likely to have responsive disease and adequate reserve capacity to tolerate and benefit from treatments. Outcomes for older adults may be enhanced by: (1) targeting unique molecular AML subtypes; (2) refining criteria for characterization of fit, vulnerable and frail; and (3) developing supportive care interventions to enhance treatment tolerance.

References

1. SEER cancer statistics review 1975–2009. Accessed 11 Apr 2013. Available from: URL: http://seer.cancer.gov/publications/.
2. Appelbaum FR, Gundacker H, Head DR, Slovak ML, Willman CL, Godwin JE, et al. Age and acute myeloid leukemia. Blood. 2006;107(9):3481–5.
3. Dohner H, Estey EH, Amadori S, Appelbaum FR, Buchner T, Burnett AK, et al. Diagnosis and management of acute myeloid leukemia in adults: recommendations from an international expert panel, on behalf of the European LeukemiaNet. Blood. 2010;115(3):453–74.
4. Grimwade D, Walker H, Harrison G, Oliver F, Chatters S, Harrison CJ, et al. The predictive value of hierarchical cytogenetic classification in older adults with acute myeloid leukemia (AML): analysis of 1065 patients entered into the United Kingdom Medical Research Council AML11 trial. Blood. 2001;98(5):1312–20.

5. van der Holt B, Breems DA, Berna BH, Van den Berg E, Burnett AK, Sonneveld P, et al. Various distinctive cytogenetic abnormalities in patients with acute myeloid leukaemia aged 60 years and older express adverse prognostic value: results from a prospective clinical trial. Br J Haematol. 2007;136(1):96–105.
6. Farag SS, Archer KJ, Mrozek K, Ruppert AS, Carroll AJ, Vardiman JW, et al. Pretreatment cytogenetics add to other prognostic factors predicting complete remission and long-term outcome in patients 60 years of age or older with acute myeloid leukemia: results from Cancer and Leukemia Group B 8461. Blood. 2006;108(1):63–73.
7. Frohling S, Schlenk RF, Kayser S, Morhardt M, Benner A, Dohner K, et al. Cytogenetics and age are major determinants of outcome in intensively treated acute myeloid leukemia patients older than 60 years: results from AMLSG trial AML HD98-B. Blood. 2006;108(10):3280–8.
8. Gupta V, Chun K, Yi QL, Minden M, Schuh A, Wells R, et al. Disease biology rather than age is the most important determinant of survival of patients > or = 60 years with acute myeloid leukemia treated with uniform intensive therapy. Cancer. 2005;103(10):2082–90.
9. Leith CP, Kopecky KJ, Godwin J, McConnell T, Slovak ML, Chen IM, et al. Acute myeloid leukemia in the elderly: assessment of multidrug resistance (MDR1) and cytogenetics distinguishes biologic subgroups with remarkably distinct responses to standard chemotherapy. A Southwest Oncology Group study. Blood. 1997;89(9):3323–9.
10. Godwin JE, Smith SE. Acute myeloid leukemia in the older patient. Crit Rev Oncol Hematol. 2003;48(Suppl):S17–26.
11. Prebet T, Boissel N, Reutenauer S, Thomas X, Delaunay J, Cahn JY, et al. Acute myeloid leukemia with translocation (8;21) or inversion (16) in elderly patients treated with conventional chemotherapy: a collaborative study of the French CBF-AML intergroup. J Clin Oncol. 2009;27(28):4747–53.
12. Mendler JH, Maharry K, Radmacher MD, Mrozek K, Becker H, Metzeler KH, et al. RUNX1 mutations are associated with poor outcome in younger and older patients with cytogenetically normal acute myeloid leukemia and with distinct gene and MicroRNA expression signatures. J Clin Oncol. 2012;30(25):3109–18.
13. Whitman SP, Caligiuri MA, Maharry K, Radmacher MD, Kohlschmidt J, Becker H, et al. The MLL partial tandem duplication in adults aged 60 years and older with de novo cytogenetically normal acute myeloid leukemia. Leukemia. 2012;26(7):1713–7.
14. Marcucci G, Metzeler KH, Schwind S, Becker H, Maharry K, Mrozek K, et al. Age-related prognostic impact of different types of DNMT3A mutations in adults with primary cytogenetically normal acute myeloid leukemia. J Clin Oncol. 2012;30(7):742–50.
15. Schwind S, Marcucci G, Kohlschmidt J, Radmacher MD, Mrozek K, Maharry K, et al. Low expression of MN1 associates with better treatment response in older patients with de novo cytogenetically normal acute myeloid leukemia. Blood. 2011;118(15):4188–98.
16. Schwind S, Marcucci G, Maharry K, Radmacher MD, Mrozek K, Holland KB, et al. BAALC and ERG expression levels are associated with outcome and distinct gene and microRNA expression profiles in older patients with de novo cytogenetically normal acute myeloid leukemia: a Cancer and Leukemia Group B study. Blood. 2010;116(25):5660–9.
17. Whitman SP, Maharry K, Radmacher MD, Becker H, Mrozek K, Margeson D, et al. FLT3 internal tandem duplication associates with adverse outcome and gene- and microRNA-expression signatures in patients 60 years of age or older with primary cytogenetically normal acute myeloid leukemia: a Cancer and Leukemia Group B study. Blood. 2010;116(18):3622–6.
18. Becker H, Marcucci G, Maharry K, Radmacher MD, Mrozek K, Margeson D, et al. Favorable prognostic impact of NPM1 mutations in older patients with cytogenetically normal de novo acute myeloid leukemia and associated gene- and microRNA-expression signatures: a Cancer and Leukemia Group B study. J Clin Oncol. 2010;28(4):596–604.
19. Rao AV, Valk PJ, Metzeler KH, Acharya CR, Tuchman SA, Stevenson MM, et al. Age-specific differences in oncogenic pathway dysregulation and anthracycline sensitivity in patients with acute myeloid leukemia. J Clin Oncol. 2009;27(33):5580–6.

20. Buchner T, Berdel WE, Wormann B, Schoch C, Haferlach T, Schnittger S, et al. Treatment of older patients with AML. Crit Rev Oncol Hematol. 2005;56(2):247–59.
21. Estey E. Acute myeloid leukemia and myelodysplastic syndromes in older patients. J Clin Oncol. 2007;25(14):1908–15.
22. Kantarjian H, O'brien S, Cortes J, Giles F, Faderl S, Jabbour E, et al. Results of intensive chemotherapy in 998 patients age 65 years or older with acute myeloid leukemia or high-risk myelodysplastic syndrome: predictive prognostic models for outcome. Cancer. 2006;106(5):1090–8.
23. Mori M, Ohta M, Miyata A, Higashihara M, Oshimi K, Kimura H, et al. Treatment of acute myeloid leukemia patients aged more than 75 years: results of the E-AML-01 trial of the Japanese Elderly Leukemia and Lymphoma Study Group (JELLSG). Leuk Lymphoma. 2006;47(10):2062–9.
24. Vey N, Coso D, Bardou VJ, Stoppa AM, Braud AC, Bouabdallah R, et al. The benefit of induction chemotherapy in patients age > or = 75 years. Cancer. 2004;101(2):325–31.
25. Oran B, Weisdorf DJ. Survival for older patients with acute myeloid leukemia: a population-based study. Haematologica. 2012;97(12):1916–24.
26. Bennett JM, Young ML, Andersen JW, Cassileth PA, Tallman MS, Paietta E, et al. Long-term survival in acute myeloid leukemia: the Eastern Cooperative Oncology Group experience. Cancer. 1997;80(11 Suppl):2205–9.
27. Mayer RJ, Davis RB, Schiffer CA, Berg DT, Powell BL, Schulman P, et al. Intensive postremission chemotherapy in adults with acute myeloid leukemia. Cancer and Leukemia Group B. N Engl J Med. 1994;331(14):896–903.
28. Rowe JM, Neuberg D, Friedenberg W, Bennett JM, Paietta E, Makary AZ, et al. A phase 3 study of three induction regimens and of priming with GM-CSF in older adults with acute myeloid leukemia: a trial by the Eastern Cooperative Oncology Group. Blood. 2004;103(2):479–85.
29. Menzin J, Lang K, Earle CC, Kerney D, Mallick R. The outcomes and costs of acute myeloid leukemia among the elderly. Arch Intern Med. 2002;162(14):1597–603.
30. Lang K, Earle CC, Foster T, Dixon D, Van Gool R, Menzin J. Trends in the treatment of acute myeloid leukaemia in the elderly. Drugs Aging. 2005;22(11):943–55.
31. O'Donnell MR, Appelbaum FR, Baer MR, Byrd JC, Coutre SE, Damon LE, et al. Acute myeloid leukemia clinical practice guidelines in oncology. J Natl Compr Canc Netw. 2006;4(1):16–36.
32. Lowenberg B, Zittoun R, Kerkhofs H, Jehn U, Abels J, Debusscher L, et al. On the value of intensive remission-induction chemotherapy in elderly patients of 65+ years with acute myeloid leukemia: a randomized phase III study of the European Organization for Research and Treatment of Cancer Leukemia Group. J Clin Oncol. 1989;7(9):1268–74.
33. Juliusson G, Antunovic P, Derolf A, Lehmann S, Mollgard L, Stockelberg D, et al. Age and acute myeloid leukemia: real world data on decision to treat and outcomes from the Swedish Acute Leukemia Registry. Blood. 2009;113(18):4179–87.
34. Rees JK, Gray RG, Wheatley K. Dose intensification in acute myeloid leukaemia: greater effectiveness at lower cost. Principal report of the Medical Research Council's AML9 study. MRC Leukaemia in Adults Working Party. Br J Haematol. 1996;94(1):89–98.
35. Tilly H, Castaigne S, Bordessoule D, Casassus P, Le Prise PY, Tertian G, et al. Low-dose cytarabine versus intensive chemotherapy in the treatment of acute nonlymphocytic leukemia in the elderly. J Clin Oncol. 1990;8(2):272–9.
36. Goldstone AH, Burnett AK, Wheatley K, Smith AG, Hutchinson RM, Clark RE. Attempts to improve treatment outcomes in acute myeloid leukemia (AML) in older patients: the results of the United Kingdom Medical Research Council AML11 trial. Blood. 2001;98(5):1302–11.
37. Lowenberg B, Suciu S, Archimbaud E, Haak H, Stryckmans P, de Cataldo R, et al. Mitoxantrone versus daunorubicin in induction-consolidation chemotherapy–the value of low-dose cytarabine for maintenance of remission, and an assessment of prognostic factors in acute myeloid leukemia in the elderly: final report. European Organization for the Research and Treatment of Cancer and the Dutch-Belgian Hemato-Oncology Cooperative Hovon Group. J Clin Oncol. 1998;16(3):872–81.

38. Bishop JF, Lowenthal RM, Joshua D, Matthews JP, Todd D, Cobcroft R, et al. Etoposide in acute nonlymphocytic leukemia. Australian Leukemia Study Group. Blood. 1990;75(1): 27–32.
39. Stone RM, Berg DT, George SL, Dodge RK, Paciucci PA, Schulman P, et al. Granulocyte-macrophage colony-stimulating factor after initial chemotherapy for elderly patients with primary acute myelogenous leukemia. Cancer and Leukemia Group B. N Engl J Med. 1995;332(25):1671–7.
40. Uyl-de Groot CA, Lowenberg B, Vellenga E, Suciu S, Willemze R, Rutten FF. Cost-effectiveness and quality-of-life assessment of GM-CSF as an adjunct to intensive remission induction chemotherapy in elderly patients with acute myeloid leukemia. Br J Haematol. 1998;100(4):629–36.
41. Lowenberg B, Suciu S, Archimbaud E, Ossenkoppele G, Verhoef GE, Vellenga E, et al. Use of recombinant GM-CSF during and after remission induction chemotherapy in patients aged 61 years and older with acute myeloid leukemia: final report of AML-11, a phase III randomized study of the Leukemia Cooperative Group of European Organisation for the Research and Treatment of Cancer and the Dutch Belgian Hemato-Oncology Cooperative Group. Blood. 1997;90(8):2952–61.
42. Baer MR, George SL, Dodge RK, O'Loughlin KL, Minderman H, Caligiuri MA, et al. Phase 3 study of the multidrug resistance modulator PSC-833 in previously untreated patients 60 years of age and older with acute myeloid leukemia: Cancer and Leukemia Group B Study 9720. Blood. 2002;100(4):1224–32.
43. van der Holt B, Lowenberg B, Burnett AK, Knauf WU, Shepherd J, Piccaluga PP, et al. The value of the MDR1 reversal agent PSC-833 in addition to daunorubicin and cytarabine in the treatment of elderly patients with previously untreated acute myeloid leukemia (AML), in relation to MDR1 status at diagnosis. Blood. 2005;106(8):2646–54.
44. Lowenberg B, Ossenkoppele GJ, van Putten W, Schouten HC, Graux C, Ferrant A, et al. High-dose daunorubicin in older patients with acute myeloid leukemia. N Engl J Med. 2009;361(13):1235–48.
45. Castaigne S, Pautas C, Terre C, Raffoux E, Bordessoule D, Bastie JN, et al. Effect of gemtuzumab ozogamicin on survival of adult patients with de-novo acute myeloid leukaemia (ALFA-0701): a randomised, open-label, phase 3 study. Lancet. 2012;379(9825):1508–16.
46. Burnett AK, Russell NH, Hills RK, Kell J, Freeman S, Kjeldsen L, et al. Addition of gemtuzumab ozogamicin to induction chemotherapy improves survival in older patients with acute myeloid leukemia. J Clin Oncol. 2012;30(32):3924–31.
47. Fenaux P, Mufti GJ, Hellstrom-Lindberg E, Santini V, Finelli C, Giagounidis A, et al. Efficacy of azacitidine compared with that of conventional care regimens in the treatment of higher-risk myelodysplastic syndromes: a randomised, open-label, phase III study. Lancet Oncol. 2009;10(3):223–32.
48. Kantarjian HM, Thomas XG, Dmoszynska A, Wierzbowska A, Mazur G, Mayer J, et al. Multicenter, randomized, open-label, phase III trial of decitabine versus patient choice, with physician advice, of either supportive care or low-dose cytarabine for the treatment of older patients with newly diagnosed acute myeloid leukemia. J Clin Oncol. 2012;30(21):2670–7.
49. Burnett AK, Milligan D, Prentice AG, Goldstone AH, McMullin MF, Hills RK, et al. A comparison of low-dose cytarabine and hydroxyurea with or without all-trans retinoic acid for acute myeloid leukemia and high-risk myelodysplastic syndrome in patients not considered fit for intensive treatment. Cancer. 2007;109(6):1114–24.
50. Milligan DW, Grimwade D, Cullis JO, Bond L, Swirsky D, Craddock C, et al. Guidelines on the management of acute myeloid leukaemia in adults. Br J Haematol. 2006;135(4):450–74.
51. Stone RM, Berg DT, George SL, Dodge RK, Paciucci PA, Schulman PP, et al. Postremission therapy in older patients with de novo acute myeloid leukemia: a randomized trial comparing mitoxantrone and intermediate-dose cytarabine with standard-dose cytarabine. Blood. 2001;98(3):548–53.
52. Wallen H, Gooley TA, Deeg HJ, Pagel JM, Press OW, Appelbaum FR, et al. Ablative allogeneic hematopoietic cell transplantation in adults 60 years of age and older. J Clin Oncol. 2005;23(15):3439–46.

53. Center for International Blood and Marrow Transplant Research (CIBMTR). Accessed 11 Apr 2013. Available from: URL: http://www.cibmtr.org.
54. Estey E, de Lima M, Tibes R, Pierce S, Kantarjian H, Champlin R, et al. Prospective feasibility analysis of reduced-intensity conditioning (RIC) regimens for hematopoietic stem cell transplantation (HSCT) in elderly patients with acute myeloid leukemia (AML) and high-risk myelodysplastic syndrome (MDS). Blood. 2007;109(4):1395–400.
55. Hegenbart U, Niederwieser D, Sandmaier BM, Maris MB, Shizuru JA, Greinix H, et al. Treatment for acute myelogenous leukemia by low-dose, total-body, irradiation-based conditioning and hematopoietic cell transplantation from related and unrelated donors. J Clin Oncol. 2006;24(3):444–53.
56. Schetelig J, Bornhauser M, Schmid C, Hertenstein B, Schwerdtfeger R, Martin H, et al. Matched unrelated or matched sibling donors result in comparable survival after allogeneic stem-cell transplantation in elderly patients with acute myeloid leukemia: a report from the cooperative German Transplant Study Group. J Clin Oncol. 2008;26(32):5183–91.
57. McClune BL, Weisdorf DJ, Pedersen TL, da Tunes SG, Tallman MS, Sierra J, et al. Effect of age on outcome of reduced-intensity hematopoietic cell transplantation for older patients with acute myeloid leukemia in first complete remission or with myelodysplastic syndrome. J Clin Oncol. 2010;28(11):1878–87.
58. Mengis C, Aebi S, Tobler A, Dahler W, Fey MF. Assessment of differences in patient populations selected for excluded from participation in clinical phase III acute myelogenous leukemia trials. J Clin Oncol. 2003;21(21):3933–9.
59. Sanz MA, Grimwade D, Tallman MS, Lowenberg B, Fenaux P, Estey EH, et al. Management of acute promyelocytic leukemia: recommendations from an expert panel on behalf of the European LeukemiaNet. Blood. 2009;113(9):1875–91.
60. Lehmann S, Ravn A, Carlsson L, Antunovic P, Deneberg S, Mollgard L, et al. Continuing high early death rate in acute promyelocytic leukemia: a population-based report from the Swedish Adult Acute Leukemia Registry. Leukemia. 2011;25(7):1128–34.
61. Lengfelder E, Hanfstein B, Haferlach C, Braess J, Krug U, Spiekermann K, et al. Outcome of elderly patients with acute promyelocytic leukemia: results of the German Acute Myeloid Leukemia Cooperative Group. Ann Hematol. 2013;92(1):41–52.
62. Kantarjian HM, O'brien S, Shan J, Aribi A, Garcia-Manero G, Jabbour E, et al. Update of the decitabine experience in higher risk myelodysplastic syndrome and analysis of prognostic factors associated with outcome. Cancer. 2007;109(2):265–73.
63. Rollig C, Thiede C, Gramatzki M, Aulitzky W, Bodenstein H, Bornhauser M, et al. A novel prognostic model in elderly patients with acute myeloid leukemia: results of 909 patients entered into the prospective AML96 trial. Blood. 2010;116(6):971–8.
64. Krug U, Rollig C, Koschmieder A, Heinecke A, Sauerland MC, Schaich M, et al. Complete remission and early death after intensive chemotherapy in patients aged 60 years or older with acute myeloid leukaemia: a web-based application for prediction of outcomes. Lancet. 2010;376(9757):2000–8.
65. Klepin HD, Geiger AM, Tooze JA, Kritchevsky SB, Williamson JD, Ellis LR, et al. The feasibility of inpatient geriatric assessment for older adults receiving induction chemotherapy for acute myelogenous leukemia. J Am Geriatr Soc. 2011;59(10):1837–46.
66. Klepin HD, Geiger AM, Tooze JA, Kritchevsky SB, Williamson JD, Pardee TS, et al. Geriatric assessment predicts survival for older adults receiving induction chemotherapy for acute myelogenous leukemia. Blood. 2013;121(21):4287–94.
67. Wedding U, Rohrig B, Klippstein A, Fricke HJ, Sayer HG, Hoffken K. Impairment in functional status and survival in patients with acute myeloid leukaemia. J Cancer Res Clin Oncol. 2006;132:665–71.
68. Etienne A, Esterni B, Charbonnier A, Mozziconacci MJ, Arnoulet C, Coso D, et al. Comorbidity is an independent predictor of complete remission in elderly patients receiving induction chemotherapy for acute myeloid leukemia. Cancer. 2007;109(7):1376–83.

69. Giles FJ, Borthakur G, Ravandi F, Faderl S, Verstovsek S, Thomas D, et al. The haematopoietic cell transplantation comorbidity index score is predictive of early death and survival in patients over 60 years of age receiving induction therapy for acute myeloid leukaemia. Br J Haematol. 2007;136(4):624–7.
70. Meyers CA, Albitar M, Estey E. Cognitive impairment, fatigue, and cytokine levels in patients with acute myelogenous leukemia or myelodysplastic syndrome. Cancer. 2005;104(4):788–93.
71. Deschler B, de Witte T, Mertelsmann R, Lubbert M. Treatment decision-making for older patients with high-risk myelodysplastic syndrome or acute myeloid leukemia: problems and approaches. Haematologica. 2006;91(11):1513–22.
72. Sekeres MA, Stone RM, Zahrieh D, Neuberg D, Morrison V, De Angelo DJ, et al. Decision-making and quality of life in older adults with acute myeloid leukemia or advanced myelodysplastic syndrome. Leukemia. 2004;18(4):809–16.
73. Gilliland DG et al. WHO classification of tumours of the haematopoietic and lymphoid tissues. Lyon: International Agency for Research on Cancer; 2008.

Chapter 5
Chronic Myelogeneous Leukemia

Andreas Hochhaus and Susanne Saussele

Abstract The impact of age as a poor prognostic factor in chronic myeloid leukemia (CML) has been well described. In the interferon era, elderly patients diagnosed with CML in chronic phase had shorter survival compared to younger patients. With the advent of targeted therapy with imatinib, studies described consistently improved responses in elderly late chronic phase patients treated with imatinib after IFN failure, with similar overall survival compared to the younger population.

Imatinib in newly diagnosed older patients showed similar rate of cytogenetic and molecular responses compared to younger patients. Few data are available relating elderly CML patients subset treated with 2nd-generation TKIs after resistance/intolerance to imatinib: both nilotinib and dasatinib have demonstrated efficacy and limited toxicity profile as in younger patients. The aim of this review is to highlight the fact that elderly CML patients can benefit from targeted therapy with limited adverse events.

Keywords Chronic myelogeneous leukemia • Tyrosine kinase inhibitors • Imatinib • Nilotinib • Dasatinib

Introduction

Chronic myeloid leukemia (CML) is a hematopoietic stem cell disorder originating from the translocation t(9;22)(q34;q11) with the resulting Philadelphia chromosome (Ph) 22q-. Juxtaposition of the ABL gene on chromosome 9 with the BCR

Disclosures AH and SS received research support and honoraria by Novartis, BMS, ARIAD and Pfizer.

Prof. Dr. A. Hochhaus (✉)
Abteilung Hämatologie/Onkologie, Klinik für Innere Medizin II,
Universitätsklinikum Jena, Erlanger Allee 101, Jena 07740, Germany
e-mail: andreas.hochhaus@med.uni-jena.de

S. Saussele, MD
III. Medizinische Universitätsklinik, Medizinische Fakultät Mannheim,
der Universität Heidelberg, Mannheim, Germany

U. Wedding, R.A. Audisio (eds.), *Management of Hematological Cancer in Older People*, DOI 10.1007/978-1-4471-2837-3_5

gene on chromosome 22 leads to a fusion gene, which is translated to a novel protein with abnormal tyrosine kinase activity. The incidence rate of CML varies from 0.6 to 2 cases per 100,000 people/year and increases with age, with a male prevalence. Median age at presentation is estimated around 65 years, but age figures differ between cancer registries and clinical trials by 10–20 years. Most clinical trials underestimate the real age of CML patients in the whole population and elderly patients are underrepresented in most studies. As a prominent example, the IRIS trial, which led to approval of imatinib for chronic phase CML, excluded patients >70 years of age [1]. A German study, aimed to determine population-based age and gender-specific incidence of CML, reported a median age of CML patients of 60.3 years, with a male/female ratio of 1.66. The crude incidence for CML was 0.79, whereas age-specific incidence was 0.57 for patients aged less than 65 years, and 1.91 for patients aged >65 years. Overall, only 64 % of patients were included in clinical trials: differences between patients who participated to trials vs patients who did not were in age (10.7 years younger), low prognostic score and management in hospital. Elderly patients had a 3.8-times lower probability to be enrolled in a clinical trial [2].

Epidemiology

The increasing age of patients is considered an important factor influencing decisions in daily clinical practice. Although there is, in principle, equal access for medical care for all patients across Europe, patients' age seems to be used as a selection criterion for treatment management [3]: An epidemiological survey in the southeast of Germany observed that only 59 % of the CML patients (median age of 64 years, no inclusion in investigational studies) received imatinib alone, 10.2 % received imatinib in combination with hydroxyurea or interferon alpha, 25.8 % were treated with hydroxyurea and 7.6 % received interferon alpha. This study, conducted in 2006, had used the database of the Bavarian association of statutory health-insurance-accredited physicians, covering 83.5 % of all patients treated outside a clinic's care in Bavaria with 10.4 million people [3]. The use of pre-imatinib-era treatment strategies such as hydroxyurea, ara-C, or interferon alpha by some physicians as salvage treatment after imatinib failure and unsuitability of stem cell transplantation (SCT) still occurs despite the growing availability of newer tyrosine kinase inhibitors (TKIs). Age is no longer a risk factor for worse outcome since the introduction of imatinib as targeted therapy [4, 5]. With imatinib therapy, older age appears to have lost much of its prognostic relevance suggesting that poor prognosis previously observed with older age was rather related to treatment-associated factors than to disease biology of CML in older patients [4]. As the long-term outcome is similar to that of younger patients [5], there is no reason to deprive older patients of the treatment with TKIs.

Furthermore, patient management by a hospital is also a significant positive factor for participation in clinical trials, as the result from epidemiological observations suggests [2]. CML patients treated in hospitals have a six-fold higher chance of being included in clinical trials than patients outside a hospital. Younger CML patients are more likely treated in university hospitals or specialized cancer treatment centers where study infrastructure for patient safety and data management are easily available. This patient group has, in general, a good prognosis and is likely to be a candidate for participation in clinical trials. In contrast, elderly patients are mainly cared for in general hospitals or in speciality practices with a reduced access to investigational therapies [6]. Reasons for non-inclusion of elderly patients in trials might also be, in some cases, immobility and comorbidities and, in others, the reluctance of physicians to admit elderly patients [2].

Current Treatment Standards

The European LeukemiaNet (ELN) has developed recommendations for medical management of patients of all ages with CML in daily clinical practice [7]. Thus, CML patients should be treated under the guidance of an experienced physician affiliated to a center with appropriate facilities for cytogenetic and molecular monitoring. Furthermore, the centers should offer and ask patients to be registered in clinical studies.

It is recommended that in practice, outside of clinical trials, the first-line treatment of chronic phase CML can be any of the three TKIs that have been approved for this indication and are available almost worldwide, namely imatinib (400 mg QD), nilotinib (300 mg BID), and dasatinib (100 mg QD). These three TKIs can be used also in second or subsequent lines, at the standard, or at a higher dose (400 mg BID for imatinib, 400 mg BID for nilotinib, and 70 mg BID or 140 mg QD for dasatinib). Bosutinib (500 mg QD) has been approved for patients resistant or intolerant to prior therapy. Ponatinib (45 mg QD) has also been approved for patients resistant or intolerant to prior TKI therapy, in particular patients with the T315I BCR-ABL mutation. Allogeneic SCT will continue to be an important treatment for patients who fail to respond durably to TKIs and are eligible for SCT. It seems reasonable that for patients in CP, transplant should be reserved for those who are resistant or intolerant to at least one 2nd generation TKI. The nature of conditioning therapy is controversial because in chronic phase there is no evidence at present that myeloablative conditioning offers any advantage over reduced intensity preparative regimens.

Current Diagnostic Approaches

A careful and close monitoring of treatment response and of prognostic factors is required to identify development of resistance to therapy, intolerance or non-compliance or progression to advanced-phase disease. Monitoring can be performed using molecular or cytogenetic tests, or both, depending on local facilities and on the degree of molecular standardization of the local laboratory.

Molecular testing should be performed by RQ-PCR to measure the BCR-ABL transcript level, that is reported on the international scale (IS). RQ-PCR should be repeated every 3 months until major molecular response (MMR, BCR-ABL IS ≤0.1 %) is achieved, then every 3–6 months. If transcript levels have increased >5 times in a single follow-up sample and MMR was lost, the test should be repeated in a shorter time interval, and patients should be questioned carefully about compliance. If cytogenetics is used, it must be performed by banding analysis of at least 20 bone marrow cell metaphases, at 3, 6, 12 months, until a CCyR is achieved.

Clonal chromosome abnormalities in Ph negative cells, which may develop in up to 10 % of responders and are more frequent in older patients, are a warning only in case of chromosome 7 involvement [7].

In routine clinical practive, however, a survey of 956 physicians in the US and in Europe suggests that treatment practices in some areas of CML management are not in line with the international recommendations [8]. Problematic areas were suboptimal timing of treatment decisions during monitoring, and unawareness of new molecular monitoring techniques and of the potential benefit of new treatment options.

Prognostic Scores

Older age was referred to be a poor prognostic variable: a negative effect on survival was reported when patients were treated with therapeutic strategies including conservative drugs (busulfan, hydroxyurea, interferon alpha) or transplant procedures. Thus, age was an important factor in the calculation of the Sokal and Euro (Hasford) scores. In the IFN era, older age was a consistently poor prognostic factor, probably related to inadequate drug delivery and treatment toxicity experienced in this setting. In the era of TKI, the outcome of elderly patients was extensively investigated. Most of the literature regarding efficacy and safety of imatinib revealed that this drug eliminated the negative effect of age on response rate and survival. Therefore, a new prognostic score was proposed (EUTOS score), based on 2,060 patients treated front-line with imatinib. A multivariate analysis was performed to identify prognostic factors at baseline with impact on the CCyR status at 18 months. The best proposed model included only basophils and spleen size. Age, as other candidate variables, such as blasts, lost their significance. The simple formula proposed was:

$$\text{EUTOS score} = (7 * \text{basophils in }\%) + (4 * \text{spleen size in cm below costal margin})$$

with indication of high risk by a score >87 and low risk by a score ≤87. Indirectly, the analysis proved that advanced age did not represent an adverse prognostic factor in the TKI era [9].

Interferon Alpha in Elderly Patients

To assess the long-term outcome of older patients with BCR-ABL positive CML, 199 patients aged ≥60 years representing 23 % of 856 patients enrolled in the German randomized CML-studies I (interferon alpha (IFN) vs hydroxyurea (HU) vs busulfan and II (IFN + HU vs HU alone) were analyzed after a median observation time of 7 years. The 5-year survival was 38 % in older and 47 % in younger patients ($P < 0.001$). Adverse effects of IFN were similar in both age groups, but IFN dosage to achieve treatment goals was lower in older patients [10].

The MD Anderson Cancer Center (MDACC) reported the experience of IFN therapy in CML patients ≥60 years. Patients were treated with IFN at a median dose of $5*10^6/m^2$ MU as single agent or in association with other substances. Older patients represented 13 % of an overall population of 274 newly diagnosed patients enrolled in trials. With IFN therapy, 51 % had a cytogenetic response with 20 % of CCyR. These results were not different from those reported in the younger population. The most frequent side effect reported was neurotoxicity in 31 % of patients [11]. In 1998, the Austrian group reported efficacy and safety data relating 41 elderly patients treated with IFN at daily dose of 3.5 MU, alone or in combination with low dose cytarabine [12]. Slight difference was reported between elderly and younger patients in terms of CCyR (10 % vs 13 %), but this was not statistically significant.

The Effect of Imatinib in Older Late Chronic Phase Patients

The first extended analysis on efficacy and safety of imatinib in older patients aged >60 years was reported by Cortes et al. of the MDACC [4]; 187 patients with newly diagnosed CML treated with imatinib first line, of whom 49 (26 %) were in the older age, were compared with 351 patients in late chronic phase after IFN failure, of whom 120 (34 %) were older than 60 years. The cut-off of 60 years was chosen because this limit was identified to be of prognostic relevance in previous multivariate analysis performed in CML cases, but also because patients aged more than 60 years were usually ineligible for transplant procedures and had also poor tolerance to IFN therapy. In early chronic phase, cytogenetic responses were similar to those of younger patients. Only two of the elderly patients were reported to suffer from transformation to advanced phases of disease compared to 5 in the younger subset. In late chronic phase patients, 120 were older (34 %), with a lower incidence of additional chromosome abnormalities compared to younger subjects, more frequent leukocytosis and bone marrow basophilia. 44 % of older patients achieved a CCyR compared to 56 % in younger patients. In multivariate analysis for predicting factors for survival, older age was in chronic and advanced disease not associated to poor outcome.

Rosti et al. reported for the GIMEMA group on 284 patients in late chronic phase CML treated with imatinib 400 mg/day. CCyR rates were lower in older patients (≥65 years) than in younger patients (<65 years) with more adverse events in older patients, but nevertheless overall survival was the same in both age groups [5]. The MDACC and the GIMEMA reports both demonstrated that the poor prognostic impact of older age was minimized by imatinib [13].

Imatinib in Newly Diagnosed Untreated Elderly Patients

Gugliotta et al. reported similar rates of CCyR and MMR in 115 patients ≥65 years among 559 patients in early CP treated with imatinib 400 or 800 mg/day. No relevant differences were observed between older and younger patients except for hemoglobin level, WBC count (median 42/nl in elderly vs 61/nl in younger) and spleen size [14].

In a multicenter study of high-dose imatinib in 115 newly diagnosed patients in chronic phase Cortes et al. reported a similar dose-intensity and no difference in adverse events at any severity for patients <65 and ≥65 years. MMR was achieved by 79 % of patients who received at least 90 % dose-intensity (RIGHT study, [15]). Latagliata et al. analyzed 117 patients in early chronic phase CML under imatinib treatment with 300–800 mg/day. No significant difference in the rate of CCyR was reported in older (≥65 years) compared to younger (<65 years) patients. Adverse events (WHO grades 3–4) were more frequent and rates of dose reduction and discontinuation of imatinib were higher in older patients [16]. Recently, the Spanish group reported the results of the observational ELDERGLI study [17]: patients age was >70 years with newly diagnosed chronic phase CML or >65 years in late chronic phase. Thirty-six patients were included with a median age of 76.6 years and a female predominance. Most frequent comorbidities reported were cardiovascular events and type II diabetes mellitus. After a median follow up of 24 months, increasing response rates were observed, with 83 % CCyR and 69 % MMR after 18 months. Only one patient progressed to blast crisis. Hematological toxicity recorded was moderate with overall 8 % anemia and thrombocytopenia and 11 % neutropenia of all grades. Most frequent non-hematological side effects were superficial edema that accounted for 44 % (grade 1/2), diarrhea (27.7 %), and infections (25 %), which caused death in two patients. The group considered imatinib a safe and effective drug also for older patients.

Strategies to Overcome Resistance in Older Patients

Few data were reported for older patients rescued with nilotinib or dasatinib after resistance or intolerance to imatinib. A subanalysis of a phase II trial with nilotinib at the dose of 400 mg BID reported on 98 patients out of 321 enrolled older patients >65 years with 8 % of these patients being >80 years of age. Baseline features were similar between younger and older patients. The rate of discontinuation was 18 %, whereas the CCyR rate was 38 % compared to 44 % in younger patients. One-year estimated overall survival was 91 % for older versus 97 % for younger patients. Similar frequencies of side effects were reported in older and younger patients: in particular, as regards biochemical abnormalities, 23 % of older patients experienced lipase elevation compared to 14 % of younger patients, while 3 % of older patients experienced total bilirubin increase compared to 9 % for younger patients. No particular differences were revealed between the age groups in terms of hematological side effects and in terms of pleuro/pericardial effusions or bleeding events. 4 % of older patients had a myocardial infarction compared to 1 % in younger patients. For the QT interval according to Fridericia formula (QTcF), prolongation higher than 500 ms was recorded in 2 % of older compared to 1 % in younger patients [18].

The expanding nilotinib access study (ENACT, [19]) enrolled 1,422 CP-CML imatinib resistant and/or intolerant patients, of whom 452 patients were aged >60 years and 165 of these were >70 years old. A higher proportion of patients aged >65 years enrolled had a longer median duration of CML and most of them were enrolled for intolerance. The results showed that about 50 % of patients aged >65 years experienced nilotinib dose interruptions and reductions due to side effects lasting more than 5 days. In this trial, 41 % of older patients achieved MCyR with 31 % achieving CCyR (33 % of elderly >70 years). In terms of safety, 56 % of older patients experienced grade 3/4 toxicity, most frequently hematological (thrombocytopenia 24 % and neutropenia 14 %). Patients who had experienced pleural effusion during dasatinib treatment did not have a recurrence of the same effect during nilotinib treatment.

Recently, a retrospective Italian analysis on 125 CP-CML patients resistant to imatinib aged >60 years was published [20]. Median age at the start of dasatinib treatment was 69 years, with a high rate of intermediate and high Sokal risk strata. Fifty-seven patients were pretreated and resistant to IFN before imatinib. Fifty-eight patients had received high-dose imatinib for resistance to the standard dose. Thirteen patients were treated with dasatinib for intolerance and 112 for resistance. The starting daily dose of dasatinib was 140 mg in 52 patients, 100 mg in 56 patients, and <100 mg in 17 patients. As to efficacy, 60 reached CCyR as best response. Four-year OS was 84.2 %. Thirty-one percent of patients experienced grade 3/4 hematological toxicity, mostly in the group of patients treated with 140 mg/day. Twenty-seven percent of patients experienced nonhematological toxicity, with no difference in the rate of events between patients treated with different dosage and schedule. Forty-one patients experienced pleuro/pericardial effusion that was of grade 3/4 in 8 % of patients, with higher frequency in the group of patients treated with 140 mg/day. Due to toxicity, 67 patients required a dose reduction and 19 patients needed permanent discontinuation. This real-life experience showed that dasatinib could be safely used in older patients.

A subanalysis of 119 patients aged >65 years treated with bosutinib was presented in 2012 and a comparison was made with 451 younger patients [21]. Bosutinib was administered at a dose of 500 mg/day. Bosutinib was discontinued in 80 % of patients over 65 years of age compared to 67 % of younger patients, in 32 % of cases being due to adverse events, mostly thrombocytopenia. Rate of treatment transformation, incidence of hematological side effects and the incidence of diarrhea were similar between patients older or younger than 65 years.

Recently, a 3rd-generation inhibitor was tested in resistant CML patients: ponatinib is a potent, oral inhibitor able to block native and mutated BCR-ABL, including T315I mutation, which are resistant to dasatinib and nilotinib. The phase II "Ponatinib Ph+ALL and CML Evaluation" (PACE) trial tested ponatinib 45 mg QD in 449 patients (median age 59 years; range 18–94) resistant or intolerant to dasatinib or nilotinib or with the T315I mutation in different phases of disease. In chronic phase patients, 46 % achieved a CCyR and 32 % MMR with 12 % $MR^{4.5}$ (BCR-ABL IS ≤0.0032 %). Similar responses were obtained in patients with or without mutations, with a higher rate in patients with the T315I mutation. However, 20 % of arterial and venous thrombotic events prompted a revision of the treatment recommendations with a lower dose recommended in good responders and precautions regarding vascular events [22].

Second Generation TKIs in First Line Use in Older Patients

The DASISION trial (Dasatinib versus Imatinib Study in Treatment-Naïve CP-CML patients) was a large phase III trial comparing dasatinib 100 mg BID versus imatinib 400 mg QD in newly diagnosed patients. A subanalysis of the study showed efficacy and safety results according to baseline comorbidity and age. In the dasatinib arm, CCyR rates were 88 % for patients aged <46 years, 78 % for those aged 46–65 years, and 85 % for those aged >65 years; the corresponding MMR rates were 45, 47, and 50 %, respectively. In the imatinib arm, CCyR rates of 70, 70, and 83 % were reported for patients <46 years, 46–65 years, and >65 years, respectively; MMR rates were 26, 30, and 29 %, respectively. Safety profiles were similar across all age groups in both treatment arms, except for fluid retention rates observed in the dasatinib arm (13, 25, and 35 %) compared to the imatinib arm (34, 45, and 67 %) for patients aged <46, 46–65, and >65 years, respectively [23].

The ENESTnd trial (Evaluating Nilotinib Efficacy and Safety in Clinical Trials of Newly Diagnosed Ph+CML Patients) is a phase III trial testing two different doses of nilotinib (300 and 400 mg BID) versus the standard dose of imatinib (400 mg QD). In this trial, 36 patients (13 %) and 28 patients (10 %) were >65 years old in the 300 and 400 mg BID nilotinib arms, respectively. Efficacy was maintained in older patients, with an MMR rate of 78 % in the nilotinib 300 mg BID arm and a $MR^{4.5}$ rate of 31 %. CCyR rates by 24 months were 83 and 68 % among older patients treated with nilotinib 300 and 400 mg, respectively, compared to 87 % in younger patients in either of the nilotinib arms. 72 and 61 % of older patients achieved MMR, respectively, whereas in younger patients, the respective rates were 71 and 67 %. As regards safety, no patients had grade 3/4 neutropenia and only one older patient reported grade 3/4 thrombocytopenia in each nilotinib arm. Transient, asymptomatic lipase elevations occurred in 11 and 16 % of older patients treated with nilotinib 300 and 400 mg, and in 7 % of younger patients in each arm.

Hyperglycemia occurred in 23 and 16 % of patients aged over 65 years on nilotinib 300 and 400 mg, respectively, and in 4 % of younger patients in either arm. Overall, the primary endpoint (MMR within 12 months) was maintained in the nilotinib 300 mg BID arm at 4-year follow-up with an MMR rate of 76 versus 56 % for imatinib; the MR^4 rates were 56 and 32 % and the $MR^{4.5}$ rates were 40 and 23 %. Statistically significant reduction of progression rate was observed in the nilotinib 300 mg BID arm (0.7 %) as compared to imatinib (4.2 %) [24].

Bosutinib was tested in a phase III randomized trial in first line versus imatinib standard dose (BELA trial). A subanalysis in older patients enrolled in the BELA trial was presented: 30 patients were treated with bosutinib and 27 with imatinib. None of the patients aged >65 years treated with bosutinib progressed. Among patients aged >65 years, grade 3/4 events were more frequently recorded (gastrointestinal events, elevated transaminases, pyrexia); 64 % of this subset required dose reduction, and 39 % required treatment discontinuation due to side effects [25]. Overall, the study did not achieve the primary endpoint (rate of CCyR) because at 12 months there was no difference between the two arms (70 % for bosutinib vs 68 % for imatinib). Despite these results, the MMR rate improved in the bosutinib arm (41 vs 21 % for imatinib arm) and responses were achieved faster with this inhibitor. Consequently, only 2 % of patients progressed to advanced phases of disease as compared to 4 % in the imatinib arm.

All studies clearly showed that efficacy was similar for the three different inhibitors tested as frontline treatment, even in patients aged >65 years, but with a specific safety profile for each one which should be carefully evaluated according to the presence of concomitant comorbidities [26].

Pharmacokinetics

For all patients, potential drug-drug interactions are a concern when multiple medications are taken, and elderly patients are more likely than younger patients to be on a multiple medication regimen. For patients aged >65 years, 90 % are taking at least one prescription drug, and 65 % are taking at least 3 prescription drugs, compared with 65 and 34 % of patients aged 45 to 64 years, respectively. All TKIs are metabolized in a similar fashion, primarily by cytochrome P450 (CYP) 3A4 (CYP3A4), a liver enzyme that is active in the metabolism of many other drugs. Other CYP enzymes and UDP-glucuronosyltransferase appear to play a minor role. Clinical recommendations for the use of TKIs with other medications, therefore, largely involve concomitant use of agents (including food, vitamins, or supplements) that are strong inducers or inhibitors of CYP3A4 or are substrates of CYP3A4. Further, the prescribing information for TKIs provides guidance for the concomitant use of antiarrhythmics or agents that prolong QTc and for the concomitant use of cumulative high-dose anthracyclines [27].

The first analysis of the effect of different imatinib dose regimens in older vs. younger patients with CML was performed using data from the German CML-

Study IV [28]. The most important finding of this analysis is that older patients on Imatinib 800 mg (IM800) had no delay in reaching MMR and MR^4 as this was the fact with standard dose imatinib where MMR and MR^4 were achieved significantly later than in younger patients. Superiority of the response rates to IM800 was more pronounced in the older than in the younger group. This effect is remarkable as the median dose for older patients on IM800 was lower than that of younger patients and only moderately higher than in older patients on Imatinib 400 mg (IM400). The result is in line with observations within this study that superior cytogenetic and molecular remission rates were reached in patients with IM800. To avoid severe adverse events on IM800, imatinib was adapted to tolerability in both age groups. Dose reductions were higher in older patients, although adverse events occurred not more frequently than in younger patients. A similar dose-intensity and no difference in adverse events was reported in high-dose imatinib therapy for patients <65 years and ≥65 years by Cortes et al. [4]. Most non-hematologic adverse events occurred more often in the IM800 arm, independent of age, but since grades 3 and 4 adverse events were similar between IM400 and IM800, this appears tolerable with regard to a potentially better outcome. The baseline characteristics beyond age seem to have no influence, but the proportion of patients with lower Karnofsky index was significantly higher in older patients. To compare survival between age groups, the German population adjusted for age and sex was taken into account. Overall survival was reduced in older compared to younger patients due to a generally reduced life expectancy of older people, whereas the five-year relative survival of older patients was comparable with that of younger patients. Nevertheless, it is important to note that a bias in favour of the study patients is likely. The relative survival estimates may be too optimistic, since the exclusion criteria of CML-Study IV prevented the participation of some of the frailest patients, e.g. those with other neoplasias in need of treatment or with conditions preventing study compliance and thus, with a supposedly reduced life expectancy. This would explain the better survival in older patients on IM800 (100.8 % at five years) than in the general population.

Comorbidities and TKI Treatment

Individual TKIs have different patterns of side-effects, and this should be considered when choosing amongst these drugs. Side effects can be divided into three general categories. The first includes major, grade 3/4, side effects that typically occur during the first phase of treatment, are manageable, but require temporary treatment discontinuation and dose reduction, and can lead to treatment discontinuation in about 10 % of patients. The second category includes minor side effects that begin early during treatment and can persist forever. They are also manageable, and tolerable, but affect negatively the quality of life, and are a cause of decreased compliance, that is a major cause of failure. Many of these side effects are common to all TKIs, with some differences in frequency and severity, so that several patients can benefit from changing the TKI. The third category includes late, "off-target" complications, that can affect the cardiovascular system, heart and blood vessels, the respiratory system, liver, pancreas, the immune defense, secondary malignancies, calcium, glucose and lipid metabolism, etc. All TKIs can be toxic to the heart and should be used with great caution in patients with heart failure. Nilotinib has been reported to be associated particularly with arterial pathology, peripheral and coronary. Dasatinib has been reported to be associated particularly with pleura effusions and lung complications. Overall, the long term off-target complications of 2nd generation TKIs are not yet fully understood. Since they are a potential cause of morbidity and mortality, continued clinical monitoring of all patients is required.

The onset of peripheral arterial occlusive disease (PAOD) was reported in selected cohorts of patients treated with nilotinib, outside clinical trials. In particular, le Coutre and colleagues [29] reported 175 patients treated with nilotinib second line and PAOD was recorded in 11 patients (6 %), of which 7 were more than 60 years old with pre-existing risk factors, such as smoking, obesity, diabetes, hypertension, and hypercholesterolemia.

Recently, the same group recommended the use of the ankle-brachial index (ABI) and duplex ultrasonography as tools to identify patients at risk of PAOD during treatment with TKIs and revealed a significantly higher frequency of this side effect in patients treated with nilotinib, although with unknown mechanisms. The coexistence of comorbidities and older age did not preclude possible treatment with this drug, but suggests that patients older than 65 years be closely monitored for early identification of this side effect. Cardiovascular morbidity and the risk for the development of PAOD should be considered in CML patients. Other potential manifestations of atherosclerosis, including fatal myocardial infarction, have been attributed to imatinib, nilotinib, and dasatinib. The authors strongly suggest to capture baseline ABI, biochemical risk factors and to monitor these parameters regularly throughout TKI therapy of CML [30].

Comorbidities are common among the elderly patients, but specific studies of TKI therapy in older patients with coexisting illnesses have not been conducted. A subanalysis of the DASISION trial of front-line dasatinib use in patients with CML-CP demonstrated no differ- ence in the outcomes for the cohort with any of the allowed comorbidities (ie, allergic, dermatologic, diabetic, endocrine, metabolic, gastrointestinal, hematologic-lymphatic, hepatobiliary, hyperlipidemic, musculoskeletal, renal, and respiratory) vs. those without comorbidities. Findings from a subanalysis of the ENESTnd trial that examined front-line nilotinib treatment in patients with preexisting type 2 diabetes suggested that the efficacy and safety of nilotinib in patients with diabetes were similar to those seen in the overall patient population. These preliminary results support the safety and efficacy of TKI therapy in patients with many comorbidities. However, patients with preexisting cardiovascular disease have been excluded from studies with nilotinib and dasatinib. The use of these agents in patients with preexisting cardiovascular disease needs to be better understood, both in the general CML population and among elderly patients with CML. The currently reported data lend further urgency to the conduct of appropriate

TKI cessation studies in patients with CML-CP who have a (yet to be defined) adequate molecular response to initial TKI therapy [31].

Lataglia et al. investigated the safety and tolerability of imatinib in very elderly CML patients in chronic phase, 211 chronic-phase CML patients aged >75 years were retrospectively analyzed using data collected from 31 institutions in Italy. Results from this large cohort of patients show that no upper age limit should be applied for the administration of imatinib to patients with chronic phase CML; the very elderly, including those with concomitant severe diseases, should be offered this treatment. The role of a reduced starting dose of imatinib warrants further studies [32].

Conclusions

Before the advent of TKIs, studies have shown that advanced age may be a negative independent factor for response in the category of elderly patients due to concomitant comorbidities and consequent increased toxicity of available agents, like interferon alpha. Any preference to avoid such therapies in elderly patients rose from lack of data due to exclusion of frail elderly patients from major clinical trials testing interferon. CML management has dramatically improved after the introduction of imatinib: in fact, this drug completely changed the way to treat and the outcome of elderly patients. It has been reported that imatinib use did not vary by race/ethnicity, socioeconomic status, geographic residence or insurance status, even after these analyses were adjusted for age at diagnosis. Imatinib has yielded promising results when used in older patients as 2nd line after IFN therapy failure or as frontline therapy; efficacy in terms of cytogenetic and molecular responses was reported similar to that described in younger patients. Imatinib has a favourable safety profile also in elderly patients, but with overall more frequent toxicity leading to high rate of discontinuation and dose reduction, probably related to the presence of concomitant comorbidities. All publications agreeing that, in the TKI era, it would be reasonable to define an elderly patient according to reproducible tools of fragility (such as comorbidity indexes) rather than simply according to years of age and physician's perception. Limited data are available for 2nd generation TKIs in older subset of patients after resistance or intolerance to imatinib: for nilotinib, no data were reported outside clinical trials, whereas for dasatinib, all data available were published in "real life" clinical practice. Few data were available for dasatinib and nilotinib in newly diagnosed elderly patients enrolled in randomized phase III trials, which selectively included only patients with limited spectrum of comorbidities. In conclusion, although lack of data exists for elderly CML subset, all published data showed that response to TKIs was not affected by age.

Several strategies have been developed to overcome the problem of imatinib resistance, including dose escalation of imatinib, combination treatments, or novel targeted agents: no different strategies were specifically applied in patients aged >65 years. This subset can be treated the same as younger patients with choice of therapy and careful monitoring in patients with specific preexisting comorbidities. Higher doses of imatinib seem to be effective in specific categories, such as resistant patients with previous cytogenetic response and no mutations, but not in patients with primary resistance or hematological failure. Trials with 2nd-generation TKIs after imatinib resistance have been shown to rescue about 50 % of resistant patients, regardless of the type of mutations and age at the time of the switch. Monitoring patients, regardless of age, according to ELN recommendations and early identification of patients with failure or suboptimal response with prompt switching to 2nd-generation TKIs could improve the outcome of patients treated with imatinib. The results of randomized trials testing safety and efficacy of 2nd-generation TKIs in first line reported a rapid reduction of leukemic burden, which translates into a reduced incidence of resistance. Even in older patients, all agents tested were effective and induced a rapid reduction of leukemic burden with limited toxicity, but until now, no clear correlation between greater molecular responses obtained with 2nd-generation TKIs and overall survival has been apparent. Longer follow-up is needed to verify whether a higher rate of deep molecular response is sustained and if a possible discontinuation of therapy, regardless of age, may be planned [26].

References

1. Druker BJ, Guilhot F, O'Brien SG, Gathmann I, Kantarjian H, Gattermann N, et al. Five-year follow-up of patients receiving imatinib for chronic myeloid leukemia. N Engl J Med. 2006;355(23):2408–17.
2. Rohrbacher M, Berger U, Hochhaus A, Metzgeroth G, Adam K, Lahaye T, et al. Clinical trials underestimate the age of chronic myeloid leukemia (CML) patients. Incidence and median age of Ph/BCR-ABL-positive CML and other chronic myeloproliferative disorders in a representative area in Germany. Leukemia. 2009;23(3):602–4.
3. Rohrbacher M, Hasford J. Epidemiology of chronic myeloid leukaemia (CML). Best Pract Res Clin Haematol. 2009;22(3):295–302.
4. Cortes J, Talpaz M, O'Brien S, Giles F, Rios MB, Shan JQ, et al. Effects of age on prognosis with imatinib mesylate therapy for patients with Philadelphia chromosome-positive chronic myelogenous leukemia. Cancer. 2003;98(6):1105–13.
5. Rosti G, Iacobucci I, Bassi S, Castagnetti F, Amabile M, Cilloni D, et al. Impact of age on the outcome of patients with chronic myeloid leukemia in late chronic phase: results of a phase II study of the GIMEMA CML Working Party. Haematologica. 2007;92(1):101–5.
6. Tardieu S, Brun-Strang C, Berthaud P, Michallet M, Guilhot F, Rousselot P, Sambuc R. Management of chronic myeloid leukemia in France: a multicentered cross-sectional study on 538 patients. Pharmacoepidemiol Drug Saf. 2005;14(8):545–53.
7. Baccarani M, Deininger MW, Rosti G, Hochhaus A, Soverini S, Apperley JF, et al. European LeukemiaNet recommendations for the management of chronic myeloid leukemia: 2013. Blood. 2013;122(6):872–84.
8. Kantarjian H, O'Brien S, Talpaz M, Borthakur G, Ravandi F, Faderl S, et al. Outcome of patients with Philadelphia chromosome-positive chronic myelogenous leukemia post-imatinib mesylate failure. Cancer. 2007;109(8):1556–60.
9. Hasford J, Baccarani M, Hoffmann V, Guilhot J, Saussele S, Rosti G, et al. Predicting complete cytogenetic response and subsequent progression-free survival in 2060 patients with CML on imatinib treatment: the EUTOS score. Blood. 2011;118(3):686–92.

10. Berger U, Engelich G, Maywald O, Pfirrmann M, Hochhaus A, Reiter A, et al. Chronic myeloid leukemia in the elderly: long-term results from randomized trials with interferon alpha. Leukemia. 2003;17(9):1820–6.
11. Cortes J, Kantarjian H, O'Brien S, Robertson LE, Pierce S, Talpaz M. Result of interferon-alpha therapy in patients with chronic myelogenous leukemia 60 years of age and older. Am J Med. 1996;100:452–5.
12. Hilbe W, Apfelbeck U, Fridrik M, Bernhart M, Niessner H, Abbrederis K, et al. Interferon-alpha for the treatment of elderly patients with chronic myeloid leukemia. Leuk Res. 1998;22:881–6.
13. Breccia M, Tiribelli M, Alimena G. Tyrosine kinase inhibitors for elderly chronic myeloid leukemia patients: a systematic review of efficacy and safety data. Crit Rev Oncol Hematol. 2012;84:93–100.
14. Gugliotta G, Castagnetti F, Palandri F, Breccia M, Intermesoli T, Capucci A, et al. Frontline imatinib treatment of chronic myeloid leukemia: no impact of age on outcome, a survey by the GIMEMA CML Working Party. Blood. 2011;117(21):5591–9.
15. Cortes JE, Kantarjian HM, Goldberg SL, Powell BL, Giles FJ, Wetzler M, Rationale and Insight for Gleevec High-Dose Therapy (RIGHT) Trial Study Group, et al. High-dose imatinib in newly diagnosed chronic-phase chronic myeloid leukemia: high rates of rapid cytogenetic and molecular responses. J Clin Oncol. 2009;27(28):4754–9.
16. Latagliata R, Breccia M, Carmosino I, Cannella L, De Cuia R, Diverio D, et al. "Real- life" results of front-line treatment with Imatinib in older patients (>=65 years) with newly diagnosed chronic myelogenous leukemia. Leuk Res. 2010;34(11):1472–5.
17. Sanchez-Gujio FM, Duran S, Galende J, Boqué C, Nieto JB, Balanzat J, et al. Evaluation of tolerability and efficacy on imatinib mesylate in elderly patients with chronic phase CML: ELDERGLI study. Leuk Res. 2011;35:1184–7.
18. Lipton JH, le Coutre PD, Wang J, Yang M, Szczudlo T, Giles F. Nilotinib in elderly chronic myeloid leukemia patients in chronic phase (CML-CP) with imatinib resistance or intolerance: efficacy and safety analysis. Blood. 2008;112:3233.
19. le Coutre PD, Turkina A, Kim DW, Ceglarek B, Alimena G, Al-Ali HK, et al. Efficacy and safety of nilotinib in elderly patients with imatinib-resistant or intolerant chronic myeloid leukemia (CML) in chronic phase: a subanalysis of the ENACT (expanding nilotinib access in clinical trials) study. Blood. 2009;114:3286.
20. Latagliata R, Breccia M, Castagnetti F, Stagno F, Luciano L, Gozzini A, et al. Dasatinib is safe and effective in unselected chronic myeloid leukemia elderly patients resistant/intolerant to imatinib. Leuk Res. 2011;35:1164–9.
21. Gambacorti-Passerini C, Brümmendorf T, Cortes J, Schafhausen P, Hochhaus A, Kindler T, et al. Efficacy and safety of bosutinib for Philadelphia chromosome-positive leukemia in older versus younger patients. Haematologica. 2012;97 Suppl 1:757.
22. Cortes JE, Kim DW, Pinilla-Ibarz J, le Coutre P, Paquette R, Chuah C, et al. A phase 2 trial of ponatinib in Philadelphia chromosome-positive leukemias. N Engl J Med. 2013;369(19): 1783–96.
23. Khoury HJ, Cortes JE, Kantarjian HM, et al. Safety and efficacy of dasatinib (DAS) vs imatinib (IM) by baseline comorbidity in patients with chronic myeloid leukemia in chronic phase (CML-CP): analysis of the DASISION trial. Blood. 2010;116:3421.
24. Larson RA, Hochhaus A, Hughes TP, Clark RE, Etienne G, Kim DW, et al. Nilotinib vs imatinib in patients with newly diagnosed Philadelphia chromosome positive chronic myeloid leukemia in chronic phase: ENESTnd 3-year follow-up. Leukemia. 2012;26:2197–203.
25. Cortes JE, Kim DW, Kantarjian HM, Brümmendorf TH, Dyagil I, Griskevicius L, et al. Bosutinib versus imatinib in newly diagnosed chronic-phase chronic myeloid leukemia: results from the BELA trial. J Clin Oncol. 2012;30:3486–92.
26. Breccia M, Alimena G. Management options for refractory chronic myeloid leukemia: considerations for the elderly. Drugs Aging. 2013;30(7):467–77.

27. Seiter K. Considerations in the management of elderly patients with chronic myeloid leukemia. Clin Lymph Myel Leuk. 2012;12(1):12–9.
28. Proetel U, Pletsch N, Lauseker M, Müller MC, Hanfstein B, Krause SW, et al. Older patients with chronic myeloid leukemia (≥65 years) profit more from higher imatinib doses than younger patients: a subanalysis of the randomized CML-Study IV. Ann Hematol. 2014;93(7): 1167–76.
29. le Coutre P, Rea D, Abruzzese E, Dombret H, Trawinska MM, Herndlhofer S, et al. Severe peripheral arterial disease during nilotinib therapy. J Natl Cancer Inst. 2011;103:1347–8.
30. Kim TD, Rea D, Schwarz M, Grille P, Nicolini FE, Rosti G, et al. Peripheral artery occlusive disease in chronic phase chronic myeloid leukemia patients treated with nilotinib or imatinib. Leukemia. 2013;27(6):1316–21.
31. Giles FJ, Mauro MJ, Hong F, Ortmann CE, McNeill C, Woodman RC, et al. Rates of peripheral arterial occlusive disease in patients with chronic myeloid leukemia in the chronic phase treated with imatinib, nilotinib, or non-tyrosine kinase therapy: a retrospective cohort analysis. Leukemia. 2013;27(6):1310–5.
32. Latagliata R. Imatinib in very elderly patients with chronic myeloid leukemia in chronic phase: a retrospective study. Drugs Aging. 2013;30(8):629–37.

Chapter 6
Myeloproliferative Neoplasms

Farah Shariff and Claire Harrison

Abstract The myeloproliferative neoplasms previously known as myeloproliferative disorders include, polycythemia vera, essential thrombocythemia and myelofibrosis and also other rarer entities such as chronic eosinophilic and neutrophilic leukemia and overlap or otherwise unclassifiable disorders. They are uncommon clonal hematological malignancies that are generally diagnosed from late middle age onwards although they may occur in children and young adults. They are increasingly common with advanced age. In this chapter we focus almost exclusively on the three commonest entities. Whilst each of these disorders usually have unique features but their clinical courses have similarities, including thrombosis, hemorrhage, a tendency for progressive myelofibrosis and the development of acute myeloid leukemia. Myelofibrosis is associated with a much poorer prognosis than the other conditions and death, usually due to progressive bone marrow failure or leukemia. Recently, mutations at position 617 in exon 14 of the JAK2 gene and exon 9 of the Calreticulin (CALR) [30] gene have has been identified in the majority of patients with polycythemia vera and half of those with essential thrombocythemia or myelofibrosis. This has improved diagnostic pathways, but challenges their current classification as separate entities. Current treatment for these patients involves aggressive management of thrombotic risk factors, aspirin for most patients unless contraindicated and cytoreductive agents such as hydroxycarbamide (hydroxyurea) for patients at highest risk of thrombosis. A new class of drugs, JAK inhibitors, have proven to be effective for symptomatic myelofibrosis and the first of these agents, ruxolitinib, has recently been licensed.

Keywords Erythrocytosis • Essential thrombocythemia • Myelofibrosis • Myeloproliferative • Polycythemia vera • Thrombocytosis • JAK inhibitors

F. Shariff, MD, MBBS, BSc (Hons), MRCP • C. Harrison, MD, DM, FRCP, FRCPath (✉)
Department of Haematology, Guy's and St Thomas' NHS Foundation Trust,
Great Maze Pond, London SE1 9RT, UK
e-mail: Claire.Harrison@gstt.nhs.uk

U. Wedding, R.A. Audisio (eds.), *Management of Hematological Cancer in Older People*, DOI 10.1007/978-1-4471-2837-3_6

Table 6.1 WHO defined myeloproliferative neoplasms

World Health Organization classification for myeloproliferative neoplasms 2008
Chronic myelogenous leukemia
Polycythemia vera
Essential thrombocythemia
Primary myelofibrosis
Chronic neutrophilic leukemia
Chronic eosinophilic leukemia, not otherwise specified
Hypereosinophilic syndrome
Mast cell disease
MPN, unclassifiable

Introduction

The myeloproliferative neoplasms (MPNs) are clonal hematological diseases characterized by overproduction of mature blood cells and, in general, a chronic course [1].The World Health Organisation has recently modified the nomenclature from myeloproliferative disorder to neoplasm to reflect the malignant nature of these diseases [2]. MPNs include polycythemia vera (PV), primary myelofibrosis (PMF) and essential thrombocythemia (ET), and the rarer entities, chronic neutrophilic leukemia, chronic eosinophilic leukemia and chronic myeloproliferative neoplasm, unclassifiable as well as mast cell diseases as summarised in Table 6.1. Here, we consider the commoner so-called classical Philadelphia-negative MPNs: ET, PV and PMF. In these entities which were all described in the last 200 years the proliferation of a single cell type defines disease phenotype: erythrocytes in PV, platelets in ET and fibroblasts in PMF.

Over the past two centuries our understanding of myeloproliferative neoplasms has evolved from their original clinical and hematopathological observations to an increasing appreciation of the molecular mechanisms underpinning the neoplastic process and their interplay with clinical phenotype and therapy. The disorders including chronic myeloid leukemia (CML), PV, and PMF were all identified as clinical and pathological entities in the nineteenth century. ET was delineated later by Epstein and Goedel in 1934, post-PV MF was described by Hirsch in 1935, and so during the first half of the twentieth century the inter-relationship between these disorders began to be defined. Dameshek however was the first author to formally articulate the idea of a common 'myeloproliferative' heritage in his landmark publication of 1951 stating: "It is possible that… 'myeloproliferative disorders' – are all… variable manifestations of proliferative activity of the bone marrow cells, perhaps due to a hitherto undiscovered stimulus" [3]. Dameshek thus importantly postulated not only the possibility of transition between these disorders, but more interestingly a common primary mechanism for all MPNs. Dameshek's proposal of a common underlying pathology began to bear fruition during the 1980s with growing evidence that tyrosine kinase (TK) activity provided the molecular mechanism for CML which is not formally discussed further in this chapter.

An acquired point mutation in the JAK 2 (JAK2 V617F) gene occurs in most patients with PV and almost half of those with ET or PMF and less prevalent mutations have been described in exon 12 of JAK2 and the transmembrane domain of the thrombopoietin receptor cMPL as well as others [4]. The JAK2 V617F mutation disrupts the secondary structure of the pseudokinase domain and then enables constitutive, cytokine-independent activation of signal transduction pathways, enhancing cell proliferation. The functional consequences of the mutations effecting exon 9 of CALR are not yet clear and they are beginning to be integrated into diagnostics. This has revolutionized the investigation and diagnosis of these conditions and has been incorporated into standard diagnostic pathways in a rational manner [5]. There have only been four large clinical trials, ECLAP [6], PT1 [7] and the COMFORT studies [8, 9] in these conditions to date, these have enabled hematologists to refine evidence-based management further, while current clinical trials focus upon novel agents used alone and in combination [10]. Each of the three commonest entities will now be considered in turn.

Polycythemia Vera

Clinical Features and Epidemiology

PV or Vasquez disease is characterized by raised red cell mass (erythrocytosis) usually but not always in combination with thrombocytosis and/or neutrophilia; pruritus, gout and splenomegaly are classical clinical features. The median age at presentation of PV is 55–60 years. Clinical events include arterial and to a lesser extent venous thromboses often at atypical sites (e.g. abdominal venous thrombosis) or rarely bleeding. Over 10–15 years, myelofibrosis occurs in 10–15 % and acute myeloid leukemia (AML) in 5–10 % of patients with this disease and as demonstrated in the ECLAP study AML is more common in patients who are older (over 65 years), treated with drugs known to increase this risk such as alkylating agents, and smokers [11].

A packed cell volume (PCV or hematocrit) persistently greater than 0.52 in a male, or 0.48 in a female, should trigger investigation, however there is a wide differential diagnosis of potential causes of an erythrocytosis as summarised in Table 6.2. Assessment of patients suspected of an erythocytosis should include a thorough history and examination, full blood count/film, haematinics, renal/liver profile, urate, JAK2 V617F screen, urinalysis and chest X-ray (especially for smokers). In the absence of an obvious secondary cause and no detectable JAK2 V617F mutation, a red cell mass may be required to identify an absolute erythrocytosis (i.e. a truly raised red cell count). Additional tests include serum erythropoietin level (suppressed in PV), bone marrow biopsy, screening for mutations in exon 12 of JAK2, truncated erythropoietin receptor, proline dehydroxylase abnormalities, abdominal ultrasound, sleep studies and screening for a high-affinity haemoglobin. The diagnostic criteria for PV are shown in Table 6.3.

Table 6.2 Causes of an erythrocytosis

Causes of absolute erythrocytosis
Primary (abnormality within RBCs)
Congenital
Truncated erythropoietin receptor
Acquired
Polycythemia vera
Secondary (abnormality outside RBCs)
Congenital
Inherited high erythropoietin levels
Abnormal hemoglobin with increased oxygen affinity
Reduced 2,3-diphosphoglycerate
Mutation in von Hippel–Lindau gene
Mutations in proline dehydroxylase genes
Acquired (increased erythropoietin)
Conditions causing low oxygen levels – high altitude, chronic lung disease, some congenital heart diseases
Renal disease – tumours (hypernephroma), cysts (usually benign), hydronephrosis, following kidney transplantation
Liver disease – hepatoma, cirrhosis, hepatitis
Tumours – bronchial cancer, fibroids in the uterus, cerebellar haemangiomata
Endocrine abnormalities – Cushing's syndrome, phaeochromocytoma
Idiopathic (undefined primary or secondary)
May resolve or pathology may be masked initially
Causes of apparent erythrocytosis
Normal variant
Early absolute erythrocytosis
Obesity, fluid loss, diuretics, smoking, hypertension, alcohol, renal disease, psychological stress

Worldwide estimates of the incidence of PV vary greatly, with the incidence thought to be between 2 and 2.8 per 100,000, with a slightly higher male preponderance.

One of the largest studies of a cohort of PV patients, the European Collaboration on Low-dose Aspirin in PV (ECLAP) over a median period of 2.8 years, revealed that the mortality of patients with PV was 2.1 times higher that of the standard population, with cardiovascular complications playing a significant role [11]. A predominance of arterial events and non-hemorrhagic cerebral vascular events was noted. Abdominal venous thrombosis such as Budd-Chiari syndrome, and obstruction of the portal, mesenteric and splenic systems have often been seen in patients with PV. A previous history of thrombotic events and a rising age are felt to independently increase the risk of further thrombotic events in this sub-group of individuals. These results were corroborated by the results of the ECLAP study whereby those over the age of 65 years and with a prior history of a thrombotic event were noted to have the highest risk of cardiac complications.

Leucocytosis appears to be another independent risk factor, whereby individuals with a WCC $>15\times10^9$ are at a higher risk of vascular events. This has been attributed to endothelial and platelet activation, leading to acceleration of arteriosclerosis

Table 6.3 Diagnostic criteria for the MPNs

Proposed diagnostic algorhythm for MPDs

Careful clinical assessment to evaluate for secondary cause and additional risk factors:

Screen for *V617F JAK2* +/- *CMPLW515L/K*

POSITIVE *V617F JAK2*

PV **-if V617F JAK2 and all of:**

1. PCV > 0.51 in ♂, 0.48♀ or raised red cell mass
2. No secondary cause of high PCV
3. Normal/low serum erythropoietin

ET **– if *V617F JAK2* & all of:**

- Platelet count > upper limit normal range
- No other myeloid disease (includes PV, MDS, MF)

MF **- if *V617F JAK2* and :**

- Reticulin> grade ¾ or presence of collagen

And any two of:

- Palpable splenomegaly
- Unexplained anaemia
- Tear drop red cells
- Leucoerythroblastic film
- Systemic symptoms (night sweats, >10% weight loss, bone pain)

6. Biopsy proven extramedullary haematopoiesis

NEGATIVE *V617F JAK2*

PV **–if 1 +2 & either one A or two B criteria:**

1. PCV > 0.6 in ♂, 0.56♀ or raised red cell mass
2. No secondary cause of high PCV & Normal erythropoietin

A Palpable splenomegaly
A Presence of acquired cytogenetic abnormality

B Neutrophila (>10 x 10^9/L; or >12.5 x 10^9/L in smokers)
B Splenomegaly on imaging
B Endogenous erythroid colonies or low erythropoietin
B Thrombocytosis (plts > 400 x 10^9/L)

ET **– if all of:**

- Platelet count > 600 x 10^9/L
- No other myeloid disease (includes CML, PV, MDS, MF)
- No reactive cause and normal iron status

MF **- if all of :**

- Reticulin> grade ¾ or presence of collagen
- Absence of *V617F JAK2* and *BCR/ABL*

And any two of:

- Palpable splenomegaly
- Unexplained anaemia
- Tear drop red cells
- Leucoerythroblastic film
- Systemic symptoms (night sweats, >10% weight loss, bone pain

6. Biopsy proven extramedullary haematopoiesis

[12]. Hypertension, hypercholesterolaemia, smoking and diabetes are independently associated with atherosclerosis, and in the context of their presence in patients with PV should be managed aggressively [13].

Management and Prognosis of PV

The risk of vascular events in treated PV patients remains raised at approximately 1.6 times normal despite optimal modern management [11]. Transformation to either Myelofibrosis or AML following PV are treated as per myelofibrosis (see below) or usually supportively, as the outlook is extremely poor; stem cell transplantation is an option in a minority of suitably fit patients who transform. Reversible factors for cardiovascular disease should be managed aggressively and low-dose aspirin considered unless contraindicated, e.g. active or previous peptic ulcer disease, prominent bleeding symptoms and presence of acquired von Willebrand's disease. The European Collaboration on Low-dose Aspirin in PV (ECLAP) study found low-dose aspirin was effective in reducing the number of thrombotic events as well as micro vascular symptoms such as erythromelagia which is associated with the spontaneous aggregation of platelets. Treatment includes repeated venesection or cytoreductive therapy to keep the PCV below 0.45 in males, and females, and in some patients the platelets less than 400×10^9/l. The target for venesection was recently confirmed in a prospective study [14].

Cytoreduction is clearly indicated if patients are intolerant of venesection or indeed if they develop thrombocytosis, symptomatic splenomegaly or a thrombosis [13]. Hydroxyurea (or hydroxycarbamide, HC) is the cytoreductive drug of first choice. Concern that it might increase the risk of leukemia is not proven but the use of phosphorus-32 (P^{32}) or busulfan is restricted because of their well-defined leukemogenic potential. Interferon alpha (IFN) is a non-leukemogenic alternative and recent data suggest that pegylated IFN may reduce JAK2 V617F levels, potentially eradicating the abnormal clone. Intermittent busulphan or P^{32} can be used in the very frail, in whom regular out-patient visits are not practical or compliance is an issue, bearing in mind their leukemogenic potential. Investigational agents include JAK inhibitors and Histone Deacetylase Inhibitors which are currently being assessed in clinical trial. A current trial is directly comparing IFN and HC.

Therapuetic Options and Considerations for the Elderly Patient with PV

Therapeutic options in managing elderly patients with PV is dependent on the use of the appropriate agent, taking into consideration the phase of the disease, age of the patient as well as their ability to tolerate or comply with therapy . Treatment affects overall survival, with those that remain untreated having an average survival of 18 months, with thrombotic events being the predominant cause of morbidity and mortality. Those who are treated have on average a median survival of 10–15 years.

The aim of cytoreduction in PV is to minimise the overall risk of thrombotic events, control disease-related symptoms and reduce the risk of disease progression. The needs of older patients are often different from those of younger patients. In particular, the impact of reduced physiological reserve as well as multiple-morbidities needs to be taken into account. Elderly patients commonly have multiple pathologies leading to polypharmacy, in addition to altered pharmacokinetics as well as pharmacodynamics. In this sub-group of patients, optimisation of their existing therapies, looking into their ability to tolerate various available therapies, and optimisation of their ability with compliance of therapy needs careful forethought. In such scenarios, a dedicated review by the elderly care team with close liaison with the treating hematologist can play a vital role in optimisation of drug use amongst this high-risk group.

Essential Thrombocythemia

Clinical Features and Epidemiology of ET

ET is characterized by a persistent thrombocytosis and recent WHO criteria suggest patients with platelets persistently over $450 \times 10^9/l$ merit investigation (see also Table 6.3) [2]. Clinical features are very similar to PV. Microvascular events are said to predominate here including erythromelalgia (asymmetric erythema, congestion and burning pain in the hands and feet) which may progress to ischaemia and gangrene, migrainous-like headaches and transient ischaemic attacks. The long-term risk of myelofibrosis and leukemia is perhaps lower than that with PV. ET is perhaps one of the most common myeloproliferative neoplasms and is thought to have an annual incidence of between 1 and 2.5 per 100,000 individuals according to the WHO. It is often identified as an incidental finding. It is predominantly diagnosed in patients between 50 and 60 years, with what appears to be an even distribution between both male and females though in younger patients there is a female preponderance [15].

The differential diagnosis of an isolated thrombocytosis includes other MPNs and reactive thrombocytosis, the causes of the latter include iron deficiency anemia, infection, chronic inflammation (e.g. rheumatoid arthritis or inflammatory bowel disease), splenectomy, acute hemorrhage and malignant disease. Such conditions may coexist with ET especially of course in the elderly, making the diagnosis difficult [16]. Investigations include full blood count/film, haematinics, renal and liver profile, C-reactive protein (CRP), anti nuclear antibody (ANA) and rheumatoid factor (RF), screening for JAK2 V617F Calreticulin [30]. MPL W515L/K mutations, chest X-ray, abdominal ultrasound scan and bone marrow examination (see Table 6.3).

Management and Prognosis of ET

Thrombosis is the major cause of morbidity and mortality for patients with ET. Hemorrhage occurs less commonly and is particularly associated with platelet counts of more than $1{,}500 \times 10^9$/l and acquired von Willebrand's disease. Most patients have a near normal life expectancy. Cytoreductive agents should be used for patients with a high risk of thrombosis (any patient of age >60 years, platelet count $>1{,}500 \times 10^9$/l, prior disease-related thrombosis or hemorrhage, treated diabetes or hypertension) [13, 16]. The total leucocyte count and allele burden of JAK2V617F are potentially useful future risk factors for thrombosis, as well as degree of reticulin deposition (fibre present in the marrow) Calreticulin [30] mutations appear to be associated with lower thrombotic risk.

In common with PV, patients with ET should be screened and aggressively managed for reversible factors for cardiovascular disease and low-dose aspirin given unless contraindicated. HC is the gold standard cytoreductive drug as has been demonstrated in the PT1 trial where it was compared with anagrelide see below [7]. Alternatives include ^{32}P and busulfan, although these agents are more leukemogenic. IFN and anagrelide have the advantage that they are probably non-leukemogenic and do not affect fertility [16]. Both control the platelet count in most patients but are poorly tolerated, with up to 30 % being unable to continue treatment in the long term. The MRC-PT1 study made a direct comparison between hydroxycarbamide and anagrelide in patients with ET at high risk of thrombosis. The results suggested that hydroxycarbamide + aspirin is a more effective first-line therapy than anagrelide + aspirin, which was associated with a higher rate of arterial thrombosis, hemorrhage and myelofibrotic transformation [7]. In those who do not respond to a single cytoreductive agent, they can be switched to an alternative combination therapy can be used where appropriate. In circumstances whereby hydroxycarbamide is used with leukemogenic agents such as Busulfan, it has the potential to potentiate the leukemogenicity of either agent. Systemic anticoagulation should be considered in individuals over the age of 60 years in those with a venous thrombosis history.

Therapuetic Options and Considerations for the Elderly Patient with ET

The comments recorded for elderly PV patients (see above) apply equally to those for elderly ET patients. Indeed a recent paper examined the management of patients over the age of 80 years with ET in total 395 patients >80 years old with ET were followed as a subgroup of an observational study the authors concluded that "Well-tolerated and effective cytoreductive therapy has been achieved in patients aged >80 years by following individual treatment modalities that appear in agreement with the recent European LeukemiaNet (ELN) guidelines" [17].

Myelofibrosis

MF may present de novo when it is known as PMF or progress from an antecedent ET or PV when it is referred to as Post-ET or Post-PV myelofibrosis [18], collectively we will refer to these conditions as MF. Fibrosis is a hallmark feature of this condition and was identified in the first description of MF by Huek in 1872 along with massive splenomegaly. This fibrosis is thought to arise from an interaction between diseased megakaryocytes, leukocytes, and bone marrow stroma which release mitogens such as platelet-derived growth factor and transforming growth factor β. The proliferating fibroblasts are polyclonal and the primary disorder affects the hematopoetic stem cell. A range of molecular abnormalities have been described in patients with MF and these are beginning to be incorporated into prognosis for these patients more so that for patients with ET or PV for example [19].

Clinical Features and Epidemiology of MF

Individuals with MF often have a significant disease burden with diverse, debilitating symptoms that are progressive in nature and severely impact on the quality of life [20, 21]. Constitutional symptoms including fevers, night sweats, pruritus and bone pain can be a prominent feature of the disease and impact significantly on quality of life. Progression to AML occurs in up to 25 % of patients. Other MPNs (PV, ET, CML) and disorders in which marrow fibrosis can develop as a secondary feature (e.g. metastatic carcinoma, lymphoma, irradiation, tuberculosis, leishmaniasis) should be excluded. Most therapies are mainly targeted at alleviating and managing symptoms though until the introduction of JAK inhibitors they were not very effective, with a delay in disease progression to the leukemic phase is the primary aim [13, 18]. The yearly calculated incidence of primary myelofibrosis (PMF) ranges from 0.4 to 1.4 per 100,000 people. A slight male preponderance exists for PMF in adults, the median age at diagnosis is 65 years and about 20 % of affected patients are aged <55 years [15].

A positive screen for JAK2 V617F Calreticulin [30] MPL W515L/K mutations is helpful in confirming the diagnosis of MF but it is important to exclude other conditions as many other conditions may be associated with marrow fibrosis including for example myelodysplasia, CML, Hodgkin's disease and other non-neoplastic conditions such as tuberculosis and leishmaniasis.

Management and Prognosis of MF

Therapeutic decisions in primary myelofibrosis depend on the stage of the disease as well as overall prognosis, whilst looking at the patient's clinical status and comorbidities as a whole. For the vast majority, medical management is the management choice. Supportive therapy with red cell transfusions and treatment of infection is often a mainstay, with androgens or erythropoietin therapy for some. (9) Several risk stratification scores have been developed for MF although they have only been validated in PMF. Of these IPSS is used at diagnosis and both DIPSS and DIPSS-Plus are the most widely used during the course of disease (these scores are discussed in detail in recent British Guidelines [18]). The overall score predicts progression and survival, and can enable a decision regarding the appropriate choice of treatment. In particular for those patients eligible for bone marrow transplantation these scores are extremely useful since international guidelines recommend consideration of this therapy when prognosis is less than 5 years and indeed outcome from transplant has been linked to IPSS as well as DIPSS [13, 22]. Transplantation has generally not been recommended for elderly patients but is being increasingly explored [22].

Conventional non-transplant related therapies for MF are diverse and are targeted usually at specific aspects of disease. Hydroxycarbamide which we have discussed in the context of ET and PV is also widely used particularly in patients with symptomatic splenomegaly and proliferative counts, with an overall response rate of ~45 % seen in a retrospective study [23]. However it may not affect prognosis. Careful dose titration is often required till clinical effect is observed. However it in itself requires patients to have regular follow up monitoring, for side effects such as cytopenias. A combination of steroids and thalidomide has been shown to be effective in some or the use of Lenalidomide in the context of those who are anaemic but have a platelet count $>100 \times 10^9$ [18]. Splenectomy is very hazardous for these patients [24] yet is sometimes effective; it is not recommended for all, and certainly in the elderly there is an added risk of complications with significant morbidity and mortality in view of existing underlying co-morbidities. Radiotherapy may be an option in those with intractable bone pain, those with evidence of extramedullary hemopoiesis in other organs or symptomatic splenomegaly deemed not suitable for surgical intervention [18]. Anemia can be managed with blood transfusions and in certain individuals with moderate anemia in the context of an erythropoietin level of <125 u/l, may benefit from recombinant treatment. Androgens such as Danazol have been seen to be an option in transfusion dependent anemia, however monitoring of liver function and prostate cancer for men is required.

The therapeutic landscape for patients with MF has been radically altered with the arrival of JAK inhibitors which have been evaluated in Phase III clinical trials (reviewed in [10, 25]). The first such agent, Ruxolitinib is now approved for use in Intermediate and high risk MF in the United States and for symptoms of MF and/or splenomegaly in the EU. Ruxolitinib has proven to be effective at relieving symptoms and reducing splenomegaly with approximately 30 % of patients achieving a 50 % or greater reduction in palpable spleen size compared to best available therapy. Exactly how these agents exert their mode of action and the relevance of trial endpoints has been debated, none of these drugs is specific to the JAK2 V617F mutation and to date they all appear equally active in patients whether they test positive for the mutation or not [26, 27]. Nonetheless there is emerging and strengthening evidence of a survival benefit and perhaps of disease modification at least with Ruxolitinib while data with other agents is thus far immature [9, 28, 29].

Therapuetic Options and Considerations for the Elderly Patient with MF

The elderly patients with MF can present a difficult challenge disease progress is inexorable and co-morbidities can rule out consideration of curative therapy such as transplantation or even clinical trials with novel agents which is an area of intense interest in this particular field. Fortuitously the JAK inhibitors are extremely well-tolerated and can be given in patients with renal, cardiac and liver impairment though with due caution.

Conclusions

The MPN are chronic neoplastic conditions characterised by a preponderance of mature blood cells, they have a central common pathogenesis with JAK/STAT activation, frequently associated with mutations in JAK2 in particular *JAK2 V617F.* The description of this mutation in 2005 has substantially modified management from diagnosis and is now influencing treatment approaches for these patients. These conditions are more prevalent in the elderly; their clinical phenotype is dominated by risk of thrombosis (so for all of them aggressive vascular risk management is mandatory); and development of either MF, after one of the more benign entities (ET or PV), or AML (which occurs after any MPN but more frequently MF). For each MPN advanced age has been shown to be a poor prognostic factor. There have been several large studies of these patients but none have systematically evaluated care for the elderly cohort. Notwithstanding these facts the evidence to date is that most elderly patients with MPN can be managed with standard therapies to which they respond as well as younger patients. The most important challenge here remaining to identify these diseases before the occurrence of a thrombosis or hemorrhage.

References

1. Campbell PJ, Green AR. The myeloproliferative disorders. N Engl J Med. 2006;355(23): 2452–66.
2. Vardiman JW, Thiele J, Arber DA, Brunning RD, Borowitz MJ, Porwit A, et al. The 2008 revision of the World Health Organization (WHO) classification of myeloid neoplasms and acute leukemia: rationale and important changes. Blood. 2009;114(5):937–51.
3. Dameshek W. Some speculations on the myeloproliferative syndromes. Blood. 1951; 6(6):372–5.
4. Vannucchi AM, Guglielmelli P. Molecular pathophysiology of Philadelphia-negative myeloproliferative disorders: beyond JAK2 and MPL mutations. Haematologica. 2008;93(7):972–6.
5. Bench AJ, White HE, Foroni L, Godfrey AL, Gerrard G, Akiki S, et al. Molecular diagnosis of the myeloproliferative neoplasms: UK guidelines for the detection of JAK2 V617F and other relevant mutations. Br J Haematol. 2013;160(1):25–34.
6. Landolfi R, Marchioli R, Kutti J, Gisslinger H, Tognoni G, Patrono C, et al. Efficacy and safety of low-dose aspirin in polycythemia vera. N Engl J Med. 2004;350(2):114–24.
7. Harrison CN, Campbell PJ, Buck G, Wheatley K, East CL, Bareford D, et al. Hydroxyurea compared with anagrelide in high-risk essential thrombocythemia. N Engl J Med. 2005;353(1): 33–45.
8. Harrison C, Kiladjian J-J, Al-Ali HK, Gisslinger H, Waltzman R, Stalbovskaya V, et al. JAK inhibition with ruxolitinib versus best available therapy for myelofibrosis. N Engl J Med. 2012;366(9):787–98.
9. Verstovsek S, Mesa RA, Gotlib J, Levy RS, Gupta V, DiPersio JF, et al. A double-blind, placebo-controlled trial of ruxolitinib for myelofibrosis. N Engl J Med. 2012;366(9): 799–807.
10. Harrison C, Verstovsek S, McMullin MF, Mesa R. Janus kinase inhibition and its effect upon the therapeutic landscape for myelofibrosis: from palliation to cure? Br J Haematol. 2012; 157(4):426–37.
11. Marchioli R, Finazzi G, Landolfi R, Kutti J, Gisslinger H, Patrono C, et al. Vascular and neoplastic risk in a large cohort of patients with polycythemia vera. J Clin Oncol. 2005;23(10): 2224–32.
12. Landolfi R, Di Gennaro L, Barbui T, De Stefano V, Finazzi G, Marfisi R, et al. Leukocytosis as a major thrombotic risk factor in patients with polycythemia vera. Blood. 2007; 109(6):2446–52.

13. Barbui T, Barosi G, Birgegard G, Cervantes F, Finazzi G, Griesshammer M, et al. Philadelphia-negative classical myeloproliferative neoplasms: critical concepts and management recommendations from European LeukemiaNet. J Clin Oncol. 2011;29(6):761–70.
14. Marchioli R, Vannucchi AM, Barbui T. Treatment target in polycythemia vera. N Engl J Med. 2013;368(16):1556.
15. McNally RJ, Rowland D, Roman E, Cartwright RA. Age and sex distributions of hematological malignancies in the U.K. Hematol Oncol. 1997;15(4):173–89.
16. Harrison CN, Bareford D, Butt N, Campbell P, Conneally E, Drummond M, et al. Guideline for investigation and management of adults and children presenting with a thrombocytosis. Br J Haematol. 2010;149(3):352–75.
17. Kiladjian JJ, Besses C, Griesshammer M, Gugliotta L, Harrison C, Coll R, et al. Efficacy and safety of cytoreductive therapies in patients with essential thrombocythaemia aged >80 years: an interim analysis of the EXELS study. Clin Drug Investig. 2013;33(1):55–63.
18. Reilly JT, McMullin MF, Beer PA, Butt N, Conneally E, Duncombe A, et al. Guideline for the diagnosis and management of myelofibrosis. Br J Haematol. 2012;158(4):453–71.
19. Vannucchi AM, Lasho TL, Guglielmelli P, Biamonte F, Pardanani A, Pereira A, et al. Mutations and prognosis in primary myelofibrosis. Leukemia. 2013;27:1861–9.
20. Emanuel RM, Dueck AC, Geyer HL, Kiladjian JJ, Slot S, Zweegman S, et al. Myeloproliferative neoplasm (MPN) symptom assessment form total symptom score: prospective international assessment of an abbreviated symptom burden scoring system among patients with MPNs. J Clin Oncol. 2012;30(33):4098–103.
21. Harrison CN, Mesa RA, Kiladjian JJ, Al-Ali HK, Gisslinger H, Knoops L, et al. Health-related quality of life and symptoms in patients with myelofibrosis treated with ruxolitinib versus best available therapy. Br J Haematol. 2013;162(2):229–39.
22. McLornan DP, Mead AJ, Jackson G, Harrison CN. Allogeneic stem cell transplantation for myelofibrosis in 2012. Br J Haematol. 2012;157(4):413–25.
23. Martinez-Trillos A, Gaya A, Maffioli M, Arellano-Rodrigo E, Calvo X, Diaz-Beya M, et al. Efficacy and tolerability of hydroxyurea in the treatment of the hyperproliferative manifestations of myelofibrosis: results in 40 patients. Ann Hematol. 2010;89(12):1233–7.
24. Tefferi A, Mesa RA, Nagorney DM, Schroeder G, Silverstein MN. Splenectomy in myelofibrosis with myeloid metaplasia: a single-institution experience with 223 patients. Blood. 2000;95(7):2226–33.
25. Cervantes F, Mesa R, Harrison C. JAK inhibitors: beyond spleen and symptoms? Haematologica. 2013;98(2):160–2.
26. Harrison CN, Kiladjian J-J, Gisslinger H, Niederwieser D, Passamonti F, Waltzman RJ, et al. Ruxolitinib provides reductions in splenomegaly across subgroups: an analysis of spleen response in the COMFORT-II study. ASH Ann Meet Abstr. 2011;118(21):279.
27. Verstovsek S, Mesa RA, Gotlib J, Levy RS, Gupta V, DiPersio JF, et al. The clinical benefit of ruxolitinib across patient subgroups: analysis of a placebo-controlled, Phase III study in patients with myelofibrosis. Br J Haematol. 2013;161(4):508–16.
28. Verstovsek S, Kantarjian HM, Estrov Z, Cortes JE, Thomas DA, Kadia T, et al. Long-term outcomes of 107 patients with myelofibrosis receiving JAK1/JAK2 inhibitor ruxolitinib: survival advantage in comparison to matched historical controls. Blood. 2012;120(6): 1202–9.
29. Cervantes F, Kiladjian J-J, Niederwieser D, Sirulnik A, Stalbovskaya V, McQuity M, et al. Long-term safety, efficacy, and survival findings from comfort-II, a phase 3 study comparing ruxolitinib with Best Available Therapy (BAT) for the Treatment of Myelofibrosis (MF). ASH Annu Meet Abstr. 2012;120(21):801.
30. Nangalia J, Massie CE, Baxter EJ, et al. Somatic CALR mutations in myeloproliferative neoplasms with nonmutated JAK2. The New England journal of medicine. 2013;369(25):2391–405.

Chapter 7
Chronic Lymphocytic Leukemia (CLL)

Valentin Goede and Michael Hallek

Abstract The majority of patients diagnosed with chronic lymphocytic leukemia (CLL) are of advanced age. These patients are markedly heterogeneous with regard to their fitness and vulnerability. A standard approach to assess fitness in older CLL patients remains to be defined. The spectrum of therapeutic options is broad and treatment should be risk- and fitness-adapted. Fit patients should be treated with the standard of care in CLL while in less fit patients alternative regimens are to be considered. Emerging new drugs (antibodies, small molecules) likely will improve the treatment of both fit and less fit older patients in the next future. This chapter reviews the current knowledge on epidemiology, biology, diagnosis, and therapy of CLL in the elderly in order to provide recommendations for the management of older CLL patients.

Keywords Chronic lymphocytic leukemia • Aging • Comorbidity • Geriatric assessment • Chemotherapy • Chemoimmunotherapy • Targeted drug

---

V. Goede, MD
German CLL Study Group (GCLLSG),
Department I of Internal Medicine,
Center of Integrated Oncology Cologne-Bonn,
University of Cologne, Kerpener Str. 62, Cologne 50924, Germany

Department of Geriatric Medicine and Research, St. Marien Hospital
and University of Cologne, Cologne, Germany
e-mail: valentin.goede@uk-koeln.de

M. Hallek, MD, PhD (✉)
German CLL Study Group (GCLLSG),
Department I of Internal Medicine,
Center of Integrated Oncology Cologne-Bonn,
University of Cologne, Kerpener Str. 62, Cologne 50924, Germany

Cluster of Excellence 'Cellular Stress Responses in Aging
Associated Diseases' (CECAD),
University of Cologne, Cologne, Germany
e-mail: michael.hallek@uni-koeln.de

U. Wedding, R.A. Audisio (eds.), *Management of Hematological Cancer in Older People*, DOI 10.1007/978-1-4471-2837-3_7

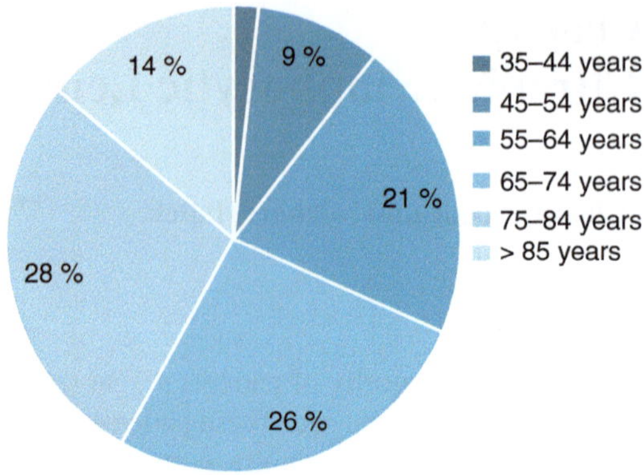

Fig. 7.1 Age-distribution among patients with newly diagnosed CLL

Epidemiology and Demographics

Chronic lymphocytic leukemia (CLL) is the most common leukemia in Europe and North America. Its incidence is 4/100,000 per year and increases significantly in older people [1]. A maximum of approximately 30/100,000 per year is reached among subjects over the age of 80 years. Because of the higher incidence of CLL late in life and the lack of symptoms at disease onset, CLL is often diagnosed at advanced age: The median age at diagnosis is 72 years. Of newly diagnosed patients, 27 % are 65–74 years old, 28 % are 75–84 years old and 14 % are 85 years old or older (Fig. 7.1) [1]. The median age of death in patients with CLL is 79 years. Because populations of the western world are aging, it is likely that these figures will change, thus leading to a constant increase of the relative and absolute numbers of older CLL patients.

Biology and Aging

The etiology of CLL is unknown and its pathogenesis is not fully understood [2]. The reason why CLL predominantly develops at an advanced age also is not clarified. Long-lasting antigen stimulation, accumulation of genomic events, and age-related changes in immunosurveillance or microenvironment potentially play a role. In some but not in all older patients, monoclonal B cell lymphocytosis (MBL) precedes CLL for many years [3].

There is no sound evidence that the clinical behaviour of CLL is significantly different in younger and older patients. At any age, CLL could stay an indolent disease for decades. Conversely, aggressive disease courses with early need of therapy and refractoriness to conventional treatment are similarly observed in both younger and older CLL patients.

Patient Heterogeneity

While biology of the disease (e.g., deletion of the short arm of the chromosome 17 or loss of the tumor suppressor p53) determines the course of the disease, CLL-unrelated though age-related changes in the host could also influence the course of CLL. Such hallmarks of aging are physiological decline of organ function (e.g., decrease in glomerular filtration rate, decrease in regenerative capacity of tissues) and pathological occurrence of comorbidities (particularly cardiovascular, neurodegenerative, and musculoskeletal diseases) that ultimately could result in the inability to manage activities of daily living, and dependency. However, these age-related changes are highly variable among individuals. Therefore, great heterogeneity is observed among older CLL patients with regard to functional organ reserve, presence of comorbidity, geriatric syndromes, disability, and dependency. For instance, severe comorbidities (i.e., cardiopulmonary disease, diabetes mellitus, other malignancy) are found in 46 % of unselected patients with newly diagnosed CLL while the remaining 54 % are either free of comorbidity (11 %) or affected with milder comorbidities (43 %, e.g. hypertension, hyperlipemia, arthritis, peptic ulcer) [4]. In another observational study of 8,343 newly diagnosed CLL patients>65 years, comorbidity was found in 45 % of the untreated CLL patients and 38 % of the treated CLL patients [5]. To date, there are no descriptive data on frequencies of geriatric syndromes (e.g., polymedication, falls, sarcopenia, dementia, delirium, depression, incontinence), disability, or dependency in older CLL patients. So far, such numbers can only be roughly extrapolated from data obtained from studies in the community-dwelling population of elderly people.

Patient Vulnerability

There is growing evidence that in older CLL patients decline of organ function and increase of comorbidity have impact on treatment tolerability and efficacy. For instance, renal impairment (reflected by a reduction in creatinine clearance) but not age is associated with greater risk of hematological toxicity upon treatment with the purine analogue fludarabine [6]. Increased comorbidity measured by Cumulative Illness Rating Scale (CIRS) has been shown to predict toxicity of combined chemotherapy and chemoimmunotherapy administered to CLL patients [7]. Higher comorbidity burden prior to treatment has also been demonstrated to be an age-independent predictor of overall survival (OS) of CLL patients [7, 8]. Underlying mechanisms are probably complex since comorbidity could affect OS of older CLL patients in multiple ways: Firstly, diseases other than CLL may cause earlier death of comorbid CLL patients. Secondly, comorbidity may facilitate occurrence of fatal treatment toxicity or make it more difficult to control adverse treatment events, hence resulting in more treatment-related deaths. Thirdly, comorbidity might enforce treating physicians to reduce the treatment dose or to interrupt therapy due to intercurrent disease, thereby limiting the treatment's benefit and offsetting control of CLL which then could result in earlier death due to CLL. Indeed, CLL-unrelated deaths, toxicity-related deaths, and CLL-related deaths all are contributors of higher mortality in comorbid CLL patients compared to more healthy subjects with CLL [9]. Potentially, characteristics of aging other than comorbidity (i.e. geriatric syndromes, disability, dependency) also have impact on treatment tolerability and survival in older CLL patients, but CLL-specific data are still lacking.

Diagnostic Options and Outcomes

Blood count including differential, blood smear microscopy, immunophenotyping, and physical examination (palpation of lymph nodes, spleen and liver) are mandatory to establish the diagnosis and to stage CLL [10, 11]. Bone marrow aspiration or biopsy is not needed to diagnose CLL and therefore is optional. All of the following diagnostic criteria must be fulfilled for establishing the diagnosis: Lymphocytosis > 5 G/L, microscopic detection of small mature lymphocytes, and a typical CLL immunophenotype (CD19+, CD20+, CD5+, CD23+). The Binet and Rai classifications are used for disease staging. Imaging could help to further quantify the extend of lymphadenopathy and organomegaly, but is not mandatory in routine practice and may put older patients at increased risk to develop renal failure if kidney function is impaired. Molecular staging could include the assessment of prognostic factors like thymidine kinase, ß2 microglobulin, ZAP70, CD38, IGHV mutational status, or FISH cytogenetics to predict time to disease progression in early-stage CLL or responsiveness to treatment in advanced-stage CLL. However, the predictive impact of such factors could differ significantly in younger and older CLL patients. In a survey of 2,487 patients diagnosed with CLL, IGHV and FISH predicted survival in younger patients (55–74 years), but failed to be prognostic in patients who were 75 years old or older [12]. In another study, expression of the CLL-specific gene CLLU1 was prognostic in CLL patients younger than 70 years, but had no prognostic impact in patients aged 70 years or older [13]. Deletion of 17p or lack or p53 function remains a significant adverse factor across age groups.

Patients above the age of 75 years with early-stage CLL were found to live as long as the age-matched general population [12]. Therefore, older patients diagnosed with CLL at an early stage (i.e., asymptomatic Binet stage A or B) usually are not in need of treatment and many of them will have indolent CLL for years [14]. For both younger and older CLL patients, treatment of CLL is indicated if signs of bone marrow failure (i.e. Binet C), severe B-symptoms (i.e., weight loss, fever, night sweats), general fatigue, symptomatic lymphadenopathy, hepatomegaly or splenomegaly, short lymphocyte doubling time, or autoimmune disorders are present [10, 11].

Additional Assessments

Treatment decisions in older CLL patients are guided by disease characteristics (i.e. detection of deletion 17p) and patient fitness (i.e. vulnerability). In principle, there are several approaches to assess patient fitness and vulnerability:

Comprehensive geriatric assessment (CGA) or use of specific scoring systems that include elements of CGA has been shown to predict toxicity and survival in older tumor patients [15–17]. However, evidence from prospective studies demonstrating that performance of a CGA in tumor patients prior to treatment will improve outcome is still very sparse. Importantly, such approach has not yet been validated in CLL. Neither it is known whether the assessment of single geriatric syndromes (e.g., polymedication, falls, loss of cognition, depression, incontinence), disability, or dependency, or whether apparatus investigations (e.g., echocardiography, stress electrocardiography) improve outcome of older CLL patients.

In contrast, comorbidity is known to be associated with treatment toxicity and reduced overall survival in older CLL patients [4, 5, 7, 8]. In clinical trials, mainly CIRS has been used to select for comorbid CLL patients and to allocate those to specific treatments although validation of the cut-offs used (e.g., total CIRS score of 6) is still incomplete.

Therapeutic Options and Outcomes

The spectrum of therapeutic options for older CLL patients is broad and ranges from intense chemoimmunotherapy to best supportive care (reviewed in [18]). In selected older patients, even allogeneic hematopoietic stem cell transplantation (HSCT) could be a reasonable treatment approach. While many of the possible treatments are approved in Europe and North America, some are still experimental and currently explored in clinical trials only (Table 7.1).

Fludarabine-Based Therapy

Chemoimmunotherapy with fludarabine, cyclophosphamide and rituximab (FCR) is the standard of care in younger and physically fit CLL patients [19]. Complete remissions (CR) are achieved in 44 % of the patients and the median progression-free survival (PFS) is 52 months. Importantly, addition of the monoclonal CD20 antibody rituximab to fludarabine and cyclophosphamide improves overall survival (OS) in CLL patients. The potential benefits of FCR treatment are coupled with a substantial risk of toxicity, however. Grade 3 or 4 neutropenia occurs in every third patients (34 %) and grade 3 or 4 infections are observed in 25 % of patients treated with FCR. Those patients with high leukocyte counts or bulky lymphadenopathy at

Table 7.1 Therapeutic options in older patients with CLL

Regimen	Evidence	Characteristics
FCR	Phase 3 trial (subgroup analysis), phase 2 trials	Equally toxic than in younger patients if patients are carefully selected for low burden of comorbidity, significant toxicity in unselected older patients.
PCR	Phase 2 trial (subgroup analysis)	Equally toxic than in younger patients if patients are carefully selected.
FCR low-dose	Phase 2 trials	Feasible in older patients with low to moderate burden of comorbidity.
FC	Phase 3 trial (subgroup analysis), phase 2 trial	Superior to CLB and F, no data for comorbid older patients, significant toxicity.
FC low-dose	Phase 2 trial	Well tolerated, but little data in comorbid older patients.
F	Phase 3 trial, phase 3 trial (subgroup analysis), phase 2 trial	Not superior to CLB, more toxic than CLB.
F low-dose	Phase 2 trial	Well tolerated, but shortened PFS.
BR	Phase 3 trial (preliminary results)	Feasible in older patients, role in comorbid older patients still unclear.
B	Phase 3 trial (subgroup analysis)	Superior to CLB, but more toxic than CLB, no data for comorbid older patients.
CLB-R	Phase 2 trial	Well tolerated, more remissions than in historical controls treated with CLB alone.
CLB	Phase 3 trial	Not inferior to F, less toxic than F.
G	Phase 3 run-in trial	Feasible in older patients, not yet approved.
O	–	No data available, not yet approved.
CAM	–	Feasible in high-risk older patients, not approved.
LEN	Phase 2 trial	Feasible in older patients, not yet approved
Ibrutinib	Phase 1/2 trial	Feasible in older patients, promising efficacy, not yet approved.
Idelalisib	–	Role in older patients unclear, not yet approved.

Abbreviations: *FCR* fludarabine, cyclophosphamide, rituximab, *PCR* pentostatin, cyclophosphamide, rituximab, *FC* fludarabine, cyclophosphamide, *F* fludarabine, *BR* bendamustine, rituximab, *B* bendamustine, *CLB-R* chlorambucil, rituximab, *CLB* chlorambucil, *G* obinutuzumab (GA101), *O* ofatumumab, *CAM* alemtuzumab, *LEN* lenalidomide

baseline are at risk to experience infusion-related reactions (IRR) during or after infusion of rituximab.

In a cohort of previously untreated CLL patients aged 70 years or older, use of FCR was associated with significant toxicity, frequent withdrawal from treatment, and early death [20]. Moreover, FCR treatment in older CLL patients was less efficacious than in younger CLL patients [21]. In the CLL8 trial of the German CLL Study Group (GCLLSG), there was no significant difference between younger patients (30–69 years) and older patients (70–80 years) treated with FCR, however. A treatment benefit was demonstrated across all age groups. Likewise, no difference in toxicity or efficacy was observed between younger and older patients in a trial investigating chemoimmunotherapy with pentostatin, cyclophosphamide and rituximab (PCR), a regimen that compares well with FCR [22]. Of note, patients in both trials had none or only mild comorbidity. It therefore can be concluded from these findings that full-dose purine analogue-based chemoimmunotherapy is feasible and beneficial in the subset of older CLL patients who are physically fit and have no major concurrent diseases.

With the goal to reduce toxicity but to keep efficacy, low-dose schedules of FCR have been proposed for older patients. A first study investigating a 'FCR lite' regimen reported impressive response rates (77 % CR), but less convincing durations of remissions (22 months) [23]. Importantly, this study was conducted in younger and not in older CLL patients (median age: 58 years). Meanwhile, first results from studies of low-dose FCR in significantly older CLL patients have been made available. In one trial in 169 patients (median age: 69 years, median total CIRS score: 5), response to treatment, grade 3–4 neutropenia and infection were observed in 81, 53 and 10 %, respectively [24]. In an Australian trial (120 patients, median age: 72 years, total CIRS score 0–6), 92 % of the patients responded to treatment and 30 % had grade 3–4 neutropenia [25]. A French study (200 patients, median age: 71 years, total CIRS score 0–6) reported a response rate of 96 % with use of G-CSF in more than half of the patients due to neutropenia [26]. FCR schedules in the three trials varied. Taken together, low-dose FCR is a treatment option in older CLL patients. Since the comorbidity burden in these phase 2 trials were relatively low, however, it is difficult to judge whether the risk-benefit ratio of this regimen will still be favorable in older CLL patients with significantly increased comorbidity. Furthermore, one has to keep in mind that so far no phase 3 trial evidence for these regimens exists.

Prior to the era of rituximab, low-dose regimens with fludarabine alone or fludarabine in combination with cyclophosphamide were explored in older CLL patients (reviewed in [18]). One phase 3 trial compared standard-dosed fludarabine with chlorambucil in older CLL patients [27]. Surprisingly and in contrast to a trial conducted in younger CLL patients, this trial failed to demonstrate superiority of fludarabine over chlorambucil in this patient population. Lack of benefit from fludarabine compared to chlorambucil treatment in older CLL patients was also observed in another large phase 3 trial [28].

Bendamustine-Based Therapy

Bendamustine is a bifunctional agent that carries a nitrogen-mustard group with alkylating properties. In a trial of previously untreated CLL patients, bendamustine was shown to be more efficacious than chlorambucil. Younger patients (35–65 years) and older patients (66–78 years) benefitted equally from the treatment with bendamustine, but the total number of enrolled patients of significantly advanced age (70 years or older) was small and the comorbidity burden of the patients was not reported [29]. Although bendamustine is frequently and often successfully used in clinical practice to treat older CLL patients, robust evidence supporting single-agent use of bendamustine in this patient population is still lacking.

Chemoimmunotherapy with bendamustine and rituximab (BR) has been suggested as a treatment option for older CLL patients. In a cohort of relapsed CLL patients which included patients of advanced age, BR proved to be safe and efficacious [30]. In a preliminary report of a randomized trial comparing BR with chlorambucil plus rituximab (CLB-R) in previously untreated and older CLL patients (median age: 74 years; burden of comorbidity not reported), BR and CLB-R yielded responses in 88 and 81 % of the patients (more CR with BR) and suggested acceptable toxicity in both treatment arms (grade 3–4 neutropenia 32 and 34 %) [31]. It therefore appears reasonable, to further develop BR as a treatment for older CLL patients including those with increased comorbidity. As with low-dose FCR, however, it remains to be determined within future trials what level of fitness and comorbidity in older CLL patients will be acceptable to apply BR in a safe and non-harming way. Final results from the trial comparing BR with CLB-R (MaBLe trial) as well as from a trial evaluating bendamustine plus the CD20 antibody ofatumumab versus chlorambucil plus ofatumumab (RIAltO trial) hopefully will help to better answer this question.

Chlorambucil-Based Therapy

For many decades, monotherapy with chlorambucil (CLB) has been the standard of care in CLL. While FCR meanwhile has replaced CLB as a new standard treatment in younger and physically fit patients, the alkylator has kept its role of a standard therapy in older and less fit patients. Indeed, so far no phase 3 trial has generated convincing evidence that a newer treatment was significantly superior to CLB in CLL patients of more advanced age and with reduced fitness. In a recent meta-analysis, single-agent therapy with CLB was confirmed to be a valuable treatment option in older CLL patients [32].

There is growing evidence, however, that chemoimmunotherapy with CLB and rituximab (CLB-R) might be superior to CLB alone in older CLL patients. In one phase 2 trial exploring CLB-R in older CLL patients (median age: 70 years, no comorbidity data provided), CR were found in 9 % of the patients and PFS was 24 months. A retrospective matched-pair comparison with patients treated with CLB alone suggested that CLB-R is more efficacious in these patients [33]. Comparable efficacy results were observed in an Italian phase 2 trial [34]. Stimulated by these encouraging results, large randomized-controlled phase 3 trials are now under way to compare chemoimmunotherapy with CLB plus CD20 antibodies with CLB alone in older and less fit CLL patients. One of those trials evaluates CLB alone versus CLB plus ofatumumab (CLB-O). The GCLLSG CLL11 trial is a three-arm phase 3 trial comparing CLB alone with CLB-R and with CLB plus the type 2 CD20 antibody obinutuzumab (CLB-G). Results of these trials are awaited soon and may replace CLB by chlorambucil-based chemoimmunotherapy as the formal standard of care in older and physically unfit or comorbid CLL patients.

Targeted Therapy

During recent years, new drugs to treat CLL have emerged. Among those are new monoclonal CD20 antibodies (obinutuzumab, ofatumumab), tyrosine kinase inhibitors (ibrutinib, idelalisib), BCL-2 inhibitors, and immunomodulators (lenalidomide). Except for ofatumumab, none of these drugs is approved in Europe or North America to be already used outside of clinical trials in CLL patients. Nevertheless, these compounds are or have been explored in clinical studies including trials designed for older CLL patients, and promising results have been reported.

Ofatumumab is a new type 1 CD20 antibody which currently is approved for the treatment of relapsed CLL refractory to fludarabine and alemtuzumab. In older CLL patients, ofatumumab in combination with CLB could be a valuable therapeutic option, but results from a large phase 3 trial have not been published yet. Obinutuzumab (GA101) is a type 2, glycoengineered CD20 antibody. Its mechanism of action is different from rituximab and ofatumumab. In preclinical experiments, GA101 was demonstrated to be more efficacious than rituximab [35]. In relapsed or refractory CLL patients, single agent treatment with GA101 resulted in rapid lymphocyte clearing from the peripheral blood [36]. In the CLL11 trial's run-in phase, six older patients (median age: 76 years) with increased comorbidity (median total CIRS score: 8, mean number of comorbidities: 5, median creatinine clearance: 60 ml/min) were treated with GA101 in combination with chlorambucil (CLB-G) [37]. All patients responded to treatment (33 % MRD negative) and after a post-therapeutic median observation period of 15 months, none of the subjects had progressed with CLL. Infusion-related reactions and transient neutropenia were identified as potential risks of CLB-G treatment in older CLL patients with increased comorbidity.

Lenalidomide is an immunomodulator with significant activity in CLL. The drug has been investigated in older CLL patients (median age: 71 years, burden of comorbidity not reported) and showed promising efficacy (15 % CR) [38]. Frequent grade 3–4 neutropenia (83 %) is a potential risk of lenalidomide therapy in older CLL patients, however.

Idelalisib (GS-1101, formerly CAL101) is an inhibitor of the phosphoinositide-3 kinase (PI3K) which is crucial for CLL cell growth and survival. The drug has been explored in CLL as single agent treatment and in combination with chemotherapy or antibodies. Pilot trials included older CLL patients but results from trials with idelalisib specifically designed for elderly patients have not been published. The Bruton's tyrosine kinase (BTK) inhibitor ibrutinib (formerly PCI32765) has already been tested in a small cohort of treatment-naïve CLL patients of advanced age (≥65 years). The drug was well tolerated (with diarrhea being the most frequent side effect). After a transient increase of lymphocytosis, oral treatment with ibrutinib resulted in sustained normalization of blood leukocytes and nodal response. PFS at 22 months in this patient population was 96 % [39]. These promising results strongly encourage researchers to further study tyrosine kinase inhibitors as well as other 'small molecules' in older CLL patients with the aim to develop 'chemotherapy-free' regimens in this patient population.

Stem Cell Therapy

Autologous HSCT in CLL does not yield better results than chemoimmunotherapy and due to its toxicity is hardly feasible in older patients. Allogeneic HSCT proved capable of completely eradicating CLL followed by long-term survival [40] but severe graft-versus-host disease and infections resulting in a high transplant-related mortality (TRM) clearly limit this approach in the elderly. Lately, TRM could be improved by the introduction of reduced-intensity conditioning (RIC) and the age limit of allogeneic HSCT in CLL has increased during recent years. Patients of up to 70 years are now offered to undergo allogeneic HSCT if there are no other reasonable alternatives to control the disease. However, older patients with a significant burden of comorbidity are unlikely to benefit from the procedure.

Current Recommendations

Based on the above mentioned and currently available evidence the following recommendations can be made for the diagnostic and therapeutic management of older patients with CLL.

Diagnostic Management

Establishment of the diagnosis and staging of CLL should be performed according to published guidelines [10, 11] and irrespective of age. Therapy of CLL is indicated in any age group if treatment criteria defined by these guidelines are met. FISH cytogenetics for 17p deletion should be done prior treatment to identify patients with a high risk of refractory disease or early relapse. Assessment of other risk factors is not relevant for the choice of treatment and these can have a different impact in older patients than in younger patients [12].

Prior therapy, older CLL patients are to be stratified into those who are fit ("go go"), those who are less fit ("slow go"), and patients who are frail ("no go"). There is no standard manner to perform this stratification which therefore is currently based on the physician's individual experience. In routine practice, the following measures could serve as a source of information and appear reasonable to create a basis for the treatment decision: Because comorbidity is a determinant of fitness, history taking in older CLL patients should not remain solely disease-specific (i.e. focus on B-symptoms, fatigue, infections etc.) but include a complete assessment of concurrent diseases plus geriatric syndromes, age-related disabilities and dependency (although the precise impact of the latter three is less clear). Physical examination could further reveal pathologies that eventually will affect the choice of treatment (e.g., decubital ulcers, sarcopenia, reduced gait speed, risk of falls, low vision). Laboratory workup should include determination of the glomerular filtration rate / calculation of the creatinine clearance enabling the physician to detect significant renal impairment and to avoid treatments with increased risk of toxicity due to drug accumulation. Other laboratory assessments (e.g., NT-Pro-BNP, HbA1c), chest X-ray, echocardiography, stress electrocardiogram, or spirometry all could be informative, but no algorithms for older CLL patients exist to decide for specific treatment regimens based on findings of such investigations. Comprehensive geriatric assessment (CGA) is helpful to systematically assess all aspects of fitness that potentially have impact on the treatment course and outcome in older CLL patients. Yet, no stratifying cut-offs have been defined for CGA to categorize older CLL patients. At the time of this publication, performance of CGA in older CLL patients therefore cannot be recommended as mandatory. In several trials, the Cumulative Illness Rating Scale (CIRS) and calculated creatinine clearance (CrCl) has been used to stratify fit (total CIRS total score ≤ 6, CrCl ≥ 70 ml/min) and less fit (total CIRS score >6, CrCl <70 ml/min) CLL patients [19, 37]. This algorithm awaits further validation. For the practitioner, use of CIRS and CrCl in older CLL patients could be a valuable tool to anticipate the fitness of older CLL patients [7], but currently could not fully replace the physician's experience when deciding for a specific treatment.

Therapeutic Management

In older CLL patients with deletion of 17p it should be evaluated whether these are eligible for allogeneic HSCT. Of course, such therapeutic manoeuver will only be feasible in a minority of older CLL patients. Older high-risk patients ineligible for allogeneic HSCT eventually will benefit from alemtuzumab-based regimens, but there is no broadly accepted therapy and treatment of these patients remains a challenge. If possible these patients should be enrolled on clinical trials. Older patients without deletion of 17p receive fitness-adapted therapy (Table 7.2):

Fit Patients

Older CLL patients who are considered fit and eligible for standard therapy should be treated with FCR chemoimmunotherapy. In the absence of significant toxicity, early withdrawal from treatment (i.e. stop of treatment before all six courses of FCR

Table 7.2 Therapeutic management of older patients with CLL

Patients	Routine practice	Clinical trial
Fit patients ("go go")		
Primary CLL	FCR	BR
Primary CLL (with loss of p53)	CAM	Targeted therapy, HSCT
Relapsed CLL	FCR[a], BR	Targeted therapy
Unfit patients ("slow go")		
Primary CLL	CLB	Low-dose FCR, BR, CLB+R, CLB+G, CLB+O, targeted therapy
Primary CLL (with loss of p53)	CAM	Targeted therapy
Relapsed CLL	Low-dose F, low-dose FC(R), B	Low-dose FCR, BR, targeted therapy
Frail patients ("no go")		
Primary & relapsed CLL	BSC	–

Abbreviations: *FCR* fludarabine, cyclophosphamide, rituximab, *BR* bendamustine, rituximab, *CAM* alemtuzumab, *HSCT* hematopoietic stem cell transplantation, *F* fludarabine, *FC* fludarabine, cyclophosphamide, *B* bendamustine, *R* rituximab, *G* obinutuzumab (GA101), *O* Ofatumumab, *BSC* best supportive care

[a]Repeat if >24 months relapse-free

have been administered) must be avoided to ensure that the regimen's unfolds its maximum efficacy. Treatment guidance by repeated assessment of minimal residual disease (MRD) is still experimental and therefore not established in routine practice. Fludarabine can be replaced by pentostatin (PCR) but without significant advantages. BR should be used within trials since non-inferiority to FCR has not yet been shown.

Unfit Patients

There are a number of approved treatments for older CLL patients considered not fit enough for standard chemoimmunotherapy with FCR. These include low-dose FCR, BR, or CLB-R as well as chemotherapy with fludarabine plus cyclophosphamide (FC), fludarabine alone (F) or bendamustine (B) alone either with normal or reduced dose. Growth factors (G-CSF, EPO) may be used according to guidelines to avoid or reduce toxicity. Since none of these regimens so far has been demonstrated in randomized phase 3 trials conducted in older unfit patients to be superior to chlorambucil, however, there is still a good rationale to treat those patients solely with the alkylator and to formally consider CLB as the standard of care in this patient population [27, 28].

Enrollment of unfit older CLL patients to clinical trials is crucial to improve the treatment of these patients. Ongoing trials are exploring chemoimmunotherapy with CLB plus CD20 antibodies in comparison with CLB alone. An increasing number of trials attempt to compare alternative regimens to CLB alone or to chlorambucil-based chemoimmunotherapy (e.g. CLB-G, CLB-O, BR, lenalidomide, ibrutinib etc.). Optimal treatment of older CLL patients with reduced fitness therefore ideally takes place within clinical trials designed for this patient population.

Frail Patients

Frail CLL patients are those patients who likely will have no benefit from any anti-leukemic therapy. These subjects should be treated with best supportive care which may include hydration, oxygen supply, administration of pain killers or sedatives.

Future Perspective

It is possible that treatment of younger patients with CLL will become less toxic in the next future whilst efficacy will be kept (i.e. by incorporating new antibodies or small molecules into treatment regimens). From such developments, both fit and less fit older CLL patients will benefit. Emerging novel drugs and new combination regimens (including chemotherapy-free treatments) will have particular impact on the treatment of older CLL patients with reduced fitness, however. Ongoing research in oncology and gerontology hopefully will enable physicians to identify these patients in a standard manner and in a more objective way or will even allow to further subdividing this patient group into different fitness levels within the "Unfit" category. Undoubtfully, all of these advances will significantly improve the management and outcome of older CLL patients in need of therapy.

References

1. Howlader N, Noone AM, Krapcho M, Neyman N, Aminou R, Altekruse SF, Kosary CL, Ruhl J, Tatalovich Z, Cho H, Mariotto A, Eisner MP, Lewis DR, Chen HS, Feuer EJ, Cronin KA, editors. SEER Cancer Statistics Review, 1975–2009 (Vintage 2009 Populations), National Cancer Institute. Bethesda, http://seer.cancer.gov/csr/1975_2009_pops09/, based on November 2011 SEER data submission, posted to the SEER web site, 2012.
2. Chiorazzi N, Ferrarini M. Cellular origin(s) of chronic lymphocytic leukemia: cautionary notes and additional considerations and possibilities. Blood. 2011;117(6):1781–91.
3. Ghia P, Caligaris-Cappio F. Monoclonal B-cell lymphocytosis: right track or red herring? Blood. 2012;119(19):4358–62.
4. Thurmes P, Call T, Slager S, Zent C, Jenkins G, Schwager S, et al. Comorbid conditions and survival in unselected, newly diagnosed patients with chronic lymphocytic leukemia. Leuk Lymphoma. 2008;49(1):49–56.
5. Reyes C, Satram-Hoang S, Hoang K, Momin F, Guduru SR, Skettino S. What is the impact of comorbidity burden on treatment patterns and outcomes in elderly chronic lymphocytic leukemia patients? Blood. 2012;120(21):758.
6. Martell RE, Peterson BL, Cohen HJ, Petros WP, Rai KR, Morrison VA, et al. Analysis of age, estimated creatinine clearance and pretreatment hematologic parameters as predictors of fluda-

rabine toxicity in patients treated for chronic lymphocytic leukemia: a CALGB (9011) coordinated intergroup study. Cancer Chemother Pharmacol. 2002;50(1):37–45.

7. Goede V, Raymonde B, Stilgenbauer S, Winter E, Fink A-M, Fischer K, et al. Cumulative Illness Rating Scale (CIRS) is a valuable tool to assess and weigh comorbidity in patients with chronic lymphocytic leukemia: results from the CLL8 trial of the German CLL Study Group. Haematologica. 2012;97(S1):0154.
8. Goede V, Cramer P, Busch R, Eichhorst B, Hallek M. Distribution and impact of comorbidity in chronic lymphocytic leukemia: meta-analysis of two phase III trials of the German CLL Study Group (GCLLSG). Leuk Lymph. 2005;46(S1):105.
9. Cramer P, Goede V, Jenke P, Busch R, Hallek M, Eichhorst B. Impact of different chemotherapy regimen in comorbid patients with advanced chronic lymphocytic leukemia: metaanalysis of two phase-III-trials of the German CLL Study Group. Blood. 2006;108(11):2840.
10. Eichhorst B, Dreyling M, Robak T, Montserrat E, Hallek M. Chronic lymphocytic leukemia: ESMO Clinical Practice Guidelines for diagnosis, treatment and follow-up. Ann Oncol. 2011;22 Suppl 6:vi50–4.
11. Hallek M, Cheson BD, Catovsky D, Caligaris-Cappio F, Dighiero G, Dohner H, et al. Guidelines for the diagnosis and treatment of chronic lymphocytic leukemia: a report from the International Workshop on Chronic Lymphocytic Leukemia updating the National Cancer Institute-Working Group 1996 guidelines. Blood. 2008;111(12):5446–56.
12. Shanafelt TD, Rabe KG, Kay NE, Zent CS, Jelinek DF, Reinalda MS, et al. Age at diagnosis and the utility of prognostic testing in patients with chronic lymphocytic leukemia. Cancer. 2010;116:4777–87.
13. Josefsson P, Geisler CH, Leffers H, Petersen JH, Andersen MK, Jurlander J, et al. CLLU1 expression analysis adds prognostic information to risk prediction in chronic lymphocytic leukemia. Blood. 2007;109(11):4973–9.
14. Bairey O, Ruchlemer R, Rahimi-Levene N, Herishanu Y, Braester A, Berrebi A, et al. Presenting features and outcome of chronic lymphocytic leukemia patients diagnosed at age 80 years or more. An ICLLSG study. Ann Hematol. 2011;90(10):1123–9.
15. Hamaker ME, Buurman BM, van Munster BC, Kuper IM, Smorenburg CH, de Rooij SE. The value of a comprehensive geriatric assessment for patient care in acutely hospitalized older patients with cancer. Oncologist. 2011;16(10):1403–12.
16. Hurria A, Togawa K, Mohile SG, Owusu C, Klepin HD, Gross CP, et al. Predicting chemotherapy toxicity in older adults with cancer: a prospective multicenter study. J Clin Oncol. 2011;29(25):3457–65.
17. Extermann M, Boler I, Reich RR, Lyman GH, Brown RH, DeFelice J, et al. Predicting the risk of chemotherapy toxicity in older patients: the Chemotherapy Risk Assessment Scale for High-Age Patients (CRASH) score. Cancer. 2012;118(13):3377–86.
18. Goede V, Hallek M. Optimal pharmacotherapeutic management of chronic lymphocytic leukaemia: considerations in the elderly. Drugs Aging. 2011;28(3):163–76.
19. Hallek M, Fischer K, Fingerle-Rowson G, Fink AM, Busch R, Mayer J, et al. Addition of rituximab to fludarabine and cyclophosphamide in patients with chronic lymphocytic leukaemia: a randomised, open-label, phase 3 trial. Lancet. 2010;376(9747):1164–74.
20. Ferrajoli A, O'Brien S, Wierda W, Lerner S, Faderl S, Kantarjian H, et al. Treatment of patients with CLL 70 years old and older: a single center experience of 142 patients. Leuk Lymph. 2005;46 Suppl 1:S87.
21. Tam CS, O'Brien S, Wierda W, Kantarjian H, Wen S, Do KA, et al. Long term results of the fludarabine, cyclophosphamide & rituximab regimen as initial therapy of chronic lymphocytic leukemia. Blood. 2008;112:975–80.
22. Shanafelt TD, Lin T, Geyer SM, Zent CS, Leung N, Kabat B, et al. Pentostatin, cyclophosphamide, and rituximab regimen in older patients with chronic lymphocytic leukemia. Cancer. 2007;109(11):2291–8.
23. Foon KA, Boyiadzis M, Land SR, Marks S, Raptis A, Pietragallo L, et al. Chemoimmunotherapy with low-dose fludarabine and cyclophosphamide and high dose rituximab in previously untreated patients with chronic lymphocytic leukemia. J Clin Oncol. 2009;27(4):498–503.

24. Smolej L, Brychtova Y, Spacek M, Doubek M, Motyckova M, Belada D, et al. Low-Dose FCR in the treatment of elderly/comorbid patients with chronic lymphocytic leukemia/small lymphocytic lymphoma (CLL/SLL): updated results of project Q-LITE by Czech CLL Study Group. Haematologica. 2012;97(S1):0151.
25. Mulligan SP, Gill DS, Turner P, Renwick WEP, Harrup R, Latimer M, et al. A Randomised Dose De-Escalation Safety Study of Oral Fludarabine, {+/-}Oral Cyclophosphamide and Intravenous Rituximab (OFOCIR) as first-line therapy of fit patients with Chronic Lymphocytic Leukaemia (CLL) aged > =65 years – end of recruitment analysis of response and toxicity of the Australasian Leukaemia and Lymphoma Group (ALLG) and CLL Australian Research Consortium (CLLARC) CLL5 Study. Blood. 2012;120(21):436.
26. Dartigeas C, Van Den Neste E, Berthou C, Maisonneuve H, Lepretre S, Dilhuydy M-S, et al. Safety and efficacy of abbreviated induction with oral Fludarabine (F) and Cyclophosphamide (C) combined with dose-dense IV Rituximab (R) in previously untreated patients with Chronic Lymphocytic Leukemia (CLL) aged > 65 years: results of a multicenter trial (LLC 2007 SA) on behalf of the French Goelams/Fcgcll-WM Intergroup. Blood. 2012;120(21):434.
27. Eichhorst BF, Busch R, Stilgenbauer S, Stauch M, Bergmann MA, Ritgen M, et al. First-line therapy with fludarabine compared with chlorambucil does not result in a major benefit for elderly patients with advanced chronic lymphocytic leukemia. Blood. 2009;114(16):3382–91.
28. Catovsky D, Richards S, Matutes E, Oscier D, Dyer MJ, Bezares RF, et al. Assessment of fludarabine plus cyclophosphamide for patients with chronic lymphocytic leukaemia (the LRF CLL4 Trial): a randomised controlled trial. Lancet. 2007;370(9583):230–9.
29. Knauf WU, Lissichkov T, Aldaoud A, Liberati A, Loscertales J, Herbrecht R, et al. Phase III randomized study of bendamustine compared with chlorambucil in previously untreated patients with chronic lymphocytic leukemia. J Clin Oncol. 2009;27(26):4378–84.
30. Fischer K, Cramer P, Busch R, Stilgenbauer S, Bahlo J, Schweighofer CD, et al. Bendamustine combined with rituximab in patients with relapsed and/or refractory chronic lymphocytic leukemia: a multicenter phase II trial of the German Chronic Lymphocytic Leukemia Study Group. J Clin Oncol. 2011;29(26):3559–66.
31. Leblond V, Laribi K, Ilhan O, Aktan M, Unal A, Rassam SMB, et al. Rituximab in combination with bendamustine or chlorambucil for treating patients with chronic lymphocytic leukemia: interim results of a Phase IIIb Study (MaBLe). Blood. 2012;120(21):2744.
32. Woyach JA, Ruppert AS, Rai K, Lin TS, Geyer S, Kolitz J, et al. Impact of age on outcomes after initial therapy with chemotherapy and different chemoimmunotherapy regimens in patients with chronic lymphocytic leukemia: results of sequential cancer and leukemia group B studies. J Clin Oncol. 2013;31(4):440–7.
33. Hillmen P, Gribben JG, Follows GA, Milligan D, Sayala HA, Moreton P, et al. Rituximab plus chlorambucil in patients with CD20-positive B-cell Chronic Lymphocytic Leukemia (CLL): final response analysis of an Open-Label Phase II Study. Blood. 2010;116(21):697.
34. Foa R, Ciolli S, Di Raimondo F, Del Poeta G, Lauria F, Forconi F, et al. Rituximab plus chlorambucil as initial treatment for elderly patients with Chronic Lymphocytic Leukemia (CLL): effect of pre-treatment biological characteristics and gene expression patterns on response to treatment. Blood. 2011;118(21):294.
35. Patz M, Isaeva P, Forcob N, Muller B, Frenzel LP, Wendtner CM, et al. Comparison of the in vitro effects of the anti-CD20 antibodies rituximab and GA101 on chronic lymphocytic leukaemia cells. Br J Haematol. 2011;152(3):295–306.
36. Morschhauser F, Cartron G, Lamy T, Milpied N-J, Thieblemont C, Tilly H, et al. Phase I Study of RO5072759 (GA101) in relapsed/refractory chronic lymphocytic leukemia. Blood. 2009;114(22):884.
37. Goede V, Fischer K, Busch R, Jaeger U, Dilhuydy MS, Wickham N, et al. Chemoimmunotherapy with GA101 plus chlorambucil in patients with chronic lymphocytic leukemia and comorbidity: results of the CLL11 (BO21004) safety run-in. Leukemia. 2013;27:1172–4.
38. Badoux XC, Keating MJ, Wen S, Lee BN, Sivina M, Reuben J, et al. Lenalidomide as initial therapy of elderly patients with chronic lymphocytic leukemia. Blood. 2011;118(13): 3489–98.

39. Byrd JC, Furman RR, Coutre S, Flinn IW, Burger JA, Blum KA, et al. The Bruton's Tyrosine Kinase (BTK) inhibitor ibrutinib (PCI-32765) promotes high response rate, durable remissions, and is tolerable in Treatment Naive (TN) and Relapsed or Refractory (RR) Chronic Lymphocytic Leukemia (CLL) or Small Lymphocytic Lymphoma (SLL) patients including patients with High-Risk (HR) disease: new and updated results of 116 patients in a Phase Ib/II Study. Blood. 2012;120(21):189.
40. Dreger P, Corradini P, Kimby E, Michallet M, Milligan D, Schetelig J, et al. Indications for allogeneic stem cell transplantation in chronic lymphocytic leukemia: the EBMT transplant consensus. Leukemia. 2007;21(1):12–7.

Chapter 8
Indolent Lymphomas in Older Patients

Andreas Viardot and Christian Buske

Abstract Indolent lymphoma is a typical cancer of older patients. The "historical" treatment approach – including a "watch and wait" period until to the appearance of lymphoma related symptoms, mild treatments in order to control disease activity or long-term maintenance therapy instead of an intensive consolidation – fits well to the requirements of the older patients and often comorbid patients. In a significant proportion of patients over 70 years, there is no need of treatment during lifetime. The development of novel therapeutic concepts such as the combination of chemotherapy with the monoclonal antibody rituximab or radioimmunotherapy are well tolerated and highly efficient, and therefore also applicable for elderly patients. The combination of rituximab and bendamustine, followed by rituximab maintenance therapy, may be one of the most attractive options in symptomatic older patients ("go-go" and partially "slow-go" patients). In patients with relapse, but also in frail patients, there are many options available ranging from different rituximab-containing chemotherapy regimens, rituximab monotherapy, radioimmunotherapy, local radiotherapy or oral drugs like chlorambucil, cyclophosphamide or prednisolone. Prognosis of indolent lymphoma is often better compared to other hematologic cancers, even in frail patients. The development of novel drugs promises new options for older patients due to their high anti-lymphoma activity accompanied by a favourable side-effect profile.

Keywords Indolent lymphoma • Follicular lymphoma • Waldenström's disease • Marginal zone lymphoma • Watch and wait • Rituximab • Radioimmunotherapy

A. Viardot, MD
Department of Internal Medicine III, Universitätsklinikum Ulm, Ulm, Germany

C. Buske, MD (✉)
Department of Internal Medicine III, Universitätsklinikum Ulm, Ulm, Germany

Comprehensive Cancer Center Ulm, Institute of Experimental Cancer Research, University Hospital Ulm, Albert-Einstein-Allee 11, Ulm 89081, Germany
e-mail: christian.buske@uni-ulm.de

U. Wedding, R.A. Audisio (eds.), *Management of Hematological Cancer in Older People*, DOI 10.1007/978-1-4471-2837-3_8

Introduction

Indolent lymphomas are typically diagnosed in older patients. The incidence is increasing due to demographic changes [1]. Therefore, physicians will face a rapidly growing number of elderly lymphoma patients in the near future. These patients often suffer from co-morbidities like renal dysfunction, cardiac diseases and physical impairment. For example 81 % of women aged 65 and above, screened for participation in the Women's Health and Aging Study, present with two or more chronic conditions [2]. Importantly, our therapeutic approaches in indolent lymphomas are based on clinical trial results, in which highly aged or frail patients are clearly underrepresented.

In contrast to other aggressive hematologic neoplasias, indolent lymphomas with their slow clinical course often do not require aggressive treatment approaches to control disease, in particular in the advanced stages, in which no curative therapy at least with conventional approaches exist. In many cases even a "watch and wait" strategy or mild single agent therapies are used in order to control symptoms. Thus, many treatment strategies are compatible to the requirements of senior patients. However, clinical trials have clearly shown that achieving a complete or even molecular remission is associated with improved disease free survival in indolent lymphoma. The emergence of novel treatment strategies, combining high anti-lymphoma activity with a favourable toxicity profile might open the door to aim at this therapeutic goal also in elderly patients. Chemotherapy-free treatment options are approved (like radioimmunotherapy) or under investigation (e.g. lenalidomide and rituximab as induction; orally available inhibitors of B-cell signalling).

Despite these promising developments and a plethora of therapeutic options for most of the patients, data from controlled clinical trials in elderly patients with co-morbidities are still rare, in particular because the vast majority of clinical trials excludes this important patient group.

Epidemiology of Lymphomas in Older Patients

Approximately 80 % of all lymphoid neoplasms are occurring in patients over 50 years [3] and the majority of lymphomas in elderly patients belong to the group of indolent lymphoma. Indolent lymphoma summarizes a heterogenous group of lymphoproliferative diseases, which share morphologic similarities including mature appearance and low proliferation of neoplastic lymphocytes as well as clinical characteristics like slow growth and long asymptomatic periods in the course of disease.

According to the WHO classification of lymphoid neoplasms [4], several entities are categorized as indolent (Table 8.1). Among them follicular lymphoma (FL) is the most frequent subentity. Other important entities, which are regarded as indolent, are the marginal zone lymphoma (extranodal and nodal), the lymphoplasmocytic lymphoma (and Waldenström's disease), the hairy cell leukemia and the small lymphocytic lymphoma.

Table 8.1 Clinically indolent lymphomas according to the WHO classification [4]

Small lymphocytic lymphoma/ chronic lymphocytic leukemia
B-cell prolymphocytic leukemia
Splenic marginal zone lymphoma
Hairy cell leukemia
Splenic B-cell lymphoma/leukemia unclassifiable[a]
Splenic red pulp small B-cell lymphoma[a]
Hairy cell leukemia-variant[a]
Lymphoplasmocytic lymphoma
Waldenström macroglobulinemia
Heavy chain diseases
Extranodal marginal zone lymphoma of the mucosa associated lymphoid tissue (MALT)
Nodal marginal zone lymphoma
Pediatric nodal marginal zone lymphoma[a]
Follicular lymphoma
Pediatric follicular lymphoma[a]
Primary cutaneous follicle center lymphoma

[a]Provisory entity

Follicular lymphoma, hairy cell leukaemia and mantle cell lymphoma are mainly diagnosed in the age between 50 and 69 years. Over half of the patients with chronic lymphocytic leukemia, immunoproliferative diseases, plasma cell neoplasms, and B-cell prolymphocytic leukemia are 70 years or older [5].

Although the incidence of lymphoid neoplasms decreased at the rate of 1 % per year among males during 1992–2001, there was an increase of follicular lymphoma at 1.8 % per year in senior people at the same time [6]. Marginal zone lymphoma and mantle cell lymphoma also increased in number in this time period, but to a lesser extent, being most likely due to improved diagnostic tools in these entities [6].

In general, advanced age is associated with an inferior prognosis and shorter survival in lymphoma, particularly beyond the age of 50 [3]. This also holds true for indolent lymphoma, but not to that extent observed in patients with precursor cell neoplasms, classical Hodgkin's lymphoma or Burkitt lymphoma [3].

The precise mechanisms, underlying the high incidence of indolent lymphomas in elderly patients, are not known. Of note, e.g. monoclonal gammopathy of unknown origin, which may precede to multiple myeloma, is rare in younger people, but occurs in 5.3 % of the population at ≥70 years old and in 7.5 % among those 85 years of age or older [7]. In a similar way, monoclonal B-lymphocytosis, which may precede to chronic lymphocytic leukemia is also associated with advanced age [8].

Age Associated Variants of Indolent Lymphomas

Usually, most indolent lymphomas are diagnosed beyond 50 years of age. However, in follicular lymphoma, a "pediatric" variant is described which occurs in patients under 40 years [9]. This variant is often localized (stage I), has a high proliferation rate (Ki-67 >30 %) and lacks a BCL2 rearrangement. This particular subset, which is otherwise morphologically not different form the "adult form", is highly indolent and does not progress or relapse. On the other hand, younger patient with typical BCL2 rearranged and advanced follicular lymphoma have an outcome comparable to elderly patients. In a similar way, the pediatric nodal marginal zone lymphoma (nMZL) was included as a provisory entity into the WHO classification. There is a male predominance (rate 20: 1) and as in pediatric FL, the disease is localized (usually head and neck lymph nodes), asymptomatic and extremely indolent [10].

Whereas pediatric FL and nMZL seem to be distinct entities with biological and clinical characteristics setting them apart from the variants at the advanced age, there are not much data about biologic differences within the age groups from 60 to 79 years versus ≥80 years of age. In general, patients ≥80 years old have a poorer performance status (PS 2–4 in 37 % in contrast to 20 % in patients between 60 and 79 years), more often B symptoms and renal failure, resulting in a slightly poorer age-adjusted International Prognostic Index (IPI) [11]. Most other risk factors are distributed equally.

The Best Starting Point for Treatment

It is generally accepted, that a careful "watch and wait" strategy is standard of care – even in younger patients – until clinical symptoms (e.g. fever, night sweat, loss in weight, local compression or hematopoietic failure) occur (Table 8.2). This approach is supported by a randomized study of the "British National Lymphoma Investigation"(BNLI) [12], providing data with a median observation time of 16 years: 309 patients were randomized either to chlorambucil or a watch and wait strategy. There was no survival benefit for one of the patient groups. Moreover, 20 % of patients did not receive any chemotherapy during the observation time. Particularly in elderly patients, this approach is appropriate since only 40 % of the patients older than 70 years required systemic treatment. A second randomized study, comparing prednimustine, interferon-γ and "watch and wait", also did not show any survival benefit for immediate treatment [13].

Table 8.2 International criteria for treatment start in follicular lymphoma

GELF criteria [13]
<u>**One or more of the following criteria:**</u>
Tumor > 7 cm in diameter
3 nodes in 3 distinct areas each > 3 cm in diameter
Symptomatic spleen enlargement
Organ compression
Ascites or pleura effusion
Presence of systemic symptoms
No leukemia
No peripheral blood cytopenia

Since more effective and importantly less toxic treatments than chlorambucil were established in the last two decades, the value of "watch and wait" is still under discussion. Particularly the monoclonal antibody rituximab, which targets CD20 – positive B – cell lymphoma cells, provides a non – toxic treatment option which is effective as monotherapy in indolent lymphomas [14]. The combination of anti-lymphoma activity with a favourable toxicity profile makes this compound highly attractive for the group of elderly patients. In a recent clinical trial of the BNLI, "watch and wait" was randomized against a monotherapy with rituximab (4 weeks induction, or 4 weeks followed by a maintenance therapy every 2 months over 2 years). The time to initiation of a new chemotherapy was much longer in the rituximab arm compared to "watch and wait". As expected, there was no significant survival benefit in all three arms after a median observation time of 3 years. In a recent non – randomized study, there was no significant difference in the freedom from treatment failure (FFTF) between patients with low tumor burden treated either with watch and wait or rituximab monotherapy [15]. Thus, although rituximab single agent therapy is effective and well tolerated first line, there are no data showing that immediate treatment with rituximab is superior to the traditional watch & wait approach. In conclusion "watch and wait" remains the most useful and cost-effective strategy, particularly in elderly patients.

Diagnostic Standards

Since therapy is guided by clinical symptoms particularly in elderly patients, medical history and physical examination is very important to guide the management of patients with indolent lymphoma. Standard laboratory analysis should contain blood count and hemogram, as well as lactate dehydrogenase. At initial diagnosis, serum immunoglobulins, immunofixation, β_2-microglobulin and serologic evaluation of HIV-, HBV- and HCV- status are recommended. Imaging studies can be used conservatively, in many cases ultrasound and conventional chest X-ray is adequate, particularly in asymptomatic patients. The intervals of examinations widely vary depending on the clinical course of the disease (every 3 months after diagnosis up to 6 months in stable patients).

Radiotherapy in Elderly Patients

Since indolent lymphomas are usually generalized at diagnosis, systemic treatment is generally preferred over local radiotherapy. However, in rare cases of localized involvement, involved-field radiotherapy is considered as standard of care according to international guidelines [16] offering the chance for a cure from lymphoma. Due to the long-term side effects of radiotherapy and the improved outcome in indolent lymphoma with systemic treatment, there may be a paradigm change in the next years, favouring mild non-toxic treatment such as rituximab single agent therapy over radiotherapy. In the prospective LYMPHOCARE registry, patients treated with systemic treatment had a significant longer progression free survival than patients with radiotherapy; there was no significant difference between patients with involved field irradiation and "watch and wait" [17]. Patients which refused radiotherapy had also an excellent long term outcome [18].

In contrast to other indolent lymphomas, extranodal marginal zone lymphoma is often localized, therefore radiotherapy is considered as standard in many cases. However, since these lymphomas have an excellent prognosis in most cases, e.g. can be successfully treated by eradication of a bacterial trigger or by treatment of an autoimmune condition, it is reasonable to abstain from radiotherapy in many elderly patients: an example for this is the localized extranodal marginal zone lymphoma of the stomach, which persists 12 months after antibacterial eradication therapy and has an excellent long – term outcome even without radiotherapy [19]. Finally, rituximab monotherapy can replace local radiotherapy in patients with need of treatment at least in several subsets of extranodal marginal zone lymphoma [20, 21]. Thus, in particular in elderly patients a watch & wait strategy or rituximab single agent might be considered as an alternative to radiotherapy. On the other hand, radiotherapy may be a useful treatment option in elderly patients with advanced and relapsed indolent lymphoma. A low-dose involved field irradiation (2×2 Gy in 4 doses, in 2 days) often provides an excellent long – term control of tumor bulk, otherwise causing local complications, and may be an ideal option for elderly patients [22].

Systemic Treatment in Elderly Patients

In the last decades, the treatment goals in younger patients with indolent lymphoma changed from supportive treatment in order to control symptoms to induction of a complete (molecular) remission as a surrogate marker for the longest progression free survival possible. Although in elderly or frail patients, the control of symptoms is still the main objective of treatment, high response rates and long progression free survival can also be achieved in this often co-morbid patient population, using new targeted treatment strategies.

An example of a targeted treatment strategy, which has dramatically changed the perspective of many patients with different types of B-cell lymphomas is the anti-CD20 monoclonal antibody Rituximab: rituximab monotherapy induces high response rate in relapsed patients (46 %) and even higher in untreated patients (67 %), which are in need of treatment [23]. The event-free survival differs from 13 months in pretreated up to 33 months in treatment naïve patients [24]. Therefore, rituximab monotherapy is an attractive treatment option in elderly patients. However, it is not approved as monotherapy in first line treatment, and may be insufficient in patients with tumor bulk or need for rapid remission. Nevertheless, rituximab monotherapy is the preferred first-line treatment in elderly patients not qualifying for chemoimmunotherapy according to the NCCN guidelines in North America [25].

In medically fit patients the standard approach is to combine rituximab with conventional cytostatic drugs. The most frequently used regimen in North America is R-CVP (Rituximab, Cyclophosphamide, Vincristine and Prednisolone) and R-CHOP (additionally Doxorubicin), whereas in Europe R-CHOP but also increasingly R – Bendamustine belongs to the most popular regimens. In elderly patients, the use of R-CHOP is limited by the neurotoxicity of vincristine, the cardiotoxicity of doxorubicine and a higher rate of febrile neutropenias. In elderly patients, qualifying for immunochemotherapy alternative schedules are more appropriate such as R – Bendamustine, R-MCP (Rituximab Mitoxantrone, Chlorambucil, Prednisolone) or R-Chlorambucil. R-MCP has shown an excellent progression free survival in patients with indolent lymphoma, but is stem cell toxic. Therefore, it is particularly appropriate for elderly patients, which are not eligible for autologous stem cell transplantation [26]. In two recent randomized clinical trials R-CVP was inferior to R-CHOP, so that R-CHOP is a valid treatment option in elderly fit patients. In the same trials fludarabine containing regimens showed a higher toxicity compared to the other arms [27, 28]. This is in line with the results of randomized clinical trials reporting a higher toxicity and survival disadvantage in elderly patients with mantle cell lymphoma [29] or chronic lymphocytic leukemia [30]. Therefore, fludarabine containing combinations (e.g. R-FC rituximab-fludarabine- cyclophosphamide or R-FM rituximab-fludarabine-mitoxantrone) should be applied with caution in elderly patients, particularly in patients with a compromised renal function.

Bendamustin was first synthesized in 1963 in East Germany and available not before 1990 in Western countries. In a randomized clinical trial, R-Bendamustin was compared with standard R-CHOP. Although initially designed to shown non-inferiority of R – Bendamustine compared to R-CHOP, this study surprisingly demonstrated a higher response rate and a impressive longer progression free survival (69.5 versus 31.2 months, hazard ratio 0.58, 95 % CI 0.44–0.74; $p<0.001$) for R – Bendamustine [31, 32]. Since Bendamustin has less toxic side-effects (e.g. no alopecia, less neutropenia and febrile neutropenia), it can probably be considered as one of the most acceptable chemoimmunotherapies in elderly patients, at least in the "go-go" and parts of the "slow-go" subgroup.

Another appealing concept in the treatment of B – cell lymphomas is radioimmunotherapy, exploiting the high radiosensitivity of lymphomas and minimizing non – targeted irradiation. In this line the conjugation of a ß-emitting radioactive particle to a monoclonal antibody against B-cell antigens provides an elegant way to deliver radiation to B – cell lymphoma cells. ^{90}Yttrium-ibritumomab (Zevalin®) and ^{131}I-Tositumomab (Bexxar®), which link ^{90}yttrium or ^{131}iodine to an anti-CD20 monoclonal antibody, are approved in Europe and U.S., respectively. Both drugs are applied as a single infusion treatment and have few non-hematologic side effects. Due to the prolonged myelosuppression which occurs between 4 and 8 weeks after treatment, a close surveillance of the patients is necessary during this period. Despite single application, the remission rates are high – between 74 % in relapsed patients [33] and 95 % in first line patients [34]. Therefore radioimmunotherapy can be considered as an alternative to multiple cycles of chemoimmunotherapy in elderly patients. In the FIT trial consolidation with Zevalin® after a chemotherapy induction provided very high remission rates, even in patients who were treated before with well – tolerable treatments like oral chlorambucil [35]. Another option to improve or at least stabilize treatment outcome of initial induction treatment is a maintenance therapy with Rituximab, which was shown to improve duration of

Table 8.3 Current recommendations for patients falling into different 'fitness categories'

Fitness	Aim of treatment	Recommended treatment
Fit – "go-go"	Complete response	Rituximab Bendamustin, rituximab CHOP
Compromised – "slow-go"	Control of symptoms	Rituximab Bendamustin, rituximab MCP, rituximab CVP, rituximab chlorambucil, rituximab monotherapy, radioimmunotherapy
Frail – "no-go"	Control of symptoms	Rituximab monotherapy Glucocorticosteroids (different schedules), vincaalcaloids, chlorambucil, bendamustin (low dose), purinethol (orally), cyclophosphamide (orally), trofosfamide (orally), low-dose radiotherapy
Patients with cardiac comorbidity	Control of symptoms	Avoid anthracyclines, avoid large fluid intake (e.g. oral therapy)
Patients with pulmonary comorbidity	Control of symptoms	Avoid bleomycin, busulfan: avoid pronounced neutropenia
Patients with renal impairment	Control of symptoms	Avoid fludarabine, dose reduction recommended for several drugs
Patients with diabetes and end-organ failure	Control of symptoms	Avoid prednisolone

response after immunochemotherapy both in first line and in relapse without major toxicities in large randomized clinical trials. In the meanwhile Rituximab maintenance was approved for follicular lymphoma after chemotherapy induction, characterizing this approach as a highly attractive option to keep elderly patients with follicular lymphoma in remission [36].

In the group of frail patients ("no-go"), there are still few data available. If in the opinion of the threating physician a chemoimmunotherapy is not feasible, rituximab monotherapy or radioimmunotherapy is recommended at least according the NCCN guidelines [25]. Another option may be the oral alkylating drugs – like chlorambucil, cyclophosphamide or trofosfamide providing control of symptoms in many cases and an objective response rate between 36 % in chlorambucil [37] and 49 % in trofosfamide [38]. However, the combination of oral chlorambucil with rituximab, which may be tolerable in many frail patients, can improve the complete response rate up to 89 % including a 63 % complete response rate in previously untreated patients [39]. In order to control symptoms in very ill patients, low dose prednisolone or dexamethason, low dose irradiation and best supportive care may be appropriate. Table 8.3 summarizes the different treatment options according to the fitness of the patient (Table 8.3).

Waldenström's Macroglobinemia

Waldenström's macroglobinemia (WM) is special within the group of indolent lymphomas, because the elevation of paraprotein IgM leads to distinct clinical symptoms like hyperviscosity, polyneuropathy, amyloidosis, cryoglobinemia or cold hemagglutinins, often requiring immediate treatment, e.g. plasmapheresis and/or rituximab/chemotherapy.

Similar to follicular lymphoma, patients with WM should be only treated if they suffer from WM related symptoms or critical cytopenias. Otherwise a watch & wait strategy is recommended. If treatment is necessary, medically fit patients should be offered a rituximab/chemotherapy. R-CHOP was shown to be effective as well as R – Bendamustine [32, 40, 41]. In the largest randomized trial so far including 418 patients with Waldenström's macroglobinemia, fludarabine was superior to oral chlorambucil with regard to the progression free survival [42]. However, fludarabine has some toxic side effects in elderly patients, particularly with impaired renal function [43]. One approach is to scale down rituximab/chemotherapy as done in the so called DRC protocol: this regimen, consisting of dexamethasone, oral cyclophosphamide and Rituximab proved to be highly effective without any major toxicity in a phase II trial in treatment naive WM patients [44].

In patients, who are not eligible for chemotherapy, rituximab single agent is effective. However, time to response is slow and sometimes exceeds 6 months. Furthermore, rituximab single agent can cause a sudden and critical increase in the IgM serum levels, triggering severe hyperviscosity symptoms. Therefore in patients at risk for hyperviscosity (e.g. IgM levels >50 g/l) plasmapheresis should precede rituximab application to lower IgM levels before initiation of treatment [45].

Experimental Therapy in Older Patients

In the recent years many attractive compounds were tested in indolent lymphomas, which are potentially of particular interest for elderly patients. In part they can be given orally and importantly they exploit different modes of actions compared to conventional chemotherapy. This opens the possibility to combine these new drugs with chemotherapy, but also to develop concepts which are not depending anymore on chemotherapy. In an ongoing phase III trial conventional chemoimmunotherapy is randomized against the chemotherapy-free combination of lenalidomide and rituximab. The latter combination induced remarkable high CR/CRu rates in untreated patients with follicular lymphoma [46]. However, due to restrictions in patients with renal insufficiency and due to hematotoxicity of the combination, this treatment may not be appropriate for all elderly patients.

The next generation of fully humanized CD20 antibodies (e.g. ofatumumab, obinutuzumab) provides a higher efficacy in vitro compared to rituximab, and is actually tested in phase III randomized studies. The side effects of these new CD20 antibodies seem to be comparable to rituximab [47, 48] and therefore applicable in older patients.

Finally, there is a new generation of orally active inhibitors of the B-cell receptor signalling. The most important representative are the BTK (bruton tyrosine kinase) inhibitor Ibrutinib and the PI3K (Phosphotadyl-inositol 3 kinase) inhibitor

CAL101, which both show promising response rates in pretreated indolent lymphoma [49, 50]. Both drugs seem to be well tolerated and have a remarkable low number of relevant adverse events in these early studies. Phase III randomized trials will define their precise role in the treatment of indolent lymphoma, but data from the aforementioned trials are encouraging and are might open the perspective to control indolent lymphomas by oral non-chemotherapy based treatment in the near future.

Geriatric Assessment

Older patients are generally underrepresented in clinical trials. Therefore, data about efficacy and toxicity of established and upcoming treatments must be considered very carefully in this subgroup. Of note, there is – to our knowledge – no publication available about the prospective evaluation of geriatric assessments in clinical trials in patients with indolent lymphomas. This is in contrast to diffuse large B-cell lymphoma of the elderly, since several prospective studies were published in elderly and high-aged patients, using distinct geriatric assessment tools (see Chap. 13). One reason for this might be that in indolent lymphomas the general practise of "watch and wait" and less toxic treatments strategies allows the treatment of elderly patients with standard approaches already today, so that physicians often do not see the medical need for geriatric assessment and age-specific adjustments of treatment in this subgroup of lymphomas. However, in a recent retrospective analysis evaluating the overall survival in patients being 80 years and older, survival was low even in indolent lymphomas (66 %), although still being superior compared to aggressive lymphomas (32 %) [51]. Furthermore, in several retrospective series of aggressive and indolent lymphomas, the instrumental activities of daily living (IADL) and comorbidity [49] or performance status [50] were independent prognostic predictors of shorter survival time. Taken together, these data underline the need to perform geriatric assessments at least within clinical trials in order to define patients who will benefit most from less dose intense treatments.

Summary

In the last decade, the chances for long term survival in patients with indolent lymphoma have significantly improved [52]. At the same time, we were able to reduce the intensity and toxicity of induction treatment by introducing novel treatment concepts as e.g. the antibody – based maintenance treatment with rituximab. There are very encouraging novel drugs at the horizon which might allow developing chemotherapy – free oral treatment concepts, which promise long-term control of advanced follicular lymphoma without compromising the quality of life in older patients.

References

1. Lichtman SM, Balducci L, Aapro M. Geriatric oncology: a field coming of age. J Clin Oncol. 2007;25(14):1821–3.
2. Fried LP, Bandeen-Roche K, Kasper JD, Guralnik JM. Association of comorbidity with disability in older women: the Women's Health and Aging Study. J Clin Epidemiol. 1999;52(1):27–37.
3. Marcos-Gragera R, Allemani C, Tereanu C, et al. Survival of European patients diagnosed with lymphoid neoplasms in 2000–2002: results of the HAEMACARE project. Haematologica. 2011;96(5):720–8.
4. Swerdlow SH, Campo E, Harris AW, et al. WHO classification of tumours of haematopoietic and lymphoid tissues. 4th ed. Lyon: IARC; 2008.
5. Sant M, Allemani C, Tereanu C, et al. Incidence of hematologic malignancies in Europe by morphologic subtype: results of the HAEMACARE project. Blood. 2010;116(19):3724–34.
6. Morton LM, Wang SS, Devesa SS, Hartge P, Weisenburger DD, Linet MS. Lymphoma incidence patterns by WHO subtype in the United States, 1992–2001. Blood. 2006;107(1): 265–76.
7. Kyle RA, Therneau TM, Rajkumar SV, et al. Prevalence of monoclonal gammopathy of undetermined significance. N Engl J Med. 2006;354(13):1362–9.
8. Rawstron AC, Bennett FL, O'Connor SJ, et al. Monoclonal B-cell lymphocytosis and chronic lymphocytic leukemia. N Engl J Med. 2008;359(6):575–83.
9. Louissaint Jr A, Ackerman AM, Dias-Santagata D, et al. Pediatric-type nodal follicular lymphoma: an indolent clonal proliferation in children and adults with high proliferation index and no BCL2 rearrangement. Blood. 2012;120(12):2395–404.
10. Taddesse-Heath L, Pittaluga S, Sorbara L, Bussey M, Raffeld M, Jaffe ES. Marginal zone B-cell lymphoma in children and young adults. Am J Surg Pathol. 2003;27(4):522–31.
11. Thieblemont C, Coiffier B. Lymphoma in older patients. J Clin Oncol. 2007;25(14):1916–23.
12. Ardeshna KM, Smith P, Norton A, et al. Long-term effect of a watch and wait policy versus immediate systemic treatment for asymptomatic advanced-stage non-Hodgkin lymphoma: a randomised controlled trial. Lancet. 2003;362(9383):516–22.
13. Brice P, Bastion Y, Lepage E, et al. Comparison in low-tumor-burden follicular lymphomas between an initial no-treatment policy, prednimustine, or interferon alfa: a randomized study from the Groupe d'Etude des Lymphomes Folliculaires. Groupe d'Etude des Lymphomes de l'Adulte. J Clin Oncol. 1997;15(3):1110–7.
14. Ardeshna KM, Qian W, Smith P. An intergroup randomised trial of rituximab versus a watch and wait strategy in patients with stage II, III, IV, asymptomatic, non-bulky follicular lymphoma (grades 1, 2 and 3a). a preliminary analysis. Blood. 2010;116:6.
15. Solal-Celigny P, Bellei M, Marcheselli L, et al. Watchful waiting in low-tumor burden follicular lymphoma in the rituximab era: results of an f2-study database. J Clin Oncol. 2012;30(31): 3848–53.
16. Zelenetz AD, Abramson JS, Advani RH, et al. Non-Hodgkin's lymphomas. J Natl Compr Canc Netw. 2011;9(5):484–560.
17. Friedberg JW, Byrtek M, Link BK, et al. Effectiveness of first-line management strategies for stage I follicular lymphoma: analysis of the National LymphoCare Study. J Clin Oncol. 2012;30(27):3368–75.
18. Advani R, Rosenberg SA, Horning SJ. Stage I and II follicular non-Hodgkin's lymphoma: long-term follow-up of no initial therapy. J Clin Oncol. 2004;22(8):1454–9.
19. Fischbach W, Goebeler ME, Ruskone-Fourmestraux A, et al. Most patients with minimal histological residuals of gastric MALT lymphoma after successful eradication of Helicobacter pylori can be managed safely by a watch and wait strategy: experience from a large international series. Gut. 2007;56(12):1685–7.
20. Else M, Marin-Niebla A, de la Cruz F, et al. Rituximab, used alone or in combination, is superior to other treatment modalities in splenic marginal zone lymphoma. Br J Haematol. 2012;159(3):322–8.

21. Valencak J, Weihsengruber F, Rappersberger K, et al. Rituximab monotherapy for primary cutaneous B-cell lymphoma: response and follow-up in 16 patients. Ann Oncol. 2009;20(2): 326–30.
22. Haas RL, Poortmans P, de Jong D, et al. High response rates and lasting remissions after low-dose involved field radiotherapy in indolent lymphomas. J Clin Oncol. 2003;21(13):2474–80.
23. Ghielmini M, Schmitz SF, Cogliatti SB, et al. Prolonged treatment with rituximab in patients with follicular lymphoma significantly increases event-free survival and response duration compared with the standard weekly x 4 schedule. Blood. 2004;103(12):4416–23.
24. Martinelli G, Schmitz SF, Utiger U, et al. Long-term follow-up of patients with follicular lymphoma receiving single-agent rituximab at two different schedules in trial SAKK 35/98. J Clin Oncol. 2010;28(29):4480–4.
25. NCCN Guidelines. Version 32012. 2012; www.nccn.org.
26. Herold M, Haas A, Srock S, et al. Rituximab added to first-line mitoxantrone, chlorambucil, and prednisolone chemotherapy followed by interferon maintenance prolongs survival in patients with advanced follicular lymphoma: an East German Study Group Hematology and Oncology Study. J Clin Oncol. 2007;25(15):1986–92.
27. Morschhauser F, Seymour J, Feugier P. Impact of induction chemotherapy regimen on response, safety and outcome in the PRIMA study. Ann Oncol. 2011;22 Suppl 4:iv88–9.
28. Federico M, Lumnari S, Dondi A. R-CVP vs. R-CHOP vs. R-FM for the initial treatment of patients with advanced stage follicular lymphoma. Preliminary results of FOLL 05 IIL trial. Ann Oncol. 2011;22 Suppl 4:iv128–9.
29. Kluin-Nelemans HC, Hoster E, Hermine O, et al. Treatment of older patients with mantle-cell lymphoma. N Engl J Med. 2012;367(6):520–31.
30. Eichhorst BF, Busch R, Stilgenbauer S, et al. First-line therapy with fludarabine compared with chlorambucil does not result in a major benefit for elderly patients with advanced chronic lymphocytic leukemia. Blood. 2009;114(16):3382–91.
31. Rummel MJ. Bendamustine plus rituximab versus CHOP plus rituximab in the first-line-treatment of patients with Waldenström's disease – first interim results of a randomized phase III study of the Studygroup Indolent Lymphomas (StiL). Vth international Workshop on Waldenström Macroglobulinemia, Stockholm. 2008.
32. Rummel MJ, Niederle N, Maschmeyer G, et al. Bendamustine plus rituximab (B-R) versus CHOP plus rituximab (CHOP-R) as first-line treatment in patients with indolent and mantle cell lymphomas (MCL): updated results from the StiL NHL1 study. J Clin Oncol. 2012;(suppl; abstr 3).
33. Witzig TE, Flinn IW, Gordon LI, et al. Treatment with ibritumomab tiuxetan radioimmunotherapy in patients with rituximab-refractory follicular non-Hodgkin's lymphoma. J Clin Oncol. 2002;20(15):3262–9.
34. Kaminski MS, Tuck M, Estes J, et al. 131I-tositumomab therapy as initial treatment for follicular lymphoma. N Engl J Med. 2005;352(5):441–9.
35. Morschhauser F, Radford J, Van Hoof A, et al. Phase III trial of consolidation therapy with yttrium-90-ibritumomab tiuxetan compared with no additional therapy after first remission in advanced follicular lymphoma. J Clin Oncol. 2008;26(32):5156–64.
36. Salles G, Seymour JF, Offner F, et al. Rituximab maintenance for 2 years in patients with high tumour burden follicular lymphoma responding to rituximab plus chemotherapy (PRIMA): a phase 3, randomised controlled trial. Lancet. 2011;377(9759):42–51.
37. Kimby E, Bjorkholm M, Gahrton G, et al. Chlorambucil/prednisone vs. CHOP in symptomatic low-grade non-Hodgkin's lymphomas: a randomized trial from the Lymphoma Group of Central Sweden. Ann Oncol. 1994;5 Suppl 2:67–71.
38. Helsing MD. Trofosfamide as a salvage treatment with low toxicity in malignant lymphoma. A phase II study. Eur J Cancer. 1997;33(3):500–2.
39. Martinelli G, Laszlo D, Bertolini F, et al. Chlorambucil in combination with induction and maintenance rituximab is feasible and active in indolent non-Hodgkin's lymphoma. Br J Haematol. 2003;123(2):271–7.

40. Buske C, Hoster E, Dreyling M, et al. The addition of rituximab to front-line therapy with CHOP (R-CHOP) results in a higher response rate and longer time to treatment failure in patients with lymphoplasmacytic lymphoma: results of a randomized trial of the German Low-Grade Lymphoma Study Group (GLSG). Leukemia. 2009;23(1):153–61.
41. Rummel MJ, Al-Batran SE, Kim SZ, et al. Bendamustine plus rituximab is effective and has a favorable toxicity profile in the treatment of mantle cell and low-grade non-Hodgkin's lymphoma. J Clin Oncol. 2005;23(15):3383–9.
42. Leblond V, Johnson S, Chevret S, Copplestone A, Rule S, Tournilhac O. Results of a randomized trial of chlorambucil versus fludarabine for patients with untreated Waldenström macroglobulinemia, marginal zone lymphoma and lymphoplasmacytic lymphoma. J Clin Oncol. 2013;31:301–7.
43. Tedeschi A, Benevolo G, Varettoni M, et al. Fludarabine plus cyclophosphamide and rituximab in Waldenstrom macroglobulinemia: an effective but myelosuppressive regimen to be offered to patients with advanced disease. Cancer. 2012;118(2):434–43.
44. Dimopoulos MA, Anagnostopoulos A, Kyrtsonis MC, et al. Primary treatment of Waldenstrom macroglobulinemia with dexamethasone, rituximab, and cyclophosphamide. J Clin Oncol. 2007;25(22):3344–9.
45. Treon SP, Branagan AR, Hunter Z, Santos D, Tournhilac O, Anderson KC. Paradoxical increases in serum IgM and viscosity levels following rituximab in Waldenstrom's macroglobulinemia. Ann Oncol. 2004;15(10):1481–3.
46. Fowler NH, McLaughlin P, Hagemeister FB. Complete response rates with lenalidomide plus rituximab for untreated indolent B-cell non-Hodgkin's lymphoma. J Clin Oncol. 2010;28(15s):(Suppl; abstr 8036).
47. Salles G, Morschhauser F, Lamy T, et al. Phase 1 study results of the type II glycoengineered humanized anti-CD20 monoclonal antibody obinutuzumab (GA101) in B-cell lymphoma patients. Blood. 2012;119(22):5126–32.
48. Czuczman MS, Fayad L, Delwail V, et al. Ofatumumab monotherapy in rituximab-refractory follicular lymphoma: results from a multicenter study. Blood. 2012;119(16):3698–704.
49. Advani RH, Buggy JJ, Sharman JP, et al. Bruton tyrosine kinase inhibitor ibrutinib (PCI-32765) has significant activity in patients with relapsed/refractory B-cell malignancies. J Clin Oncol. 2013;31:88–94.
50. Castillo JJ, Furman M, Winer ES. CAL-101: a phosphatidylinositol-3-kinase p110-delta inhibitor for the treatment of lymphoid malignancies. Expert Opin Investig Drugs. 2012;21(1):15–22.
51. Nabhan C, Smith SM, Helenowski I, et al. Analysis of very elderly (>/=80 years) non-hodgkin lymphoma: impact of functional status and co-morbidities on outcome. Br J Haematol. 2012;156(2):196–204.
52. Liu Q, Fayad L, Cabanillas F, et al. Improvement of overall and failure-free survival in stage IV follicular lymphoma: 25 years of treatment experience at The University of Texas M.D. Anderson Cancer Center. J Clin Oncol. 2006;24(10):1582–9.

Chapter 9
The Challenge of Treating Elderly Patients with Mantle Cell Lymphoma

Simone Ferrero and Martin Dreyling

Abstract Treatment of elderly patients with mantle cell lymphoma is considered a major challenge, due to the peculiar chemorefractory features and continuous relapse pattern of this neoplasm. With a median age of 65 years at presentation, more than half of the patients with newly diagnosed mantle cell lymphoma fall into the category 'elderly'. The most effective treatment for this type of lymphoma consists of high dose cytarabine followed by upfront autologous stem cell transplantation, but such a therapeutic option is not feasible for the higher age category, due to limiting toxicity. Nevertheless, patients obtaining a complete molecular response, independent of age, can enjoy longstanding event-free survival and even improved overall survival. Thus, it is important to obtain a complete response also in the elderly patients: these considerations justify more intensive approaches.

However, it is fundamental to classify these patients in geriatric categories, objectively identifying those able to receive a chemotherapy aiming at long term control of the disease and patients appropriate only for a palliative therapy, primarily mitigating lymphoma symptoms. Therefore, treatment of elderly patient with mantle cell lymphoma should be individualized, and benefits and possible side effects should be carefully balanced.

Keywords Mantle cell lymphoma • Elderly • Tailored treatment • Therapeutic algorithm • New drugs • Clinical trials • Prognostic factors • Diagnostic procedures

---

S. Ferrero, MD (✉)
Division of Hematology, Department of Molecular Biotechnologies and Health Sciences, University of Torino, Torino, Italy
e-mail: simone.ferrero@unito.it

M. Dreyling, MD, PhD
Department of Medicine III, University Hospital Großhadern/LMU München, Munich, Germany

U. Wedding, R.A. Audisio (eds.), *Management of Hematological Cancer in Older People*, DOI 10.1007/978-1-4471-2837-3_9

Introduction and Epidemiology

With an incidence of about 2 per 100,000 per year, mantle cell lymphoma (MCL) is a relatively rare entity and accounts for 6–8 % of all malignant lymphoma subtypes in USA and Western Europe. This disease is predominantly found in the elderly male population, since the median age at diagnosis is 65 years and the male/female ratio about 3–4/1 [1].

The majority of patients presents with advanced stage disease (Ann Arbor stage III/IV) and generalized lymphadenopathies at initial diagnosis. More than 90 % of patients display also extranodal manifestations, with bone marrow involvement most frequent (60–80 %, with circulating MCL cells detected in the peripheral blood smear or by flow cytometry), followed by gastrointestinal tract (lymphomatous polyposis up to 60 %) and liver (25 %). In relapsed disease, central nervous system may be involved in 4–8 % of large patients series [2, 3], and is usually associated with neurologic symptoms. B-symptoms with fever, weight loss and night sweats are present in less than the half of patients.

While a minority of MCL cases (10–15 %), generally characterized by leukemic disease, splenomegaly and absence of significative adenopathies, show a more indolent behaviour and may not need therapy for several years [4–6], most patients with MCL follow an aggressive clinical course, associated with rapid progression, only temporary responses to chemotherapy, and a high recurrence rate, resulting in incurable disease with poor long-term prognosis and reported median survival time of approximately 3–4 years [1, 7].

Whereas the prognosis of younger patients (<65 years) has significantly improved in the last years due to the introduction of high-dose cytarabine chemotherapy (± autologous stem cell transplantation) and anti-CD20 antibody therapy with rituximab, this therapeutic option is in general not feasible for the advanced age patients, accounting for the majority of MCL cases [8–12]. Thus, even considering the rituximab-linked survival advantage achieved also in the elderly population [13, 14], the treatment of these MCL patients remains a challenge for the clinician.

However, in the last years the growing number of molecular targeted drugs (some of them showing striking antitumor activity), along with the interesting data of combinations with conventional chemotherapy and rituximab, are completely changing the therapeutic scenario for older MCL patients. In this chapter we describe the most efficient currently available treatments in this patients subset, focusing on the balance of expected treatment efficacy against the risk of therapy-related toxicity, as well as impaired quality of life, (which is particularly relevant in such an elderly population). Finally, we will offer a practical therapeutic algorithm, based on the specific patients features, to determine the most appropriate treatment for elderly patients presenting with MCL.

Biological and Clinical Risk Factors

MCL uniformly poor outcome has limited the efforts to identify prognostic parameters up to the end of the millennium [1, 15, 16]. Conversely, the improved outcome obtained in the last decade also among elderly patients and the perception that the clinical history of MCL was even more heterogeneous than that of most other lymphoproliferative disorders, prompted investigational efforts to identify biological and clinical prognostic markers. Although several candidate markers were tested, only the following have been more extensively investigated, potentially allowing a more individualized therapeutic approach in MCL patients:

- molecular risk factors, particularly proliferative index [17]
- MCL International Prognostic Index (MIPI) [18]
- minimal residual disease (MRD) [19]

Molecular Risk Factors

The initial event in molecular pathogenesis of MCL is the juxtaposition of the cyclin D1 gene to the immunoglobulin heavy chain locus, t(11;14)(q13;q32) [15], resulting in aberrant overexpression of cyclin D1, a key regulator of cell cycle. In addition to the t(11;14) translocation, several secondary genetic events are required for lymphomagenesis [20, 1, 21] and some of these have been associated with clinical outcome. Features associated with worse prognosis include genetic aberrations that lead to further disturbances of cell cycle regulation, including truncation of the cyclin D1 transcript, mutation of genes involved in DNA damage response (deletions and mutations of ATM and/or TP53), and dysregulated cell survival pathways [22, 23].

However, the most consistent biological prognostic parameter remains the proliferative activity of the tumours. Different measurements of proliferation such as the mitotic index, Ki-67 index, gene expression proliferation signature or other proliferation-related markers have revealed their prognostic value in patients with MCL with different discriminative power [24]. Most other biological predictors are usually related to proliferation and lose their independent significance in multivariate analysis when compared with cell proliferation, or have not been adequately evaluated in comparison to proliferation [23–25]. The percentage of dividing cells by Ki67 immunostaining seems to be the most applicable and discriminative method to evaluate proliferation [26, 27] and has been confirmed, independently of clinical prognostic factors, in the context of several clinical trials [11, 17, 28]. However, the major limitation of this marker in clinical routine is the low reproducibility of quantitative scores among different pathologists [29].

Nevertheless, some studies have reported genetic alterations that maintain their prognostic prediction independently of cell proliferation. TP53 mutations have been confirmed to be of prognostic significance in large series of patients. The quantitative evaluation of the expression of small panels of genes, including MYC, seems to improve the prognostic value of cell proliferation [30, 31]. Similarly, the concomitant inactivation of the two regulatory pathways INK4a/CDK4 and ARF/TP53 in MCL was associated with a poor survival that was independent of Ki-67 proliferation index [32]. Interestingly, the impact of the chromosome 3q gains and 9q losses on survival is independent of the microarray proliferation signature [33]. However, these results have not been confirmed by independent studies in larger series of patients and therefore are not recommended for clinical routine [34].

Finally, a genetic signature identifying the indolent forms of MCL has been recently investigated: in fact it would be worthwhile to recognize this patients subset upfront, especially in those frail elderly patients for whom a watch and wait approach is considered a serious option [4]. Indolent MCLs predominantly show hypermutated immunoglobulin genes, noncomplex karyotypes and a peculiar gene expression profile (with a signature of 13 genes underexpressed in comparison to typical MCL) [35, 36]. In contrast, the role of the transcription factor SOX11 expression is still controversial and should not be applied to predict prognosis [5, 6]. However, the clinical and biological studies on indolent MCL are still limited and further investigations are needed to clarify these issues [34].

MCL International Prognostic Index (MIPI)

As the predictive value of prognostic scores transferred from other lymphomas was sub-optimal [37–39, 26], a new dedicated prognostic score was established in 2008, the MCL International Prognostic Index (MIPI) [18]. This score, taking into account four parameters (age, performance status, lactate dehydrogenase and leukocyte count), was originally constructed using a mathematical algorithm to balance the weight of different predictors, but proved effective also in a simplified categorized version (Table 9.1) [18, 40]. The MIPI score allows to discriminate three prognostic subgroups: the low risk group with a 5-year median overall survival (OS) of 60 %, and the intermediate and the high-risk group with a median OS of 51 and 29 months, respectively. Moreover, several independent studies succeeded in validating the MIPI score in different clinical and therapeutic settings [40–43]. As MIPI is highly applicable and has been validated in most independent series, its use should be routinely applied clinical practice [34].

Minimal Residual Disease

PCR-based evaluation of MRD has shown remarkable predictive value in MCL. Starting from the first prognostic demonstrations in autologous transplantation (auto-SCT) field [44], the value of MRD as powerful independent outcome predictor

Table 1 Simplified MIPI calculation

Points	Age (years)	ECOG performance status	LDH/ULN	Leukocytes ($\times 10^9$/L)
0	<50	0–1	<0.670	6,700
1	50–59	–	0.670–0.999	6,700–9,999
2	60–69	2–4	1.000–1.499	10,000–14,999
3	>69	–	>1.499	>14,999

Risk stratification	
0–3 points	Low risk
4–5 points	Intermediate risk
6–11 points	High risk

For each prognostic factor, 0–3 points are given to each patient and points are summed up to define a category of risk was prospectively validated in two large European MCL Network trials [19]. Most notably the predictive value of MRD detection was observed both in young patients treated intensively and in elderly patients receiving conventional treatment and maintenance either with interferon-alpha or rituximab. Those patients who obtained a complete molecular response (defined as negativity of an allele-specific Real Time PCR analysis, having a minimal sensitivity of 1 neoplastic cell per 10^4 healthy cells) demonstrated a significantly longer remission duration versus those patients who did not obtain such MRD levels. The differences were impressive also for elderly patients: the 2-years rate of ongoing remissions differed from 76 to 36 % for patients with molecular remission versus non-molecular responsive patients, respectively. Thus, MRD negativity may be obtained also in elderly patients and the achievement of molecular remission is meaningful for the long-term outcome.

On the other hand the limitations to a widespread use of MRD analysis in the clinical practice are that MRD detection by PCR is not devoid of costs and should be only performed in centralized experienced laboratories, despite a considerable standardization effort is ongoing [45].

Based on the reliability of MRD detection in MCL, tailored treatment driven by PCR results has been employed, mainly targeting molecular relapses of autografted MCL patients [46–48]. Rituximab monotherapy led to re-induction of molecular remission in the majority of patients and, based on the larger Nordic study, seemed to provide clinical benefit, too [47]. However, the broad applicability of such approaches still needs to be proven, in particular among elderly patients receiving conventional treatment only.

Thus MRD detection, despite being a powerful independent predictor, is not yet recommended in clinical routine outside of clinical trials, due to its limitations of applicability, reproducibility and validation [34].

Current Diagnostic Standards

The diagnosis of MCL is established according to the criteria of the WHO classification of hematological neoplasms. In general histologic confirmation of diagnosis is mandatory and a lymph node biopsy is strongly recommended. In contrast, fine-needle biopsy is not appropriate. Bone marrow aspiration alone is not sufficient but should be complemented by flow cytometry to identify the typical lymphoma immunophenotype and bone marrow biopsy to quantify the percentage of infiltration [49]. Most tumours have a classic morphology of small-medium sized cells with irregular nuclei, dense chromatin, and unapparent nucleoli. In addition to classic MCL, a blastoid variant of this disease has been described that is characterized by high mitotic rate and particularly aggressive behaviour and is associated with INK4a/ARF deletions, TP53 mutations, and complex karyotypes [15, 32, 50, 51]. However, the tumour cells may present with a spectrum of morphological variants that may raise some difficulties in the differential diagnosis with chronic lymphocytic leukaemia, marginal zone lymphomas, large B-cell lymphomas, or blastic hematological proliferations. Because an accurate histologic diagnosis is essential, second opinion by an experienced hematopathologist is advisable [34].

Beside the classical immunophenotype (immunoglobulin M/D, CD19, CD20, CD22, CD43, CD79a, CD5 positive and CD23, CD10, CD200, BCL6 usually negative), the detection of cyclin D1 overexpression or the t(11;14) translocation is essential, since histo-morphological phenotypes may differ significantly [5, 15, 52, 53]. Nevertheless, rare cases of cyclin D1-negative variant of MCL has been recognized [54], characterized by the same gene expression profiling and genomic alterations as classical MCL and showing in 50 % of cases a cyclin D2 translocation [33, 55, 56]. SOX11, a transcription factor expressed in 90 % of MCL, may be applied to identify this variant [57, 58]. Moreover, as already stated, Ki67 proliferative index staining is recommended as a strong prognostic indicator of long term outcome [34].

The laboratory evaluation comprises differential blood count and standard serum chemistry analysis, including the determination of LDH as one of the major risk parameters. Abdominal CT of the neck, chest, abdomen, and pelvis is mandatory. Cerebrospinal fluid evaluation and cranial imaging with MRI is not usually required at first presentation, unless neurologic symptoms are present [3]. PET scan is not included in the consensus recommendations based on scarce data and especially limited therapeutic consequences [59–62]. Additional diagnostics depends on the clinical presentation and includes an ear-nose-throat consultation and gastroscopy/colonoscopy, based on up to 60 % asymptomatic infiltration of the bowel [63, 64]. As the results from upper and lower endoscopy have generally only a modest impact on therapeutic decisions, they are mandatory only in limited stages symptomatic patients [64] or as confirmation of complete responses within clinical trials [65].

Moreover, PET scan and gastrointestinal tract endoscopy examination may be particularly useful for clinical stage I–II patients, in order to confirm the early stage and better define the indication to localized treatment [66, 67].

Current Treatment Concepts

Given the high median age of MCL patients and considering that no curative treatment is available so far, toxicity of induction therapy is a major concern. Thus, it is essential to define the therapeutic goal, which may be long term control of the disease, balancing the expected treatment efficacy (remarkable lifespan prolongation) against the risk of impairing toxicity and reduced quality of life. Consequently, it may be important to obtain a complete response (CR) also in elderly patients. Given that a good performance status and the absence of comorbidities are required for any intensified treatment aiming at CR, a common approach consists of an upfront stratification of patients into elderly fit and elderly frail categories [68]. Comprehensive Geriatric Assessment (CGA) was demonstrated as a reliable tool to objectively identify patients eligible for a chemotherapy targeting at long term control of the disease or patients for palliative approaches only [69–71].

A summary of the most important recently published clinical studies involving elderly MCL patients is shown in Table 9.2.

Table 2 Recent published clinical studies involving elderly MCL patients

	Author	Study features	Evaluable MCL patients	Therapeutic regimen	ORR% (CR%)	Median PFS (months)	Median OS (months)
Conventional immuno chemotherapy	Kluin-Nelemans et al. (2012) [79]	Phase III, first-line, randomized	485	Induction: R-CHOP vs R-FC	86 (34) vs 78 (40)	28 vs 26 (TTF)	62 % vs 47 % (4-year OS)
				Maintenance: rituximab vs interferon alpha	–	58 % vs 29 % (4-year DOR)	79 % vs 67 % (4-year OS)
	Rummel et al. (2013) [82]	Phase III, first-line, randomized	94	R-CHOP vs rituximab-bendamustine	na	21.1 vs 35.4	na
	Visco et al. (2013) [84]	Phase II first-line/relapse	40	Rituximab. bendamustine. cytarabine	90 (83)	First-line 95 % relapse 70 % (2-y PFS)	na
Proteasome inhibitors	Ruan et al. (2010) [90]	Phase II, first-line	36	R-CHOP+bortezomib	91 (72)	44 % (2-year PFS)	86 % (2-year OS)
	Houot et al. (2012) [91]	Phase II, first-line	39	Rituximab. doxorubicin, dexamethasone, chlorambucil, bortezomib	79 (59)	26	69 % (2-year OS)
	Goy et al. (2009) [85]	Phase II, relapse	141	Bortezomib	33 (8)	6.7 (TTP)	23.5
	Lamm et al. (2011) [104]	Phase II, relapse	16	Bortezomib, rituximab, dexamethasone	81 (44)	12.1	38.6
	Kouroukis et al. (2011) [108]	Phase II, relapse	25	Bortezomib, gemcitabine	60 (11)	11.4	na

(continued)

Table 2 (continued)

	Author	Study features	Evaluable MCL patients	Therapeutic regimen	ORR% (CR%)	Median PFS (months)	Median OS (months)
mTOR inhibitors	Hess et al. (2009) [109]	Phase III, relapse, randomized	54	Temsirolimus 175/75	22 (2)	4.8	12.8
			54	Temsirolimus 175/25	6 (0)	3.4	10
			53	Investigator's choice	2 (2)	1.9	9.7
	Ansell et al. (2011) [110, 111]	Phase II, relapse	69	Temsirolimus. rituximab	59 (19)	9.7	29.5
	Renner et al. (2012) [112]	Phase II, relapse	35	Everolimus	20 (6)	5.5	na
Immunomodulatory drugs	Witzig et al. (2011) [89]	Phase II, relapse	57	Lenalidomide	42 (21)	5.7	na
	Eve et al. (2012) [113]	Phase II, relapse	26	Lenalidomide	31 (8)	3.9	10
	Wang et al. (2012) [114]	Phase II, relapse	44	Lenalidomide, rituximab	57 (36)	11.1	24.3
	Zaja et al. (2012)	Phase II, relapse	33	Lenalidomide, dexamethasone	52 (24)	12	20
	Harel et al. (2010) [116]	retrospective, relapse	58	Thalidomide ±bortezomib±rituximab	50 (21)	29 % (1-year TTF)	62 % (1-year OS)
	Ruan et al. (2010) [101]	Phase II, relapse	22	RT-PEPC	73 (32)	10	45 % (2-year OS)
Antibody-based approaches	Smith et al. (2012) [95]	Phase II. first-line	50	R-CHOP +^{90}γ-ibriturnurnab tiuxetan	64 (46)	30.8 (TTF)	73 % (5-year OS)
	Wang et al. (2009) [118]	Phase II. relapse	32	^{90}γ-ibritumumab tiuxetan	31 (16)	6 (EFS)	21
	Cartron et al. (2010) [122]	Phase II. relapse	15	GA-101	27 (na)	2.5	na
B-cell receptor signalling inhibitors and other targeted approaches	Wang et al. (2012) [120]	Phase II, relapse	110	Ibrutinib	68 (22)	13.9	na
	Kahl et al. (2010) [121]	Phase I, relapse	16	Cal-101	62 (na)	3 (DOR)	na
	Lin et al. (2010) [128]	Phase I, first-line/relapse	10	Flavopiridol, fludarabine, rituximab	80 (70)	21.9	na
	Evens et al. (2012) [132]	Phase II, relapse	11	Abexinostat	27 (na)	4	na

Studies involving at least 10 MCL patients are shown

First-Line Treatment of Elderly Fit Patients

Conventional Immunochemotherapy

Thus far, the most frequently applied chemotherapy schedules for elderly fit patients consist of 3-weekly R-CHOP (rituximab, cyclophosphamide, doxorubicin, vincristine and prednisone) or R-CVP (rituximab, cyclophosphamide, vincristine and prednisone) depending on cardiac comorbidities [1, 65]. The anti-CD20 monoclonal antibody rituximab should always be added to induction therapy, as it results in improvement of overall response rate (ORR) and even OS in the absence of significant toxicity [14, 65, 72, 73].

Alternatively, fludarabine-containing schemes have been explored as well achieving high response rates, with or without cyclophosphamide and mitoxantrone (FC or FCM) [74–78]. On these basis the European MCL Network conducted a large international phase III trial comparing R-CHOP with R-FC (followed by a second randomization between maintenance phase with interferon alpha versus rituximab) for elderly patients. Unexpectedly, the outcome of the fludarabine-containing regimen was disappointing and accordingly this trial established R-CHOP immunochemotherapy followed by rituximab maintenance as the "gold standard" first-line therapy for elderly MCL [79]. In fact, although CR rates after R-FC and R-CHOP were similar (40 % versus 34 %), progressive disease was more frequent during R-FC (14 % versus 5 %). The median OS was also significantly inferior after R-FC (4-year survival rate, 47 % vs. 62 %) and more patients in the experimental arm died due to lymphoma or infections. In addition to lower efficacy, haematologic grade 3–4 toxicity was more frequent during R-FC. Thus, the use of upfront R-FC in elderly MCL patients is discouraged [34].

Alternative chemotherapy regimens have been also explored. An important candidate is bendamustine, showing excellent responses in patients with relapsed MCL [80, 81]. Notably, in a randomized trial with 94 MCL patients, the schema rituximab-bendamustine (BR) compared favourably with R-CHOP in first-line treatment, achieving a prolonged progression-free survival (PFS: 35.4 vs 22.1 months) and fewer toxic effects (lower neutropenia, infections, polyneuropathy and alopecia) [82]. Bendamustine also performed well in first-line treatment of MCL if combined with vincristine and prednisone (BOP regimen) [83]. Moreover, the promising activity of a new regimen combining rituximab, bendamustine and cytarabine (R-BAC) has been recently confirmed in primary and relapsed MCL (90 % ORR with 83 % CR on the total series of 40 patients), resulting in an excellent 2-years PFS of 70 % for relapsed and 95 % for first-line patients, respectively [84]. Currently, a phase II study of R-BAC accruing untreated elderly "fit" (according to CGA) MCL patients is ongoing (EudraCT Number: 2011-005739-23, Table 9.3).

Table 3 Ongoing clinical trials accruing elderly MCL patients

NCT code	Study features	Estimated enrollment (patients)	Estimated primarycompletion date (month/year)	Therapeutic regimen	Sponsor	Location countries
EudraCT Number: 2012-002542-20	Phase III, randomized, first-line	633	06/2019	R-CHOP vs R-CHOP/R-HAD + maintenance rituximab vs rituximab/lenalidomide	LYSARC & EuMCLNet	France, Belgium Germany, Italy, Netherlands, Portugal
01776840	Phase III, randomized, first-line	520	03/2018	BR vs BR + ibrutinib	Janssen Research & Development LLC	Worldwide
01415752	Phase II, randomized, first-line	332	04/2015	BR ± bortezomib + rituximab maintenance ± lenalidomide	ECOG	USA
01662050	Phase II, single arm, first-line	57	01/2014	R-BAC	FIL	Italy
00963534	Phase II, single arm, first-line	60	09/2014	BR + lenalidomide	NLG	Denmark, Finland, Norway, Sweden
01449344	Phase III, randomized, relapse	175	09/2016	R-HAD vs R-HADB	EuMCLNet	France, Germany
01646021	Phase III, randomized, relapse	280	08/2014	Ibrutinib vs temsirolimus	Janssen Research & Development LLC	Worldwide
01078142	Phase I/II, single arm, relapse	72	03/2014	BERT	GLSG & EuMCLNet	Germany
01389427	Phase I/II, single group assignment, relapse	63	06/2013	R-CHOP or R-FC or R-HAD + temsirolimus	GOELAMS	France
01737177	Phase II, single arm, relapse	42	07/2014	R-2B	FIL	Italy

New Targeted Drugs Combinations

Other promising candidates for combination with immunochemotherapy are bortezomib and lenalidomide, both effective as single agents in relapse setting [85–89]. R-CHOP combined with bortezomib achieved highly promising response rates in a phase II study of 36 primary MCL patients (ORR 91 % with 72 % CR/unconfirmed CR and a 2-year PFS of 44 %) [90]. A recent phase II study for newly diagnosed elderly patients with MCL treated with bortezomib in combination with doxorubicin, dexamethasone, chlorambucil and rituximab (RiPAD+C regimen) showed a ORR of 79 % with 51 % CR and a median PFS of 26 months. The scheme was toxic, however, with 2 treatment-related deaths (5 %), 4 patients (10 %) discontinuing the treatment because of severe toxicity and 7 patients (18 %) experienced grade 3 neurotoxicity [91]. Moreover, two clinical trials are currently ongoing, assessing the combination of BR plus bortezomib or lenalidomide in first-line treatment of MCL patients (NCT01415752 and NCT00963534, respectively, Table 9.3).

First-Line Treatment for Elderly Frail Patients

If treatment of elderly frail patients is considered, this should consist of mild immunochemotherapy, as chlorambucil combined with rituximab, which is usually very well tolerated [92, 65]. All treatments should be given with the perspective that cure will not be obtained, and that palliation should aim at improvement of quality of life [34].

Bendamustine is also an active monotherapy that is well tolerated in older or frail patients and may be discussed in combination with rituximab in selected cases of this patients subset [80–82].

Single agent therapy with rituximab (four gifts at weekly intervals) for treatment-naive patients is not recommended, as only very low ORR of 27 % with 3 % CR have been obtained. Continuation of maintenance therapy with rituximab did not further contribute and caused up to 13 % grade 3–4 hematologic toxicity [93].

Consolidation and Maintenance Therapy

Although high response rates have been achieved by the discussed therapeutic approaches, survival curves do not show any plateau, as almost all patients will finally relapse after induction treatment and most likely die of recurrent disease. Thus it is crucial to implement additional consolidation concepts (e.g. rituximab maintenance, radioimmunotherapy –RIT- consolidation, new molecules within studies) to maintain long lasting remissions.

In the past, maintenance therapy with interferon-alpha has been applied in several studies, but the beneficial effects on PFS did not reach the statistical significance [7, 94].

In the abovementioned European MCL Network Elderly trial, responding patients were randomized between a maintenance phase with interferon alpha or rituximab. In fact, rituximab maintenance reduced the risk of progression or death by 45 % (58 % patients in remission after 4 years vs. 29 % with interferon alpha), almost doubled duration of remission and significantly improved OS among patients responsive to R-CHOP [79]. Thus, rituximab maintenance (1 dose every 2 months until progression) should be offered to all patients responding upon R-chemotherapy, especially R-CHOP induction [34].

In addition to rituximab, various other candidates might be suitable for maintenance therapy. Lenalidomide seems attractive, either alone or combined with rituximab, and is currently being tested in the Italian randomized trial FIL-MCL0208 for young patients after auto-SCT (EudraCT Number 2009-012807-25). A comparison in older patients of additional lenalidomide with rituximab maintenance versus rituximab alone is being investigated in the current European MCL Network "MCL R2 Elderly" randomized trial (EudraCT Number 2012-002542-20, Table 9.3).

Despite some concerns about its cumulative neurotoxicity, bortezomib maintenance is currently also being tested in the Dutch-Belgian HOVON 75 trial for young patients after high dose induction therapy and auto-SCT (EudraCT Number 2006-000386-11).

Finally, promising data have been achieved by RIT consolidation in elderly patients, too. Four cycles of R-CHOP followed by yttrium-90 (^{90}Y)-ibritumomab tiuxetan (an anti-CD20 radio-immunoconjugate antibody) compared favourably with historical results of six cycles of R-CHOP in patients with previously untreated MCL. This regimen was well tolerated and may be applicable to most patients [95].

A list of the main ongoing clinical trials for elderly MCL patients is shown in Table 9.3.

Treatment of Limited Stage Disease

Similarly to other non-Hodgkin lymphomas, one might consider to treat localized disease (stage I/II) with limited immunochemotherapy followed by involved field radiotherapy [65]. Stage I disease is, however, rare in MCL, with the large majority of patients presenting with advanced stage IV disease and usually bone marrow involvement. Moreover, no reliable data of randomized clinical trials are available. Two retrospective Canadian analyses, each accounting for 26 patients with limited disease treated with various combinations of radiotherapy and/or chemotherapy, suggested an important role for radiotherapy [66, 96]. Radiotherapy alone by applying involved field or even extended field radiotherapy might be considered for frail elderly patients with limited stage I/II disease [68], but achieved only temporary remissions in an ongoing trial of the German Lymphoma Study Group (Martin Dreyling, personal communication 2013).

Treatment of Relapsed Disease

Almost all patients will finally relapse after induction therapy. In younger patients relapsed lymphoma may have a curative approach based on allogeneic transplantation [97, 98]. Given the difficulties to offer elderly patients dose-intensified salvage therapy with or without stem cell transplantation (autologous or allogeneic), the therapeutic goal of relapsed MCL should be the prolonged disease control. For selection of optimal treatment, efficacy versus toxicity, but also the ease of administration (for example orally versus intravenously) have to be balanced and discussed with the patient. In addition, new treatment modalities should be offered in the context of clinical trials, especially to the elderly patients, as they have a very poor outcome once relapsed [68]. Therefore (if not in a palliative situation) these patients should be generally referred to experienced centers to determine the optimal therapeutic strategy. A list of the major current clinical trials for elderly MCL patients is provided in Table 9.3. In general, treatment strategies should depend on the individual risk profile and patients fitness: hence a CGA should be always performed to define the best treatment option for relapsed patients, too. In this regard the most recent data of salvage regimens are discussed below (Table 9.2).

Immunochemotherapy Combinations

Most elderly patients received R-CHOP as first line treatment. A well established salvage regimen, based on purine analogues, is R-FC or R-FCM [78]. Conversely, if a purine analogue was included in the first line treatment, an anthracycline based regimen at relapse may be considered (R-CHOP) [68]. However, although the addition of rituximab to conventional chemotherapy (R-FCM, R-GEMOX, R-DHAP) increased response rates up to 60–70 %, the duration of response in relapsing disease remains limited (mainly less than 1 year) and such treatment options should be considered basically palliative [78, 99, 100].

As already discussed before, more promising data have been recently achieved by the combined regimens with bendamustine, such as the well tolerated BR and the even more effective but also more toxic R-BAC regimen [80, 84]. Thus, depending on patients performance status and comorbidities, a treatment comprising bendamustine should be preferred in relapse setting for elderly patients.

Finally, for a palliative approach, the efficacy, feasibility and low toxicity of an oral low-dose metronomic polichemotherapy combination (PEP-C) is noteworthy and such well tolerable regimens should be always considered for elderly patients, optionally in combination with rituximab and thalidomide [101, 102].

Established Molecular Targeted Approaches

The first "new drug" to be registered in relapsed MCL in US has been bortezomib, based on its selective and reversible proteasome 26S inhibitor efficacy [85–87]. Although the combination of bortezomib with rituximab and chemotherapy showed high response rates (up to 60–70 %), median PFS rates among heavily pre-treated patients were only in the range of 12 months. The published regimens encompass both combinations with rituximab and steroids [103, 104], as well as combinations with immunochemotherapies such as rituximab, dexamethasone and high dose-cytarabin (R-HAD), rituximab, prednisone and cyclophosphamide (R-CP), rituximab-bendamustine (BR) and gemcitabine [105–108]. The toxicity profile predominantly consists of polyneuropathy and neutro-thrombocytopenia. A phase III clinical trial is currently ongoing, randomizing MCL relapsed patients to receive either R-HAD ± bortezomib (NCT01449344).

Temsirolimus, an intravenous mammalian target of rapamycin (mTOR) inhibitor, received the European Medicines Agency approval in 2009, due to its single-agent activity in patients with relapsed MCL. Temsirolimus induced a significant improvement in median PFS and ORR, compared with investigator's choice monotherapy (4.8 vs. 1.9 months and 22 % vs 2 %, respectively) [109]. Hematological adverse events were generally well managed by dose reductions or treatment delay. Temsirolimus should be considered in advanced relapses (greater than second line), especially for non fit patients [34]. The addition of rituximab to temsirolimus was subsequently tested in a phase II study on 71 patients. An increased ORR of 59 %, with up to 19 % CR was observed, with a median time to progression (TTP) of about 10 months [110]; the toxicity profile was similar to temsirolimus monotherapy. To further improve its efficacy, temsirolimus is being currently investigated in combination with BR in a phase II clinical trial (NCT01078142) [111].

Another well tolerated oral mTOR inhibitor is Everolimus [112], but further studies in combination with chemotherapy or other biological drugs are warranted.

A number of phase II trials have confirmed the promising response rates of the immunomodulatory compound lenalidomide in relapsed MCL [88, 89, 113]. Recently a phase II study in 52 patients with relapsed MCL confirmed the impact of a chemo-free lenalidomide-rituximab combination with high response rates (57 % ORR, 36 % CR) and impressive response durations up to 19 months [114]. The manageable toxicity (mainly mild hematological) and the oral formulation make this drug an attractive option also in the context of maintenance regimens. A phase II trial of the rituximab-lenalidomide-bendamustine combination + lenalidomide maintenance is ongoing for relapsed MCL (NCT01737177).

Largely overshadowed by its subsequent follower lenalidomide, thalidomide is an active compound in relapsed MCL, with a favourable side effect profile (7 % grade 3–4 adverse events, including thromboembolism), with an interesting ORR up to 50 % (plus 29 % SD, stable disease) and a time to treatment failure (TTF) of 29 % and 11 % at 1 and 2 years, respectively [115, 116]. Thus, thalidomide might offer a cost-effective alternative to more expensive targeted agents, especially in countries with limited health-care resources [117].

In contrast to its favorable safety profile (mainly manageable thrombocytopenia and neutropenia) and promising data in other types of lymphoma, monotherapy RIT with ^{90}Y-ibritumomab tiuxetan does not impact substantially the prognosis of relapsed MCL, with an ORR of 32 % and a EFS (event free survival) of 6 months [118]. Thus recent studies are exploring its combination with others efficient targeted drug, such as bortezomib. [119]

Innovative Molecular Targeted Approaches

The growing insights into the underlying molecular biology of MCL form the basis for the ongoing exploration of targeted approaches [21]. A number of new compounds are currently being tested in MCL and are available for the application within clinical trials.

The most convincing data come for the oral Bruton's tyrosine kinase (BTK) inhibitor ibrutinib that specifically blocks the B-cell receptor (BCR) signaling survival pathway. In an international phase II trial on refractory/relapsed MCL patients ibrutinib monotherapy showed impressive efficacy and excellent tolerability with an impressive ORR of 68 %, 22 % CR and a PFS of around 14 months. Noteworthy is the favorable safety profile, with less than 15 % grade 3/4 hematological toxicity and mainly mild gastro-intestinal symptoms, fatigue and infections in a population of heavily pre-treated patients [120]. Two phase III trials are currently ongoing, the first comparing ibrutinib versus temsirolimus in relapsed patients (NCT01646021) and the second investigating a BR schedule ± ibrutinib as first line treatment (NCT01776840).

Another antagonist of the BCR signal cascade, CAL-101, a specific inhibitor of phosphatidylinositol 3-kinase delta isoform, is currently being tested in phase I/II trials: [121], however, preliminary results are less promising than ibrutinib.

New monoclonal antibodies (mAB), such as GA101 (obinutuzumab) and ofatumumab, targeting a variety of epitopes in addition to CD20 are currently investigated in preclinical and clinical trials, but data on MCL are still scarce [122–124]. Other interesting approaches are the bispecific anti-CD19/anti-CD3 mAB, which showed a high efficacy in a phase I/II trial particularly in the MCL patients [125, 126] and the toxin-immunoconjugated mAB, such as the anti-CD79b DCDS4501A [127]. Nevertheless, additional studies on larger patients cohorts are warranted.

Two cell cycle targeted drugs (direct inhibitors of cyclin-dependent kinase 4 and 6, flavopiridol and PD0332991), showed activity in relapsed MCL alone in combination with fludarabine, rituximab or bortezomib. [128–130]

Finally, promising results come also from oral second generation BCL-2 specific BH3 mimetic ABT-199 and a novel oral pan Histone Deacetylase Inhibitor Abexinostat [131, 132].

Current Therapeutic Recommendations for Elderly Patients

Because MCL is as yet regarded as incurable and mostly affects elderly individuals, the toxic effects of treatment regimens are of particular concern, as underlying comorbidities or decreased organ function may compromise the eligibility for cytotoxic chemotherapy.

Older patients have highly variable physiologic ages, and their treatment should be individualized for optimal outcomes. Treatment paradigms should also take into account the diversity of patients' life expectancy, functional reserve, social support, and personal preference. A CGA is a useful tool for estimating life expectancy and tolerance of treatment and for identifying reversible factors that may interfere with cancer treatment, including depression, malnutrition, anemia, neutropenia, and lack of caregiver support [69–71]. The most common instrument of the CGA are the following tests: Activities of Daily Living (ADL), Instrumental Activities of Daily Living (IADL), Performance status (PS), Charlson Comorbidity Index Cumulative Illness Rating Scale—Geriatrics (CIRS-G), Mini Nutritional Assessment (MNA), Geriatric Depression Scale (GDS) and Folstein Mini Mental Status (MMS). Through these practical tools elderly patients can be divided in three geriatric groups, allowing the healthcare providers to tailor to each patient the most appropriate therapies, using different drugs in the context of different treatment aims.

As regards to MCL, the following patients and treatment classification are suggested (Fig. 9.1):

1. For the "fit" patients the treatment aim should be the achievement of the CR, with a potential of long-term control of the disease. The recommended induction schedule is R-CHOP plus rituximab maintenance. At relapse a regimen containing bendamustine (such as BR or R-BAC) and eventually new drugs in context of clinical trials (R-HAD plus bortezomib, BR plus lenalidomide or temsirolimus) are advisable.
2. For the "compromised" patients the treatment should aim to a medium-term control of the disease, well balancing the expected therapy efficacy against the known toxicities. Thus, a suggested upfront schedule may be the well tolerated and effective BR regimen. Alternative mild chemotherapy schemes are R-CVP or R-chlorambucil. At relapse the repetition of the prior induction regimen could be an appropriate approach, if a longstanding remission (>1–2 years) was previously achieved. Otherwise, monotherapies with targeted drugs (in particular temsirolimus, bortezomib, lenalidomide, thalidomide or ibrutinib in the context of a clinical trial), as well as tolerable combinations with rituximab, steroids or low-dose chemotherapy should be preferred. Oral palliative combinations, such as the metronomic PEP-C, could be also useful options in this setting. At the same time a multidisciplinary palliative support should be started.
3. For the "frail" patients the preservation of the quality of life should be the primary objective of the clinical care. Therefore mild, basically oral, chemotherapy schemes such as R-chlorambucil or PEP-C are recommended. At progression alternative oral chemotherapy combinations, steroids, radiotherapy and also molecular approaches in selected cases represent the standard of care. An adequate palliative support is crucial.

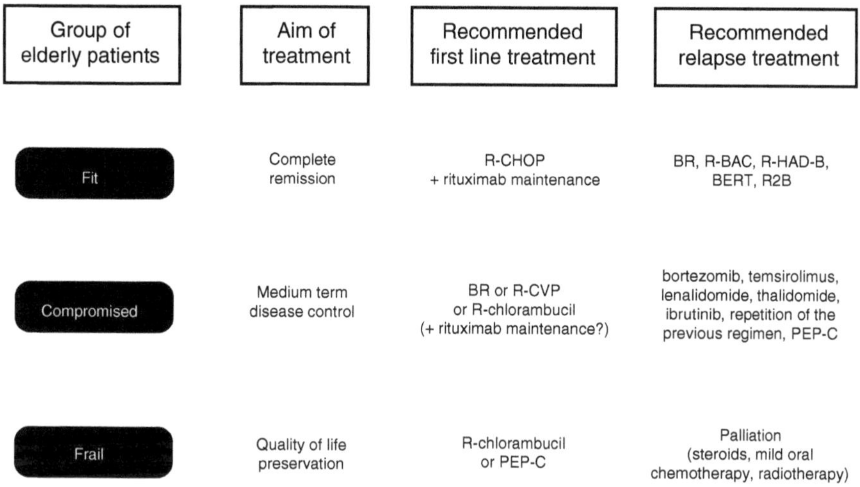

Fig. 9.1 Therapeutic recommendations for different groups of elderly MCL patients. Abbreviations: *R-CHOP* rituximab-cyclophosphamide-doxorubicin-vincristine-prednisone, *BR* bendamustine-rituximab, *R-CVP* rituximab-cyclophosphamide-vincristine-prednisone, *R-chlorambucil* rituximab-chlorambucil, *PEP-C* metronomic prednisone-etoposide-procarbazine-cyclophosphamide, *R-BAC* rituximab-bendamustine-cytarabine, *R-HAD-B* rituximab-high-dose cytarabine-dexamethasone-bortezomib, *BERT* bendamustine-rituximab-temsirolimus, *R-2B* rituximab-lenalidomide-bendamustine + lenalidomide maintenance

Concerning patients with specific comorbidities there are no established recommendations. In general anthracyclines should be avoided in patients with cardiac comorbidities, preferring e.g. a bendamustine based regimen. Similarly, a bendamustine combination may replace R-CHOP in patients with uncontrolled diabetes. In relapsed disease neither platinum derivatives nor fludarabine or lenalidomide should be applied in patients with renal impairment.

In addition an appropriate pre-emptive use of growth factors, according to the major guidelines [133–135], should be strongly encouraged.

Abbreviations

^{90}Y	Yttrium-90
ADL	Activities of Daily Living
ATM	Ataxia-telangiectasia mutated kinase
Auto-SCT	Autologous stem cell transplantation
BCL-2	B-cell lymphoma 2
BCR	B-cell receptor
BH3	BCL-2 homology 3
BERT	Bendamustine-rituximab-temsirolimus
BOP	Bendamustine, vincristine, prednisone
BR	Rituximab, bendamustine

BTK	Bruton's tyrosine kinase inhibitor
CD	Cluster of differentiation
CDK	Cyclin dependent kinase
CGA	Comprehensive Geriatric Assessment
CIRS-G	Charlson Comorbidity Index Cumulative Illness Rating Scale—Geriatrics
CR	Complete response
CT	Computed tomography
DNA	Deoxyribonucleic acid
EFS	Event free survival
FC(M)	Fludarabine, cyclophosphamide, (mitoxantrone)
FIL	Italian Lymphoma Foundation
GDS	Geriatric Depression Scale
HOVON	The Haemato Oncology Foundation for Adults in the Netherlands
IADL	Instrumental Activities of Daily Living
LDH	Lactate dehydrogenase
mAB	Monoclonal antibody
MCL	Mantle cell lymphoma
MIPI	Mantle cell lymphoma International Prognostic Index
MMS	Folstein Mini Mental Status
MNA	Mini Nutritional Assessment
MRD	Minimal residual disease
MRI	Magnetic resonance imaging
mTOR	Mammalian target of rapamycin
NCT	National clinical trial
ORR	Overall response rate
OS	Overall survival
PCR	Polymerase chain reaction
PEP-C	Metronomic prednisone-etoposide-procarbazine-cyclophosphamid
PET	Positron emission tomography
PFS	Progression free survival
PS	Performance status
R-2B	Rituximab-lenalidomide-bendamustine + lenalidomide maintenance
R-BAC	Rituximab-bendamustine-cytarabine
R-CHOP	Rituximab, cyclophosphamide, doxorubicin, vincristine and prednisone
R-CP	Rituximab, prednisone and cyclophosphamide
R-CVP	Rituximab, cyclophosphamide, vincristine and prednisone
R-DHAP	Rituximab, dexamethasone, high-dose cytarabine, cisplatin
R-GEMOX	Rituximab, gemcitabine, oxaliplatin
R-HAD-B	Rituximab-high-dose cytarabine-dexamethasone-bortezomib
RiPAD + C	Rituximab, bortezomib, doxorubicin, dexamethasone, chlorambucil
RIT	Radioimmunotherapy
SD	Stable disease
SOX11	SOY(sex determining region Y)-box 11
TP	Tumor protein
TTF	Time to treatment failure

TTP	Time to progression
USA	United States of America
WHO	World Health Organization

References

1. Dreyling M, Hiddemann W. Current treatment standards and emerging strategies in mantle cell lymphoma. Hematology Am Soc Hematol Educ Program. 2009. p.542–51.
2. Cheah CY, George A, Giné E, et al. Central nervous system involvement in mantle cell lymphoma: clinical features, prognostic factors and outcomes from the European Mantle Cell Lymphoma Network. Ann Oncol. 2013;24(8):2119–23.
3. Conconi A, Franceschetti S, Lobetti-Bodoni C, et al. Risk factors of central nervous system relapse in mantle cell lymphoma. Leuk Lymphoma. 2013;54(9):1908–14.
4. Martin P, Chadburn A, Christos P, et al. Outcome of deferred initial therapy in mantle-cell lymphoma. J Clin Oncol. 2009;27(8):1209–13. doi:10.1200/JCO.2008.19.6121.
5. Fernandez V, Salamero O, Espinet B, et al. Genomic and gene expression profiling defines indolent forms of mantle cell lymphoma. Cancer Res. 2010;70:1408–18.
6. Nygren L, Baumgartner Wennerholm S, Klimkowska M, et al. Prognostic role of SOX11 in a population-based cohort of mantle cell lymphoma. Blood. 2012;119(18):4215–23. doi:10.1182/blood-2011-12-400580.
7. Hiddemann W, Unterhalt M, Herrmann R, et al. Mantle-cell lymphomas have more widespread disease and a slower response to chemotherapy compared with follicle-center lymphomas: results of a prospective comparative analysis of the German Low-Grade Lymphoma Study Group. J Clin Oncol. 1998;16:1922–30.
8. Gianni AM, Magni M, Martelli M, et al. Long-term remission in mantle cell lymphoma following high-dose sequential chemotherapy and in vivo rituximab-purged stem cell autografting (R-HDS regimen). Blood. 2003;102(2):749–55.
9. Dreyling M, Lenz G, Hoster E, et al. Early consolidation by myeloablative radiochemotherapy followed by autologous stem cell transplantation in first remission significantly prolongs progression-free survival in mantle-cell lymphoma: results of a prospective randomized trial of the European MCL Network. Blood. 2005;105(7):2677–84.
10. Romaguera JE, Fayad L, Rodriguez MA, et al. High rate of durable remissions after treatment of newly diagnosed aggressive mantle-cell lymphoma with rituximab plus hyper-CVAD alternating with rituximab plus high-dose methotrexate and cytarabine. J Clin Oncol. 2005;23(28):7013–23.
11. Geisler CH, Kolstad A, Laurell A, et al. Long-term progression-free survival of mantle cell lymphoma after intensive front-line immunochemotherapy with in vivo-purged stem cell rescue: a nonrandomized phase 2 multicenter study by the Nordic Lymphoma Group. Blood. 2008;112(7):2687–93. doi:10.1182/blood-2008-03-147025.
12. Hermine O, Hoster E, Walewski J, et al. Alternating courses of 3x CHOP and 3x DHAP plus Rituximab followed by a high dose ARA-C containing myeloablative regimen and autologous stem cell transplantation (ASCT) increases overall survival when compared to 6 courses of CHOP plus Rituximab followed by myeloablative radiochemotherapy and ASCT in mantle cell lymphoma: final analysis of the MCL younger trial of the European Mantle Cell Lymphoma Network (MCL net). Blood. 2012;120:151.
13. Herrmann A, Hoster E, Zwingers T, et al. Improvement of overall survival in advanced stage mantle cell lymphoma. J Clin Oncol. 2009;27(4):511–8. doi:10.1200/JCO.2008.16.8435.
14. Griffiths R, Mikhael J, Gleeson M, et al. Addition of rituximab to chemotherapy alone as first-line therapy improves overall survival in elderly patients with mantle cell lymphoma. Blood. 2011;118(18):4808–16. doi:10.1182/blood-2011-04-348367.
15. Swerdlow SH, Campo E, Harris NL, et al. WHO classification of tumours of haematopoietic and lymphoid tissues. 4th ed. Lyon: IARC Press; 2008. p. 233–7.

16. Nickenig C, Dreyling M, Hoster E, et al. Combined cyclophosphamide, vincristine, doxorubicin, and prednisone (CHOP) improves response rates but not survival and has lower hematologic toxicity compared with combined mitoxantrone, chlorambucil, and prednisone (MCP) in follicular and mantle cell lymphomas: results of a prospective randomized trial of the German Low-Grade Lymphoma Study Group. Cancer. 2006;107(5):1014–22.
17. Determann O, Hoster E, Ott G, et al. Ki-67 predicts outcome in advanced-stage mantle cell lymphoma patients treated with anti-CD20 immunochemotherapy: results from randomized trials of the European MCL Network and the German Low Grade Lymphoma Study Group. Blood. 2008;111(4):2385–7.
18. Hoster E, Dreyling M, Klapper W, et al. A new prognostic index (MIPI) for patients with advanced-stage mantle cell lymphoma. Blood. 2008;111(2):558–65.
19. Pott C, Hoster E, Delfau-Larue MH, et al. Molecular remission is an independent predictor of clinical outcome in patients with mantle cell lymphoma after combined immunochemotherapy: a European MCL intergroup study. Blood. 2010;115(16):3215–23. doi:10.1182/blood-2009-06-230250.
20. Jares P, Colomer D, Campo E. Genetic and molecular pathogenesis of mantle cell lymphoma: perspectives for new targeted therapeutics. Nat Rev Cancer. 2007;7(10):750–62.
21. Pérez-Galán P, Dreyling M, Wiestner A. Mantle cell lymphoma: biology, pathogenesis, and the molecular basis of treatment in the genomic era. Blood. 2011;117(1):26–38. doi:10.1182/blood-2010-04-189977.
22. Navarro A, Royo C, Hernández L, et al. Molecular pathogenesis of mantle cell lymphoma: new perspectives and challenges with clinical implications. Semin Hematol. 2011;48(3):155–65.
23. Royo C, Salaverria I, Hartmann EM, et al. The complex landscape of genetic alterations in mantle cell lymphoma. Semin Cancer Biol. 2011;21(5):322–34.
24. Jares P, Campo E. Advances in the understanding of mantle cell lymphoma. Br J Haematol. 2008;142(2):149–65. doi:10.1111/j.1365-2141.2008.07124.x.
25. Rosenwald A, Wright G, Wiestner A, et al. The proliferation gene expression signature is a quantitative integrator of oncogenic events that predicts survival in mantle cell lymphoma. Cancer Cell. 2003;3(2):185–97.
26. Tiemann M, Schrader C, Klapper W, et al. Histopathology, cell proliferation indices and clinical outcome in 304 patients with mantle cell lymphoma (MCL): a clinicopathological study from the European MCL Network. Br J Haematol. 2005;131(1):29–38.
27. Klapper W, Hoster E, Determann O, et al. Ki-67 as a prognostic marker in mantle cell lymphoma-consensus guidelines of the pathology panel of the European MCL Network. J Hematop. 2009;2(2):103–11. doi:10.1007/s12308-009-0036-x.
28. Hoster E, Klapper W, Rosenwald A, et al. Cell proliferation (Ki-67) as prognostic marker in mantle cell lymphoma. Blood. 2012;120:2677.
29. de Jong D, Rosenwald A, Chhanabhai M, et al. Immunohistochemical prognostic markers in diffuse large B-cell lymphoma: validation of tissue microarray as a prerequisite for broad clinical applications–a study from the Lunenburg Lymphoma Biomarker Consortium. J Clin Oncol. 2007;25(7):805–12.
30. Kienle D, Katzenberger T, Ott G, et al. Quantitative gene expression deregulation in mantle-cell lymphoma: correlation with clinical and biologic factors. J Clin Oncol. 2007;25(19):2770–7.
31. Hartmann E, Fernàndez V, Moreno V, et al. Five-gene model to predict survival in mantle-cell lymphoma using frozen or formalin-fixed, paraffin-embedded tissue. J Clin Oncol. 2008;26(30):4966–72. doi:10.1200/JCO.2007.12.0410.
32. Hernández L, Beà S, Pinyol M, et al. CDK4 and MDM2 gene alterations mainly occur in highly proliferative and aggressive mantle cell lymphomas with wild-type INK4a/ARF locus. Cancer Res. 2005;65(6):2199–206.
33. Salaverria I, Zettl A, Beà S, et al. Specific secondary genetic alterations in mantle cell lymphoma provide prognostic information independent of the gene expression-based proliferation signature. J Clin Oncol. 2007;25(10):1216–22.

34. Dreyling M, Thieblemont C, Gallamini A, et al. ESMO Consensus conferences: guidelines on malignant lymphoma. part 2: marginal zone lymphoma, mantle cell lymphoma, peripheral T-cell lymphoma. Ann Oncol. 2013;24(4):857–77.
35. Orchard J, Garand R, Davis Z, et al. A subset of t(11;14) lymphoma with mantle cell features displays mutated IgVH genes and includes patients with good prognosis, nonnodal disease. Blood. 2003;101(12):4975–81.
36. Royo C, Navarro A, Clot G, et al. Non-nodal type of mantle cell lymphoma is a specific biological and clinical subgroup of the disease. Leukemia. 2012;26(8):1895–8. doi:10.1038/leu.2012.72.
37. Velders GA, Kluin-Nelemans JC, De Boer CJ, et al. Mantle-cell lymphoma: a population-based clinical study. J Clin Oncol. 1996;14(4):1269–74.
38. Argatoff LH, Connors JM, Klasa RJ, et al. Mantle cell lymphoma: a clinicopathologic study of 80 cases. Blood. 1997;89(6):2067–78.
39. Møller MB, Pedersen NT, Christensen BE. Mantle cell lymphoma: prognostic capacity of the Follicular Lymphoma International Prognostic Index. Br J Haematol. 2006;133(1):43–9.
40. Geisler CH, Kolstad A, Laurell A, et al. The Mantle Cell Lymphoma International Prognostic Index (MIPI) is superior to the International Prognostic Index (IPI) in predicting survival following intensive first-line immunochemotherapy and autologous stem cell transplantation (ASCT). Blood. 2010;115(8):1530–3. doi:10.1182/blood-2009-08-236570.
41. van de Schans SA, Janssen-Heijnen ML, Nijziel MR, et al. Validation, revision and extension of the Mantle Cell Lymphoma International Prognostic Index in a population-based setting. Haematologica. 2010;95(9):1503–9. doi:10.3324/haematol.2009.021113.
42. Chiappella A, Puccini B, Ferrero S, et al. Retrospective analysis of 206 mantle cell lymphoma patients at diagnosis: mantle cell International Prognostic Index (MIPI) Is a good predictor of death event In patients treated either with Rituximab-chemotherapy or Rituximab-high-dose-chemotherapy. Blood. 2010;116:1784.
43. Budde LE, Guthrie KA, Till BG, et al. Mantle cell lymphoma international prognostic index but not pretransplantation induction regimen predicts survival for patients with mantle-cell lymphoma receiving high-dose therapy and autologous stem-cell transplantation. J Clin Oncol. 2011;29(22):3023–9. doi:10.1200/JCO.2010.33.7055.
44. Pott C, Schrader C, Gesk S, et al. Quantitative assessment of molecular remission after high-dose therapy with autologous stem cell transplantation predicts long-term remission in mantle cell lymphoma. Blood. 2006;107(6):2271–8.
45. van der Velden VH, Cazzaniga G, Schrauder A, et al. Analysis of minimal residual disease by Ig/TCR gene rearrangements: guidelines for interpretation of real-time quantitative PCR data. Leukemia. 2007;21(4):604–11.
46. Ladetto M, Magni M, Pagliano G, et al. Rituximab induces effective clearance of minimal residual disease in molecular relapses of mantle cell lymphoma. Biol Blood Marrow Transplant. 2006;12:1270–6.
47. Andersen NS, Pedersen LB, Laurell A, et al. Pre-emptive treatment with rituximab of molecular relapse after autologous stem cell transplantation in mantle cell lymphoma. J Clin Oncol. 2009;27:4365–70.
48. Ferrero S, Monitillo L, Mantoan B, et al. Pre-emptive rituximab-based treatment of molecular relapses in follicular and mantle cell lymphoma. Ann Hematol. 2013;92(11):1503–11.
49. Schmidt C, Dreyling M. Therapy of mantle cell lymphoma: current standards and future strategies. Hematol Oncol Clin North Am. 2008;22(5):953–63. doi:10.1016/j.hoc.2008.07.001, ix.
50. Hernandez L, Fest T, Cazorla M, et al. p53 gene mutations and protein overexpression are associated with aggressive variants of mantle cell lymphomas. Blood. 1996; 87(8):3351–9.
51. Pinyol M, Bea S, Plà L, et al. Inactivation of RB1 in mantle-cell lymphoma detected by nonsense-mediated mRNA decay pathway inhibition and microarray analysis. Blood. 2007; 109(12):5422–9.
52. Zanetto U, Dong H, Huang Y, et al. Mantle cell lymphoma with aberrant expression of CD10. Histopathology. 2008;53(1):20–9. doi:10.1111/j.1365-2559.2008.03060.x.

53. Palumbo GA, Parrinello N, Fargione G, et al. CD200 expression may help in differential diagnosis between mantle cell lymphoma and B-cell chronic lymphocytic leukemia. Leuk Res. 2009;33(9):1212–6. doi:10.1016/j.leukres.2009.01.017.
54. Fu K, Weisenburger DD, Greiner TC, et al. Cyclin D1-negative mantle cell lymphoma: a clinicopathologic study based on gene expression profiling. Blood. 2005;106(13):4315–21.
55. Hartmann EM, Campo E, Wright G, et al. Pathway discovery in mantle cell lymphoma by integrated analysis of high-resolution gene expression and copy number profiling. Blood. 2010;116(6):953–61. doi:10.1182/blood-2010-01-263806.
56. Salaverria I, Royo C, Carvajal-Cuenca A, et al. CCND2 rearrangements are the most frequent genetic events in cyclin D1(−) mantle cell lymphoma. Blood. 2013;121(8):1394–402. doi:10.1182/blood-2012-08-452284.
57. Mozos A, Royo C, Hartmann E, et al. SOX11 expression is highly specific for mantle cell lymphoma and identifies the cyclin D1-negative subtype. Haematologica. 2009;94(11): 1555–62. doi:10.3324/haematol.2009.010264.
58. Dictor M, Ek S, Sundberg M, et al. Strong lymphoid nuclear expression of SOX11 transcription factor defines lymphoblastic neoplasms, mantle cell lymphoma and Burkitt's lymphoma. Haematologica. 2009;94(11):1563–8. doi:10.3324/haematol.2009.008474.
59. Cheson BD, Pfistner B, Juweid ME, et al. Revised response criteria for malignant lymphoma. J Clin Oncol. 2007;25(5):579–86.
60. Brepoels L, Stroobants S, De Wever W, et al. Positron emission tomography in mantle cell lymphoma. Leuk Lymphoma. 2008;49(9):1693–701. doi:10.1080/10428190802216707.
61. Hosein PJ, Pastorini VH, Paes FM, et al. Utility of positron emission tomography scans in mantle cell lymphoma. Am J Hematol. 2011;86(10):841–5. doi:10.1002/ajh.22126.
62. Cohen JB, Hall NC, Ruppert AS, et al. Association of pre-transplantation positron emission tomography/computed tomography and outcome in mantle cell lymphoma. Bone Marrow Transplant. 2013. doi:10.1038/bmt.2013.46.
63. Romaguera JE, Medeiros LJ, Hagemeister FB, et al. Frequency of gastrointestinal involvement and its clinical significance in mantle cell lymphoma. Cancer. 2003;97(3):586–91.
64. Salar A, Juanpere N, Bellosillo B, et al. Gastrointestinal involvement in mantle cell lymphoma: a prospective clinic, endoscopic, and pathologic study. Am J Surg Pathol. 2006;30(10):1274–80.
65. Ghielmini M, Zucca E. How I treat mantle cell lymphoma. Blood. 2009;114(8):1469–76. doi:10.1182/blood-2009-02-179739.
66. Bernard M, Tsang RW, Le LW, et al. Limited-stage mantle cell lymphoma: treatment outcomes at the Princess Margaret Hospital. Leuk Lymphoma. 2013;54(2):261–7. doi:10.3109/1042819 4.2012.711828.
67. Li ZM, Zucca E, Ghielmini M. Open questions in the management of mantle cell lymphoma. Cancer Treat Rev. 2013. doi:10.1016/j.ctrv.2012.12.013. pii: S0305-7372(13)00008-X. [Epub ahead of print].
68. Kluin-Nelemans HC, Doorduijn JK. Treatment of elderly patients with mantle cell lymphoma. Semin Hematol. 2011;48(3):208–13. doi:10.1053/j.seminhematol.2011.03.008.
69. Balducci L, Extermann M. Management of cancer in the older person: a practical approach. Oncologist. 2000;5(3):224–37.
70. Repetto L, Fratino L, Audisio RA, et al. Comprehensive geriatric assessment adds information to Eastern Cooperative Oncology Group performance status in elderly cancer patients: an Italian Group for Geriatric Oncology Study. J Clin Oncol. 2002;20(2):494–502.
71. Balducci L. New paradigms for treating elderly patients with cancer: the comprehensive geriatric assessment and guidelines for supportive care. J Support Oncol. 2003;1(4 Suppl 2): 30–7.
72. Lenz G, Dreyling M, Hoster E, et al. Immunochemotherapy with rituximab and cyclophosphamide, doxorubicin, vincristine, and prednisone significantly improves response and time to treatment failure, but not long-term outcome in patients with previously untreated mantle cell lymphoma: results of a prospective randomized trial of the German Low Grade Lymphoma Study Group (GLSG). J Clin Oncol. 2005;23(9):1984–92.
73. Schulz H, Bohlius J, Skoetz N, et al. Chemotherapy plus Rituximab versus chemotherapy alone for B-cell non-Hodgkin's lymphoma. Cochrane Database Syst Rev. 2007;(4):CD003805.

74. Zinzani PL, Magagnoli M, Moretti L, et al. Fludarabine-based chemotherapy in untreated mantle cell lymphomas: an encouraging experience in 29 patients. Haematologica. 1999;84(11):1002–6.
75. Foran JM, Rohatiner AZ, Coiffier B, et al. Multicenter phase II study of fludarabine phosphate for patients with newly diagnosed lymphoplasmacytoid lymphoma, Waldenström's macroglobulinemia, and mantle-cell lymphoma. J Clin Oncol. 1999;17(2):546–53.
76. Zinzani PL, Magagnoli M, Moretti L, et al. Randomized trial of fludarabine versus fludarabine and idarubicin as frontline treatment in patients with indolent or mantle-cell lymphoma. J Clin Oncol. 2000;18(4):773–9.
77. Hiddemann W, Dreyling M. Mantle cell lymphoma: therapeutic strategies are different from CLL. Curr Treat Options Oncol. 2003;4(3):219–26.
78. Forstpointner R, Dreyling M, Repp R, et al. The addition of rituximab to a combination of fludarabine, cyclophosphamide, mitoxantrone (FCM) significantly increases the response rate and prolongs survival as compared with FCM alone in patients with relapsed and refractory follicular and mantle cell lymphomas: results of a prospective randomized study of the German Low-Grade Lymphoma Study Group. Blood. 2004;104(10):3064–71.
79. Kluin-Nelemans HC, Hoster E, Hermine O, et al. Treatment of older patients with mantle-cell lymphoma. N Engl J Med. 2012;367(6):520–31. doi:10.1056/NEJMoa1200920.
80. Rummel MJ, Al-Batran SE, Kim SZ, et al. Bendamustine plus rituximab is effective and has a favorable toxicity profile in the treatment of mantle cell and low-grade non-Hodgkin's lymphoma. J Clin Oncol. 2005;23(15):3383–9.
81. Robinson KS, Williams ME, van der Jagt RH, et al. Phase II multicenter study of bendamustine plus rituximab in patients with relapsed indolent B-cell and mantle cell non-Hodgkin's lymphoma. J Clin Oncol. 2008;26(27):4473–9. doi:10.1200/JCO.2008.17.0001.
82. Rummel MJ, Niederle N, Maschmeyer G, et al. Bendamustine plus rituximab versus CHOP plus rituximab as first-line treatment for patients with indolent and mantle-cell lymphomas: an open-label, multicentre, randomised, phase 3 non-inferiority trial. Lancet. 2013. doi:10.1016/S0140-6736(12)61763-2. pii: S0140-6736(12)61763-2.
83. Herold M, Schulze A, Niederwieser D, et al. Bendamustine, vincristine and prednisone (BOP) versus cyclophosphamide, vincristine and prednisone (COP) in advanced indolent non-Hodgkin's lymphoma and mantle cell lymphoma: results of a randomised phase III trial (OSHO# 19). J Cancer Res Clin Oncol. 2006;132(2):105–12.
84. Visco C, Finotto S, Zambello R, et al. Combination of rituximab, bendamustine, and cytarabine for patients with mantle-cell non-Hodgkin lymphoma ineligible for intensive regimens or autologous transplantation. J Clin Oncol. 2013;31(11):1442–9. doi:10.1200/JCO.2012.45.9842.
85. Goy A, Younes A, McLaughlin P, et al. Phase II study of proteasome inhibitor bortezomib in relapsed or refractory B-cell non-Hodgkin's lymphoma. J Clin Oncol. 2005;23(4):667–75.
86. O'Connor OA, Wright J, Moskowitz C, et al. Phase II clinical experience with the novel proteasome inhibitor bortezomib in patients with indolent non-Hodgkin's lymphoma and mantle cell lymphoma. J Clin Oncol. 2005;23(4):676–84.
87. Fisher RI, Bernstein SH, Kahl BS, et al. Multicenter phase II study of bortezomib in patients with relapsed or refractory mantle cell lymphoma. J Clin Oncol. 2006;24(30):4867–74.
88. Wiernik PH, Lossos IS, Tuscano JM, et al. Lenalidomide monotherapy in relapsed or refractory aggressive non-Hodgkin's lymphoma. J Clin Oncol. 2008;26(30):4952–7. doi:10.1200/JCO.2007.15.3429.
89. Witzig TE, Vose JM, Zinzani PL, et al. An international phase II trial of single-agent lenalidomide for relapsed or refractory aggressive B-cell non-Hodgkin's lymphoma. Ann Oncol. 2011;22(7):1622–7. doi:10.1093/annonc/mdq626.
90. Ruan J, Martin P, Furman RR, et al. Bortezomib plus CHOP-rituximab for previously untreated diffuse large B-cell lymphoma and mantle cell lymphoma. J Clin Oncol. 2011;29(6):690–7. doi:10.1200/JCO.2010.31.1142.
91. Houot R, Le Gouill S, Ojeda Uribe M, et al. Combination of rituximab, bortezomib, doxorubicin, dexamethasone and chlorambucil (RiPAD+C) as first-line therapy for elderly mantle cell lymphoma patients: results of a phase II trial from the GOELAMS. Ann Oncol. 2012;23(6):1555–61. doi:10.1093/annonc/mdr450.

92. Bauwens D, Maerevoet M, Michaux L, et al. Activity and safety of combined rituximab with chlorambucil in patients with mantle cell lymphoma. Br J Haematol. 2005;131(3):338–40.
93. Ghielmini M, Schmitz SF, Cogliatti S, et al. Effect of single-agent rituximab given at the standard schedule or as prolonged treatment in patients with mantle cell lymphoma: a study of the Swiss Group for Clinical Cancer Research (SAKK). J Clin Oncol. 2005;23(4):705–11.
94. Teodorovic I, Pittaluga S, Kluin-Nelemans JC, et al. Efficacy of four different regimens in 64 mantle-cell lymphoma cases: clinicopathologic comparison with 498 other non-Hodgkin's lymphoma subtypes. European Organization for the Research and Treatment of Cancer Lymphoma Cooperative Group. J Clin Oncol. 1995;13(11):2819–26.
95. Smith MR, Li H, Gordon L, et al. Phase II study of rituximab plus cyclophosphamide, doxorubicin, vincristine, and prednisone immunochemotherapy followed by yttrium-90-ibritumomab tiuxetan in untreated mantle-cell lymphoma: Eastern Cooperative Oncology Group Study E1499. J Clin Oncol. 2012;30(25):3119–26. doi:10.1200/JCO.2012.42.2444.
96. Leitch HA, Gascoyne RD, Chhanabhai M, et al. Limited-stage mantle-cell lymphoma. Ann Oncol. 2003;14(10):1555–61.
97. Tam CS, Bassett R, Ledesma C, et al. Mature results of the M.D. Anderson Cancer Center risk-adapted transplantation strategy in mantle cell lymphoma. Blood. 2009;113(18):4144–52. doi:10.1182/blood-2008-10-184200.
98. Hamadani M, Saber W, Ahn KW, et al. Allogeneic hematopoietic cell transplantation for chemotherapy-unresponsive mantle cell lymphoma: a cohort analysis from the center for international blood and marrow transplant research. Biol Blood Marrow Transplant. 2013;19(4):625–31. doi:10.1016/j.bbmt.2013.01.009.
99. Rodríguez J, Gutierrez A, Palacios A, et al. Rituximab, gemcitabine and oxaliplatin: an effective regimen in patients with refractory and relapsing mantle cell lymphoma. Leuk Lymphoma. 2007;48(11):2172–8.
100. Witzig TE, Geyer SM, Kurtin PJ, et al. Salvage chemotherapy with rituximab DHAP for relapsed non-Hodgkin lymphoma: a phase II trial in the North Central Cancer Treatment Group. Leuk Lymphoma. 2008;49(6):1074–80. doi:10.1080/10428190801993470.
101. Ruan J, Martin P, Coleman M, et al. Durable responses with the metronomic rituximab and thalidomide plus prednisone, etoposide, procarbazine, and cyclophosphamide regimen in elderly patients with recurrent mantle cell lymphoma. Cancer. 2010;116(11):2655–64. doi:10.1002/cncr.25055.
102. Coleman M, Ruan G, Elstrom RL, et al. Metronomic therapy for refractory/relapsed lymphoma: the PEP-C low-dose oral combination chemotherapy regimen. Hematology. 2012;17 Suppl 1:S90–2. doi:10.1179/102453312X13336169155970.
103. Baiocchi RA, Alinari L, Lustberg ME, et al. Phase 2 trial of rituximab and bortezomib in patients with relapsed or refractory mantle cell and follicular lymphoma. Cancer. 2011;117(11):2442–51.
104. Lamm W, Kaufmann H, Raderer M, et al. Bortezomib combined with rituximab and dexamethasone is an active regimen for patients with relapsed and chemotherapy-refractory mantle cell lymphoma. Haematologica. 2011;96(7):1008–14. doi:10.3324/haematol.2011.041392.
105. Weigert O, Weidmann E, Mueck R, et al. A novel regimen combining high dose cytarabine and bortezomib has activity in multiply relapsed and refractory mantle cell lymphoma - long-term results of a multicenter observation study. Leuk Lymphoma. 2009;50(5):716–22. doi:10.1080/10428190902856790.
106. Gerecitano J, Portlock C, Hamlin P, et al. Phase I trial of weekly and twice-weekly bortezomib with rituximab, cyclophosphamide, and prednisone in relapsed or refractory non-Hodgkin lymphoma. Clin Cancer Res. 2011;17(8):2493–501. doi:10.1158/1078-0432.CCR-10-1498.
107. Friedberg JW, Vose JM, Kelly JL, et al. The combination of bendamustine, bortezomib, and rituximab for patients with relapsed/refractory indolent and mantle cell non-Hodgkin lymphoma. Blood. 2011;117(10):2807–12. doi:10.1182/blood-2010-11-314708.
108. Kouroukis CT, Fernandez LA, Crump M, et al. A phase II study of bortezomib and gemcitabine in relapsed mantle cell lymphoma from the National Cancer Institute of

Canada Clinical Trials Group (IND 172). Leuk Lymphoma. 2011;52(3):394–9. doi:10.3109/10428194.2010.546015.

109. Hess G, Herbrecht R, Romaguera J, et al. Phase III study to evaluate temsirolimus compared with investigator's choice therapy for the treatment of relapsed or refractory mantle cell lymphoma. J Clin Oncol. 2009;27(23):3822–9. doi:10.1200/JCO.2008.20.7977.
110. Ansell SM, Tang H, Kurtin PJ, et al. Temsirolimus and rituximab in patients with relapsed or refractory mantle cell lymphoma: a phase 2 study. Lancet Oncol. 2011;12(4):361–8. doi:10.1016/S1470-2045(11)70062-6.
111. Hess G, Keller H, Atta J, et al. Temsirolimus in Combination with Bendamustine and Rituximab for the Treatment of Relapsed Mantle Cell and Follicular Lymphoma: Report on An Ongoing Phase I/II Trial. Blood (ASH Annual Meeting Abstracts). 2011;118:2697.
112. Renner C, Zinzani PL, Gressin R, et al. A multicenter phase II trial (SAKK 36/06) of single-agent everolimus (RAD001) in patients with relapsed or refractory mantle cell lymphoma. Haematologica. 2012;97(7):1085–91. doi:10.3324/haematol.2011.053173.
113. Eve HE, Carey S, Richardson SJ, et al. Single-agent lenalidomide in relapsed/refractory mantle cell lymphoma: results from a UK phase II study suggest activity and possible gender differences. Br J Haematol. 2012;159(2):154–63. doi:10.1111/bjh.12008.
114. Wang M, Fayad L, Wagner-Bartak N, et al. Lenalidomide in combination with rituximab for patients with relapsed or refractory mantle-cell lymphoma: a phase 1/2 clinical trial. Lancet Oncol. 2012;13(7):716–23. doi:10.1016/S1470-2045(12)70200-0.
115. Kaufmann H, Raderer M, Wöhrer S, et al. Antitumor activity of rituximab plus thalidomide in patients with relapsed/refractory mantle cell lymphoma. Blood. 2004;104(8):2269–71.
116. Harel S, Bachy E, Haioun C, et al. Efficacy and safety of thalidomide in mantle cell lymphoma: results of the French ATU Program. Blood. 2010;116:1794.
117. Dreyling M, Kluin-Nelemans HC, Beà S, et al. Update on the molecular pathogenesis and clinical treatment of mantle cell lymphoma: report of the 11th annual conference of the European Mantle Cell Lymphoma Network. Leuk Lymphoma. 2013;54(4):699–707. doi:10.3109/10428194.2012.733882.
118. Wang M, Oki Y, Pro B, et al. Phase II study of yttrium-90-ibritumomab tiuxetan in patients with relapsed or refractory mantle cell lymphoma. J Clin Oncol. 2009;27(31):5213–8. doi:10.1200/JCO.2009.21.8545.
119. Beaven AW, Shea TC, Moore DT, et al. A phase I study evaluating ibritumomab tiuxetan (Zevalin®) in combination with bortezomib (Velcade®) in relapsed/refractory mantle cell and low grade B-cell non-Hodgkin lymphoma. Leuk Lymphoma. 2012;53(2):254–8. doi:10.3109/10428194.2011.608445. Epub 2011 Sep 19.
120. Wang M, Rule SA, Martin P, et al. Interim results of an international, multicenter, Phase 2 study of Bruton's tyrosine kinase (BTK) inhibitor, ibrutinib (PCI-32765), in relapsed or refractory mantle cell lymphoma (MCL): durable efficacy and tolerability with longer follow-up. Blood. 2012;120:904.
121. Kahl B, Byrd JC, Flinn IW, et al. Clinical safety and activity in a Phase 1 study of CAL-101, an isoform-selective inhibitor of phosphatidylinositol 3-kinase P110{delta}, in patients with relapsed or refractory non-Hodgkin lymphoma. Blood. 2010;116:1777.
122. Cartron G, Thieblemont C, Solal-Celigny P, et al. Promising efficacy with the new anti-CD20 antibody GA101 in heavily pre-treated NHL patients – first results from a Phase II study in patients with relapsed/refractory DLBCL and MCL. Blood. 2010;116:2878.
123. Magni M, Di Nicola M, Carlo-Stella C, et al. Safety, tolerability and activity of Ofatumumab, Bendamustine and Dexamethasone combination as first-line treatment of mantle-cell lymphoma in the elderly: a Multicenter Study. Blood. 2011;118:1647.
124. Vose JM, Loberiza FR, Bociek RG, et al. Phase I/II trial of Ofatumumab/Lenalidamide for patients with relasped/refractory B-cell non-Hodgkin lymphoma: high response rate in indolent lymphoma. Blood. 2012;120:3692.
125. Bargou R, Leo E, Zugmaier G, et al. Tumor regression in cancer patients by very low doses of a T cell-engaging antibody. Science. 2008;321(5891):974–7. doi:10.1126/science.1158545.

126. Viardot A, Goebeler M, Scheele JS, et al. Treatment of patients with non-Hodgkin lymphoma (NHL) with CD19/CD3 bispecific antibody blinatumomab (MT103): double-step dose increase to continuous infusion of 60 μg/m^2/d is tolerable and highly effective. Blood. 2010;116:2880.
127. Palanca-Wessels MC, Flinn IW, Sehn LH, et al. A Phase I study of the anti-CD79b antibody-drug conjugate (ADC) DCDS4501A targeting CD79b in relapsed or refractory B-cell non-Hodgkin's lymphoma (NHL). Blood. 2012;120:56.
128. Lin TS, Blum KA, Fischer DB, et al. Flavopiridol, fludarabine, and rituximab in mantle cell lymphoma and indolent B-cell lymphoproliferative disorders. J Clin Oncol. 2010;28(3):418–23. doi:10.1200/JCO.2009.24.1570.
129. Holkova B, Perkins EB, Ramakrishnan V, et al. Phase I trial of bortezomib (PS-341; NSC 681239) and alvocidib (flavopiridol; NSC 649890) in patients with recurrent or refractory B-cell neoplasms. Clin Cancer Res. 2011;17(10):3388–97. doi:10.1158/1078-0432.CCR-10-2876.
130. Leonard JP, LaCasce AS, Smith MR, et al. Selective CDK4/6 inhibition with tumor responses by PD0332991 in patients with mantle cell lymphoma. Blood. 2012;119(20):4597–607. doi:10.1182/blood-2011-10-388298.
131. Davids MS, Roberts AW, Anderson MA, et al. The BCL-2-specific BH3-Mimetic ABT-199 (GDC-0199) is active and well-tolerated in patients with relapsed non-Hodgkin lymphoma: interim results of a Phase I study. Blood. 2012;120:304.
132. Evens AM, Vose JM, Harb W, et al. A Phase II multicenter study of the histone deacetylase inhibitor (HDACi) abexinostat (PCI-24781) in relapsed/refractory follicular lymphoma (FL) and mantle cell lymphoma (MCL). Blood. 2012;120:55.
133. Rizzo JD, Brouwers M, Hurley P, et al. American Society of Clinical Oncology/American Society of Hematology clinical practice guideline update on the use of epoetin and darbepoetin in adult patients with cancer. J Clin Oncol. 2010;28(33):4996–5010. doi:10.1200/JCO.2010.29.2201.
134. Aapro MS, Bohlius J, Cameron DA, et al. 2010 update of EORTC guidelines for the use of granulocyte-colony stimulating factor to reduce the incidence of chemotherapy-induced febrile neutropenia in adult patients with lymphoproliferative disorders and solid tumours. Eur J Cancer. 2011;47(1):8–32. doi:10.1016/j.ejca.2010.10.013.
135. NCCN guidelines for supportive care: http://www.nccn.org

Chapter 10
Hodgkin Lymphoma in the Elderly

Paul Fields

Abstract The treatment of Hodgkin Lymphoma has continued to improve, however the advances achieved in younger patients have not been replicated in elderly group affected with this disease. The reasons for this are multifactorial, and in part due to the presence of co-morbid illness, the inability to tolerate therapies which are curative in younger age cohorts, poor functional status and intrinsic biological disease characteristics which differ between the older and younger patient. As a result fewer elderly patients are entered into clinical trials, and there exists no uniform consensus as how to treat the elderly patient off trial. Because of this, urgent new therapies are required to treat the elderly patient, which still may offer the chance of long term survival whilst minimising particularly for the elderly patient, any attendant short term toxicities. This review examines the results of previous chemotherapy directed approaches, summarises the results of more recent chemotherapeutic approaches, and finally examines the encouraging recent results incorporating targeted biological approaches which may ultimately deliver improved outcomes for the elderly patient affected with this disease.

Keywords Hodgkin • Lymphoma • RS Cell • Eldery • Cancer

Introduction

In recent years there has been significant success in the treatment of younger patients with Hodgkin lymphoma (HL); however these treatment successes have not been replicated in the older patient affected with Hodgkin Lymphoma. This is, in part, due to presence of co-morbid illnesses, the inability to tolerate therapies which are curative in younger age cohorts, poor functional status and different adverse biological disease characteristics. As a result fewer proportionate elderly patients enter clinical trials and there remains no uniform consensus approach on how to treat the elderly patient off trial. In the next few years the proportion of patients over 80 years

P. Fields, MD
Department of Haematology, Guy's and St Thomas' and Kings College Hospitals, Kings Health Partners AHSC, London, UK
e-mail: Paul.Fields@gstt.nhs.uk

U. Wedding, R.A. Audisio (eds.), *Management of Hematological Cancer in Older People*, DOI 10.1007/978-1-4471-2837-3_10

is expected to double and this renders the need to develop more optimal treatment strategies imperative. The current gold standard in younger patients such as ABVD is not readily applicable to the elderly patient. This review examines the results of previous elderly studies and summarise newer chemotherapy approaches and recent developments incorporating targeted biological approaches which may help circumvent the requirement for combination chemotherapy in the elderly patient.

Pathology and Morphological Diagnosis

The classical malignant cell in Hodgkin Lymphoma is the Reed Sternberg cell (RS cell) and is typically a large cell with two or more nuclear lobes containing separate nucleoli creating an "owl's eye appearance". Reed Sternberg cells are derived are derived from B lymphocytes. The tumour itself may only contain 1 % malignant cells surrounded by varying proportions of infiltrating monoclear cells including T lymphocytes , macrophages , neutrophils, eosinophils and plasma cells and this may lead to difficulty in securing a definitive histological diagnosis. Histological subtypes of classical HL are described according to the morphological features and are termed Nodular sclerosis (NS, the majority of cases in the younger cohort), mixed cellularity, lymphocyte rich and lymphocyte depleted and these variants constitute classical Hodgkin Lymphoma. Although stage distribution is similar in young and elderly patients, the proportion of patients with mixed cellularity morphological type is higher in the elderly cohorts [1, 2].

Immunohistostaining for cell markers in classical Hodgkin lymphoma reveals RS cells as CD30+ve and usually CD15+ve while Lymphocyte predominant (LP) cells are CD30-ve, CD15- but CD45+ve and CD20+ve. Cell of origin molecular studies reveal both RS and LP cells have undergone immunoglobulin gene rearrangements in keeping with B cell lineage derivation. The less common Nodular Lymphocyte predominant Hodgkin Lymphoma subtype (NLPHL) characteristically displays a nodular morphological architecture and the malignant cells are again infrequent and large, typically with single but multilobated nuclei that often contain multiple small nucleoli. These cells have popcorn like appearance and have been termed lymphocyte predominant cells (LP cells).

Biological Characteristics

The biology of elderly HL is different in that the mixed cellularity subtype predominates histologically, and there is an increased association with EBV when compared to younger cohorts and this is also a poor prognostic factor in the elderly cohort but not for other groups. In a retrospective analysis by Diepstra et al., Epstein Barr (EBV) positivity was associated with a decreased failure free survival in the elderly and retained its poor prognostic status on a multivariate analysis [3].

In a series of 922 patients with classical Hodgkin's lymphoma between 1988 and 1997 biopsy specimens were retrieved and assayed for EBV with immunohistochemistry and insitu hybridisation [4]. From the result of this series, in older patients aged between 45 and 96 years with the Nodular Sclerosis subtype (NS), the presence of EBV nearly doubled the risk of overall and HL specific mortality even after adjustment for age, stage at diagnosis and other factors. Two further prior population based studies of adults greater than 60 years demonstrated poor overall survival and disease specific survival in EBV + ve HL compared with EBV-ve patients similar to the findings observed in the Keegan study of patients aged greater than 45 years [5, 6].

The mechanisms by which EBV promote cellular survival are multiple, including pathways which increase cell proliferation, decrease apoptosis and enhanced evasion of the immune response in part caused by down regulation of HLA presentation of viral peptides. The variation and impact of tumour cell EBV on Hodgkin's lymphoma in different patient groups suggests that these may represent different biological disease entities and is founded upon epidemiological evidence and the changes observed between EBV cellular immunity status in young and old patients. In general immune senescence in the elderly may facilitate a more active proliferation in EBV + ve tumours [7] than that which occurs in children and young adults where EBV antigens might stimulate a more potent anti-EBV or anti-tumour immune response. It is interesting that EBV HL tumour cells may escape immune surveillance. LMP1 expression may alter the immune response in that the viral protein induces expression of interleukin-10 or interleukin-6 which are cytokines that pertubate cellular immune responses [8, 9], and high tumour concentrations of IL-10 are noted to suppress local EBV specific cellular cytoxicity to permit local proliferation of the tumour, particularly in patients with age related decline in immune competence. These mechanisms and the interaction of tumour cells with the microenvironment deserve more scientific investigation in future studies which may lead to the design of more rationale biological targeted interventions in patients who are unable to undergo treatment with conventional chemotherapy.

Disease Staging

Disease stage at presentation predicts outcome with early stage disease achieving a better prognosis than presentation with advanced stage disease. The disease assessment at diagnosis and restaging has evolved from simple X ray imaging in conjunction with laparotomy and often splenectomy with lymphangiography in the 1970s, to full body CT scanning routinely and more recently the introduction of the use of positron emission tomography in combination with CT (PET/CT). The sensitivity of PET/CT is greater than that of conventional CT for identifying both nodal and extra nodal disease [10, 11] and prospective studies are addressing its utility in patient outcome both as a diagnostic modality and at restaging to evaluate response to treatment [12].

Clinical Features of Elderly Hodgkin's

In numerous early studies elderly patients were often noted to present with advanced disease, but more recent studies from the German Hodgkin Study Group (GHSG) of 372 patients documented a high incidence of very early as well as very late disease which echoed previous studies [5, 13, 14]. Elderly patients tended to show a female preponderance, present more often with B symptoms and higher ECOG scores, and interestingly elderly patients less often present with mediastinal masses as observed in younger cohorts.

Prognostic Factors

In elderly Hodgkin's increasing age >70 has been shown to be associated with inferior survival rates [15, 16]. Multiple retrospective studies have stressed the presence of co–morbidities and func-tional impairment which correlate with poorer outcome [17–19]. In an early study by Levis et al. in patients treated with VEPEMB, multivariate analysis showed that in addition to advanced stage and the presence of B symptoms the presence of co-morbidity associated with inferior disease specific survival [18].In a large US series, loss of ADL, and age greater than 70 years were the most significant prognostic factors in a multivariate analysis [16].It is clear that more elderly patients are unable to tolerate multi agent chemotherapy regimens as well as younger patients, and this in part results in suboptimal dose intensity being delivered. In elderly patients with ABVD, Landren et al. reported that relative dose intensity of >65 % was required to achieve significantly improved OS as compared to less <65 %, and unfortunately this is rarely only ever achieved [15]. Importantly as with other forms of Lymphoma, achievement of CR status to induction therapy is important to predict long term outcome. Proctor et al. reported in patients treated with the VEPMB regimen, that achievement of CR was the only factor which predicted for enhanced OS in a multivariate analysis [17]. For patients presenting with advanced stage disease the clinical characteristics defined in the international prognostic index have enabled upfront risk stratification to be made. However it is noteworthy in the original Hasenclever classification, only 9 % patients over the age of 55 years and none older than 65 years were included in the series making applicability to elderly Hodgkin patients uncertain [16].

Co-Morbidity and Hodgkin Lymphoma

The incidence of co-morbidity rises with age and this is an important factor in accounting for poor treatment outcome in Hodgkin lymphoma. In a Dutch population study by Van Sprosen et al., 194 HL patients were registered with assessment of age specific co –morbid illnesses and their impact on outcome was reported [20]. 56 % of patients who were 60 years or older suffered with severe co-morbidity with no differences observed in prevalence between early or advanced disease presentation. The most frequent co-morbidities observed cardiovascular disease (18 %), hypertension (13 %), COPD (13 %), and diabetes mellitus (10 %). In the presence of co-morbidity 50 % less chemotherapy was administered to patients with HL which resulted in poorer OS particularly within 4 months after diagnosis [20]. Further studies confirmed the high incidence of co-morbid illness in older HL patients, with Levis et al. reporting 37 % of 105 elderly HL patients treated with VEPEMB carried attendant co-morbid illness [18].

Treatment

The aim of treatment in HL in all patient groups is to maximise the chance of cure whilst limiting both immediate and long term complications of therapy. However in the elderly population early toxicity is of more immediate concern as it is heavily impacted by the condition of the patient at presentation in terms of functional status, critical organ integrity, and the presence of attendant co–morbid illness. The treatment decision needs therefore to minimise these factors whilst aiming to deliver maximal therapeutic benefit. For the elderly patient there have been few age directed Hodgkin studies, and many of the lessons learned about the issues treating the more elderly patient have evolved from studies in which all age ranges and groups were treated in a similar fashion. Patients with classical HL are divided into three treatment groups; early favourable, early unfavourable (intermediate) which comprise early stage disease and patients in the advanced disease category.

Early Stage Disease: Fit Patients

In a recent publication by Boll et al., the use of ABVD in early stage HL was analysed from German Study Group HD 10 and HD 11 trials [21]. In total 1,299 patients of which 117 aged 60–75 years, were treated with 4 cycles of ABVD followed by either 30 Gy or 20 Gy involved field radiotherapy (IFTR). In 14 % of the patients treatment was not administered according to protocol because of excessive toxicity. The mean delay in treatment was twice as high for elderly patients, and 59 % achieved a dose intensity of >80 % compared to 85 % of younger patients. WHO 3 and 4 for leucopoenia, nausea, and infection was recorded in 68 % of patients with a treatment related mortality of 5 % as compared to 0.3 % for those aged <60 years. At a median follow up of 92 months, 28 % of patients had died and the 5 year PFS and OS estimate was 75 and 81 %. In this series of patients 7 % mortality was attributed to cardiac causes, which may in part be due to toxicity induced by chemotherapy or radiotherapy. Compared to earlier trials, the survival rates are higher compared to patients with early stage treated with chemotherapy and extended field radiotherapy alone with a 5 year survival rate of 55 %. Further data on the use of VEPMB in early stage disease reported a 5 year FFS and OS of 79 and 94 % respectively and in another study of 3 cycles of VEPMB followed by radiation a 3 year PFS and OS of 74 and 81 % was attained [17].

Advanced Stage Disease: Fit Patients

Definitive treatment algorithms for HL in the elderly are lacking and there is no world-wide consensus approach to the treatment of the elderly patient with advanced disease. Due to increased age, presence of co-morbidities and impaired functional status it is difficult to administer adequate dose intense aggressive regimens to such groups of patients. In elderly patients considerations such as development of secondary malignancies and infertility are not as important as in younger populations and more aggressive regimens are not likely to be tolerated by the more elderly patients. Therefore there is an urgent clinical need to discover age appropriate regimens which can still deliver with curative intent.

ABVD and BEACOPP Based Regimens (Table 10.1)

In younger patients ABVD has been very successful treatment for advanced stage disease however in the more elderly population results with the regimen are inferior. The regimen includes Doxorubicin and Bleomycin and this is of concern in patients who carry attendant cardiorespiratory co-morbid illness. The CALBG group reported 5 years OS of 31 % versus 79 % for patients less than 40 years. In a further study Levis et al. comparing ABVD vs. hybrid regimen of ABVD/MOPP found results in patients >65 years with 8 year event free survival (EFS) of 41 % and overall survival of 46 %. Importantly these poor survival rates were in part due to the high reported a treatment related mortality TRM of 23 % observed with the use of ABVD/MOPP like chemotherapy [26].

In a further study reporting [24] the American intergroup trial E2496 44 patients aged >60 years were entered into the study and received either ABVD or the Stanford V regimen. No survival difference was reported between the ABVD and Stanford V arms. However the incidence of Bleomycin lung toxicity was reported to be as high as 24 %, of which the majority occurred in the ABVD arm and an resultant associated Bleomycin mortality rate of 18 % was observed [24]. Exploratory analyses compared outcomes on the basis of age, which confirmed a higher treatment related mortality rate in more elderly patients of 9 % vs. 0.3 % for patients <60 years ($p<0.001$) and reported a 5 years OS of 58 % compared to 90 % for younger patients ($p<0.0001$). When a competing risk analysis model was performed, the results suggested a major component of age dependent survival in HL was due to non- HL related events which emphasises the need for optimal co-morbid disease control in more elderly patients being treated for HL.

High intensity regimens such as escalated BEACOPP were tested in the GHSG HD9 prospective elderly trial and were randomised to receive either eight course of BEACOPP or eight courses of COPP-ABVD. The disease free specific freedom from treatment failure at 5 years was 74 % for BEACOPP and 55 % for COPP-ABVD. However the high toxic TRM rate of 21 % in patients greater than 60 years treated with BEACOPP resulted in equivalence in OS rates of 50 % in both arms,

Table 10.1 Selected early studies elderly Hodgkin lymphoma

Year Author	Number Median age	Treatment	Outcome	Therapy associated death rate	Comment
1994 Levis et al. [27]	65 72 years	ABVD; MOPP/ABVD	CR 67 % 8 year OS 46 % 8 year EFS 41 %	23 %	Elderly treatment related mortality 23 % in ABVD regimens
2002 Weekes et al. [2]	56	ChlVPP (31) ChlVPP/ABV (25) 25	5 year OS 30 % 5 year EFS 24 % 5 year OS 67 % 5 year EFS 52 %	13 % 16 %	Inclusion of an Anthracycline important to better outcomes in the elderly
2005 Ballova et al. [25]	68 70 years	COPP/ABVD BEACOPP baseline	CR 77 % 5 year OS 50 % CR 76 % 5 year 50 %	8 % 21 %	High TRM with dose intensive regimens Note Limited efficacy ABVD in elderly populations
2013 Evens et al. [24]	44 65 years	Stanford V/ABVD	5 Year OS Young 90 % Elderly 58 %	0.3 % young 9 % elderly	Outcome older versus younger significantly worse 24 % Bleomycin toxicity in the elder group

negating any benefit derive from dose intensification in this group [25]. As would be predicted the main cause of mortality in these patients was neutropaenic sepsis and in subsequent studies the use of antibiotic prophylaxis was mandated. In a subsequent multivariate analysis conducted to define factors associated with TRM, a simple algorithm to define a risk score identified the major risk factors as increased age ≥40 years and poor performance status (≥2) [26] and this underscores the toxicity and futility of intensive regimens like this in the more elderly patient.

Lower Intensity Regimens

In an effort to limit ABVD toxicity other less intensive regimens have been tried but with limited success. Levis et al. tested the CVP/CEB regimen which although producing less treatment related mortality resulted in higher relapse rates and a 5 year relapse free survival of 43 % [27]. A further retrospective study carried out by the Nebraska Lymphoma Study Group investigated the importance of anthracyline in drug combinations and randomised ChlVPP (Chlorambucil, vinblastine, procarbazine and prednisolone) versus the combination of ChlVPP/ABV. The 5 year event free survival (EFS) was 24 % treated with ChlVPP alone versus 52 % for those treated with the combination regimen (p=0.011) and 5 Year OS was 30 % versus 67 %. In a subsequent multivariate analysis the use of Doxorubicin was the only factor associated with superior outcomes and therefore remains important in the treatment of elderly HL patients [2]. A further study tested the VEPMB regimen (Vinblastine, cyclosphamide, procarabazine, etoposide, mitoxoantrone, Bleomycin) in which 57/105 patients with advanced disease received 6 cycles of treatment with consolidation radiotherapy to either bulky disease or residual mass. A reported a CR rate of 58 % at the end of treatment was noted with a 5 year FFS and OS of 34 and 32 % [18]. A further study randomised VEPEMB against ABVD and reported a 3 Year OS and EFS for ABVD and VEPMB of 79 % vs. 60 % (p=ns) and 52 % vs. 24 % (p=0.08) [28].

Tailored Specific Elderly Directed Treatment Regimens (Table 10.2)

In a search to develop tailor made elderly specific regimens to aim to deliver with curative intent, the GHSG have reported on two newer regimens in the elderly; BACOPP (Bleomycin, doxorubicin, cyclophosphamide, vincristine, procarbazine and prednisolone and PVAG (prednisolone, vinblastine, doxorubicin, and gemcitabine) in elderly untreated patients with HL. In the BACOPP regimen where etoposide was omitted to improve treatment related mortality the CR rate attained was 85 % and the 3 year PFS and OS 60 and 71 % respectively. However the regimen was associated with significant toxicity with 30 % of patient experiencing early termination (87 % with adverse grade III-IV adverse events) and a still reported TRM of 12 % making the regimen unsuitable [23]. The PVAG regimen replaced the

Table 10.2 Selected results Elderly directed non ABVD regimens

Name	Number Median age	Regimen	Outcome	Therapy associated death rate	Comment
2007 Kolstad et al. [30]	29 71 years	CHOP-21	CR 72 % 3 year OS 79 % 3 PFS 76 %	7.0 %	Small numbers
2010 Halbsguth et al. [23]	65 67 years	BACOPP	CR 88 % 3 year OS 71 % 3 year PFS 60 %	12 %	Still unacceptable TRM
2011 Boll et al. [29]	59 68 years	PVAG	CR 78 % 3 year OS 66 % 3 year PFS 58 %	1.7 %	Low TRM
2012 Proctor et al. [17]	103 73 years	VEPEMB + radiotherapy Early stage VEPEMB × 6 Advanced stage	Early stage CR 74 % 3 year OS 81 % 3 year PFS 74 % Advanced stage CR 61 % 3 year OS 66 % 3 year PFS 58 %	7.0 %	Achievement of CR significant for OS CR, co-morbidity, age, significant for PFS EBV status no significant effect on outcome

Bleomycin and Dacarabazine in ABVD with Gemcitabine and Prednisolone. A CR rate of 78 % was achieved and the 3 year PFS and OS of 58 and 66 % was achieved with a lower TRM of 2 % [29].

Kolstad and colleagues reported excellent results using the NHL regimen CHOP for elderly patients. 29 patients were treated with CHOP-21 for both early stage (2–4 cycles with IFRT) and advanced stage (6–8 cycles +/– IFTR). The CR rate was an impressive 93 % with a median follow up of 41 months and 3 year PFS and OS for advanced stage patients of 67 and 72 % respectively. This regimen may be useful in elderly patients where significant pulmonary co-morbidity is present and where avoidance of Bleomycin is desirable [30]. In a further effort to reduce cardiotoxicity, the use of VEPEMB (vinblastine, cyclosphosphamide, procacarabazine, etoposide, mitoxoantrone, bleomycin) regimen was tested in early and late stage disease reporting a CR rate of 98 % for early stage disease and 58 % for advanced stage patients. Five year FFS was 79 and 34 % for early and late stage disease respectively [18]. In a multivariate analysis stage, B symptoms and co morbidity maintained their independent prognostic value in affecting OS, DSS, and FFS. A follow on UK phase II study further tested the VEPEMB protocol and incorporated a co-morbidity assessment to define patients into a curative treatment approach (non-frail group) or define those as too frail to enter the treatment arm. This study permitted treating centres to record "all" patients in a population based study. A total of 103 patients of which 72 with advanced disease were designated non frail and eligible for VEPMB treatment. The reported CR rate was 61 % and 3 year PFS and OS for the advanced stage patients was 58 and 66 % respectively. Overall treatment related mortality was 7 %. A further 54 non frail patients either received ABVD, or ChlVPP chemotherapy. In all arms of the study with treatment with curative intent (n = 157), achievement of CR remained significant for OS and CR plus co-morbidity and age for PFS. Although the regimen contains Bleomycin pulmonary toxicity demonstrated was minimal [17]. None of those designated as frail completed or responded to chemotherapy, and the authors concluded that a novel agent approach may afford better outcomes in this group compared to chemotherapy. A further advance afforded by this study is that the suitability of patients to receive curative multi [31] agent chemotherapy was stratified by co-morbid assessment and other well defined measures such as ADL, IADL and ECOG which ensured a consistent assessment to stratify patient groups.

Newer Paradigms: Novel Targeted Approaches and Strategies to Improve Outcomes in the Elderly Population (Table 10.3)

Due to the toxicity encountered with chemotherapeutic regimens in the elderly as observed from previous studies, the development of novel agents which minimise these risks are desirable. Adcetris (Brentuximab vedotin, BV) is an innovative targeted antibody drug conjugate which targets the CD30, a cell surface antigen which is expressed on Hodgkin Reed Sternberg cells [35]. The antibody binds to CD30 on the cell surface and delivers the drug to CD30 positive cells. Upon internalisation

Table 10.3 New agents tested in relapsed/refractory Hodgkin lymphoma

Name	Number	Mechanism	Outcomes	Toxicity	Comment
Brentuximab Vedotin [32] 2012	102	Antibody drug conjugate	ORR 75 % CR 34 %	Neuropathy 42 % typically grade I/II Grade ≥3 Thrombocytopaenia 8 % Neutropaenia 20 %	Being tested as single agent/combination studies
HDAC Inhibitors [33] Panobinostat 2012	129	Anti proliferative/immune perturbation	27 % ORR CR 4 % PR 23 % Median response duration 6.9/12	Thrombocytopaenia 79 % Grade III/IV	Studies on going
Lenalidomide [22] 2011	36	Multiple: Ant proliferative/ microenvironment alterations	19 % ORR 1 CR 6 PR	Grade III, IV Neutropaenia 47 % Anaemia 29 % Thrombocytopaenia 18 %	Studies ongoing Combination with MTOR and HDAC inhibitors
Bendamustine [34] 2013	36	Bifunctional alkylator/ purine analogue	ORR 53 % CR 33 % PR 19 % Median duration of response 5/12	Grade ≥3 Thrombocytopaenia 20 % Anaemia 14 %, Infection 14 %	75 % failed ASCT Ongoing studies

and migration to the lysosome, monomethyl auristatin (MMAE) the antibody conjugate, is released into the cells and directly inhibits the microtubule network of dividing cells. When this occurs the cells undergo apoptosis. Recent phase I and Phase II studies in relapsed and refractory HL [31] has revealed excellent overall response rates with evidence of minimal toxicity in the cardiovascular and respiratory systems. In a pivotal phase II study of 102 patients with relapsed or refractory disease after autologous stem cell transplant, overall response was observed in 75 % of patients with CRs recorded in 34 % [32]. The median duration of response for responding patients was 6.7 and 20.5 months for patients who achieved CR. The most common adverse events were typically grade or 1 or 2 and were managed with standard supportive care. The most common side effect was cumulative peripheral neuropathy, typically sensory which improved or resolved in 80 % of patients during the study. Because of the toxicity particularly cardiac and pulmonary encountered with chemotherapy such as ABVD, the use of agents such as BV should be tested in elder frailer patients with HL who are considered unfit for chemotherapy. A trial is underway in the UK which tests this hypothesis (Brevity Study, Chief investigator J Radford). Further combination studies with AVD are underway in frontline HL studies (NCT 01476410). The use of CT-PET to permit response adaptive designs in these studies is advantageous. Further useful other novel agents include HDAC inhibitors [33] which exert direct antiproliferative effects on HRS cells and also perturbation of the cytokine and chemokine secretion leading to disrupted microenvironment milieu [36]. Several studies are underway evaluating the role of HDAC inhibitors in association with MTOR inhibitors and chemotherapy. Lenalidomide in phase II studies has demonstrated activity in relapsed refractory HL with ORR of 19.5 % with a cytostatic response rate of 33.3 % [22]. Because of the knowledge accrued through the prognostic significance of interim CT-PET in large prospective studies multivariate analysis has shown that interim PET response is the single most important prognostic feature in response adaptive therapies for advanced Hodgkin's Lymphoma [12]. These response adaptive strategies will be incorporated into the use of treatment of elderly HL in prospective studies testing novel agents such as BV.

Future Perspectives: Elderly Hodgkin Lymphoma

The treatment of HL has improved immeasurably over last two decades where large randomized clinical trials have led to defined standards of care for early and late forms of the disease. However the improvements made in the younger cohorts of the disease are not readily translated to success in the more elderly patient. To achieve success with ABVD required a minimum threshold RDI to be achieved and the inclusion of an Anthracycline. In the more elderly patient, the presence of attendant cardio respiratory co-morbidity and poor functional status may contraindicate the former approach and as such new forms of treatment are urgently required. In the good risk elderly patient who demonstrates no co-morbid illness, in particular no cardio-respiratory contra-indication, a standard approach is still to recommend ABVD. However in the higher risk patients where there exists suboptimal cardio-respiratory reserve, newer elderly regimens which have demonstrated therapeutic efficacy should be considered i.e. PVAG or VEPMB regimens. In order to improve outcomes further for older patients with Hodgkin's disease new clinical trials will have to be designed which particularly address the specific patient needs of the elderly population. Design of clinical trials which prospectively evaluate functional, co-morbid status will allow a more risk stratified approach to allow appropriate therapies to be administered. As a result, those aspects of patient's status which previously excluded patients from a clinical trial can be tested. The use of response adapted therapies incorporating CT-PET scanning may also be advantageous to the elderly population where escalation and de-escalation of therapy can be tailored into the therapeutic journey. The use of full supportive care measures is imperative, but caution should be applied when using GCSF growth factor support to Bleomycin regimens as evidence exists that Bleomycin lung toxicity is enhanced with GCSF [37].

The exciting development of new therapeutic agents such as Brentuximab Vedotin either being used alone or in combination with standard chemotherapy may help to improve outcome in elderly patients with HL and define new standards of care. The results of whether novel agents can be combined safely either with chemotherapy or other novel agents in the elderly population are eagerly waited. Given the potency of these novel agents observed in the relapse or refractory setting, testing them alone in frail elderly patients is underway and may provide a suitable replacement for chemotherapy. Finally the challenges and opportunity offered by new discoveries in the differences in disease biology according to age, may lead to the development of newer more efficacious therapeutic avenues in the future.

- Better understanding of the biology of Elderly disease
- Response adaptive strategies incorporating CT-PET in escalation and de-escalation treatment strategies
- Recognition, assessment and optimisation of co-morbid and functional status.
- Further improvements in supportive care , prediction of treatment toxicity
- Incorporation of non-toxic novel agents to the therapeutic armamentarium

References

1. Erdkamp FL, Breed WP, Bosch LJ, Wijnen JT, Blijham GB. Hodgkin disease in the elderly. A registry-based analysis. Cancer. 1992;70(4):830–4. Epub 1992/08/15.
2. Weekes CD, Vose JM, Lynch JC, Weisenburger DD, Bierman PJ, Greiner T, et al. Hodgkin's disease in the elderly: improved treatment outcome with a doxorubicin-containing regimen. J Clin Oncol. 2002;20(4):1087–93. Epub 2002/02/15.
3. Diepstra A, van Imhoff GW, Schaapveld M, Karim-Kos H, van den Berg A, Vellenga E, et al. Latent Epstein-Barr virus infection of tumor cells in classical Hodgkin's lymphoma

predicts adverse outcome in older adult patients. J Clin Oncol. 2009;27(23):3815–21. Epub 2009/05/28.
4. Keegan TH, Glaser SL, Clarke CA, Gulley ML, Craig FE, Digiuseppe JA, et al. Epstein-Barr virus as a marker of survival after Hodgkin's lymphoma: a population-based study. J Clin Oncol. 2005;23(30):7604–13. Epub 2005/09/28.
5. Stark GL, Wood KM, Jack F, Angus B, Proctor SJ, Taylor PR, et al. Hodgkin's disease in the elderly: a population-based study. Br J Haematol. 2002;119(2):432–40. Epub 2002/10/31.
6. Enblad G, Sandvej K, Sundstrom C, Pallesen G, Glimelius B. Epstein-Barr virus distribution in Hodgkin's disease in an unselected Swedish population. Acta Oncol. 1999;38(4):425–9. Epub 1999/07/27.
7. Gandhi MK, Tellam JT, Khanna R. Epstein-Barr virus-associated Hodgkin's lymphoma. Br J Haematol. 2004;125(3):267–81. Epub 2004/04/17.
8. Herbst H, Samol J, Foss HD, Raff T, Niedobitek G. Modulation of interleukin-6 expression in Hodgkin and Reed-Sternberg cells by Epstein-Barr virus. J Pathol. 1997;182(3):299–306. Epub 1997/07/01.
9. Herbst H, Foss HD, Samol J, Araujo I, Klotzbach H, Krause H, et al. Frequent expression of interleukin-10 by Epstein-Barr virus-harboring tumor cells of Hodgkin's disease. Blood. 1996;87(7):2918–29. Epub 1996/04/01.
10. Friedberg JW, Fischman A, Neuberg D, Kim H, Takvorian T, Ng AK, et al. FDG-PET is superior to gallium scintigraphy in staging and more sensitive in the follow-up of patients with de novo Hodgkin lymphoma: a blinded comparison. Leuk Lymphoma. 2004;45(1):85–92. Epub 2004/04/06.
11. Hutchings M, Loft A, Hansen M, Pedersen LM, Berthelsen AK, Keiding S, et al. Position emission tomography with or without computed tomography in the primary staging of Hodgkin's lymphoma. Haematologica. 2006;91(4):482–9. Epub 2006/04/06.
12. Hutchings M, Loft A, Hansen M, Pedersen LM, Buhl T, Jurlander J, et al. FDG-PET after two cycles of chemotherapy predicts treatment failure and progression-free survival in Hodgkin lymphoma. Blood. 2006;107(1):52–9. Epub 2005/09/10.
13. Engert A, Ballova V, Haverkamp H, Pfistner B, Josting A, Duhmke E, et al. Hodgkin's lymphoma in elderly patients: a comprehensive retrospective analysis from the German Hodgkin's Study Group. J Clin Oncol. 2005;23(22):5052–60. Epub 2005/06/16.
14. Enblad G, Glimelius B, Sundstrom C. Treatment outcome in Hodgkin's disease in patients above the age of 60: a population-based study. Ann Oncol. 1991;2(4):297–302. Epub 1991/04/01.
15. Landgren O, Algernon C, Axdorph U, Nilsson B, Wedelin C, Porwit-MacDonald A, et al. Hodgkin's lymphoma in the elderly with special reference to type and intensity of chemotherapy in relation to prognosis. Haematologica. 2003;88(4):438–44. Epub 2003/04/19.
16. Evens AM, Helenowski I, Ramsdale E, Nabhan C, Karmali R, Hanson B, et al. A retrospective multicenter analysis of elderly Hodgkin lymphoma: outcomes and prognostic factors in the modern era. Blood. 2012;119(3):692–5. Epub 2011/11/26.
17. Proctor SJ, Wilkinson J, Jones G, Watson GC, Lucraft HH, Mainou-Fowler T, et al. Evaluation of treatment outcome in 175 patients with Hodgkin lymphoma aged 60 years or over: the SHIELD study. Blood. 2012;119(25):6005–15. Epub 2012/05/12.
18. Levis A, Anselmo AP, Ambrosetti A, Adamo F, Bertini M, Cavalieri E, et al. VEPEMB in elderly Hodgkin's lymphoma patients. Results from an Intergruppo Italiano Linfomi (IIL) study. Ann Oncol. 2004;15(1):123–8.
19. Guinee VF, Giacco GG, Durand M, van den Blink JW, Gustavsson A, McVie JG, et al. The prognosis of Hodgkin's disease in older adults. J Clin Oncol. 1991;9(6):947–53. Epub 1991/06/01.
20. van Spronsen DJ, Janssen-Heijnen ML, Breed WP, Coebergh JW. Prevalence of co-morbidity and its relationship to treatment among unselected patients with Hodgkin's disease and non-Hodgkin's lymphoma, 1993–1996. Ann Hematol. 1999;78(7):315–9. Epub 1999/08/31.

21. Boll B, Gorgen H, Fuchs M, Pluetschow A, Eich HT, Bargetzi MJ, et al. ABVD in older patients with early-stage Hodgkin lymphoma treated within the German Hodgkin Study Group HD10 and HD11 trials. J Clin Oncol. 2013;31(12):1522–9. Epub 2013/03/20.
22. Fehniger TA, Larson S, Trinkaus K, Siegel MJ, Cashen AF, Blum KA, et al. A phase 2 multicenter study of lenalidomide in relapsed or refractory classical Hodgkin lymphoma. Blood. 2011;118(19):5119–25. Epub 2011/09/23.
23. Halbsguth TV, Nogova L, Mueller H, Sieniawski M, Eichenauer DA, Schober T, et al. Phase 2 study of BACOPP (bleomycin, adriamycin, cyclophosphamide, vincristine, procarbazine, and prednisone) in older patients with Hodgkin lymphoma: a report from the German Hodgkin Study Group (GHSG). Blood. 2010;116(12):2026–32. Epub 2010/06/17.
24. Evens AM, Hong F, Gordon LI, Fisher RI, Bartlett NL, Connors JM, et al. The efficacy and tolerability of adriamycin, bleomycin, vinblastine, dacarbazine and Stanford V in older Hodgkin lymphoma patients: a comprehensive analysis from the North American intergroup trial E2496. Br J Haematol. 2013;161(1):76–86. Epub 2013/01/30.
25. Ballova V, Ruffer JU, Haverkamp H, et al. A prospectively randomized trial carried out by the German Hodgkin Study Group (GHSG) for elderly patients with advanced Hodgkin`s disease coamparing BEACOPP baseline and COPP-ABVD (study $HD9_{eldery}$). Ann Oncol. 2005;16:124–31.
26. Wongso D, Fuchs M, Plutschow A, Klimm B, Sasse S, Hertenstein B, et al. Treatment-related mortality in patients with advanced-stage Hodgkin lymphoma: an analysis of the German Hodgkin Study Group. J Clin Oncol. 2013;31(22):2819–24. Epub 2013/06/26.
27. Levis A, Depaoli L, Urgesi A, Bertini M, Orsucci L, Vitolo U, et al. Probability of cure in elderly Hodgkin's disease patients. Haematologica. 1994;79(1):46–54. Epub 1994/01/01.
28. Levis A, Merli F, Tamiazzo S, et al. ABVD versus VEPEMB in elderly Hodgkin`s lymphoma patient [Abstract]. Blood. 2007;110:2322.
29. Boll B, Bredenfeld H, Gorgen H, Halbsguth T, Eich HT, Soekler M, et al. Phase 2 study of PVAG (prednisone, vinblastine, doxorubicin, gemcitabine) in elderly patients with early unfavorable or advanced stage Hodgkin lymphoma. Blood. 2011;118(24):6292–8. Epub 2011/09/16.
30. Kolstad A, Nome O, Delabie J, Lauritzsen GF, Fossa A, Holte H. Standard CHOP-21 as first line therapy for elderly patients with Hodgkin's lymphoma. Leuk Lymphoma. 2007;48(3): 570–6. Epub 2007/04/25.
31. Younes A, Bartlett NL, Leonard JP, Kennedy DA, Lynch CM, Sievers EL, et al. Brentuximab vedotin (SGN-35) for relapsed CD30-positive lymphomas. N Engl J Med. 2010;363(19): 1812–21. Epub 2010/11/05.
32. Younes A, Gopal AK, Smith SE, Ansell SM, Rosenblatt JD, Savage KJ, et al. Results of a pivotal phase II study of brentuximab vedotin for patients with relapsed or refractory Hodgkin's lymphoma. J Clin Oncol. 2012;30(18):2183–9. Epub 2012/03/29.
33. Younes A, Sureda A, Ben-Yehuda D, Zinzani PL, Ong TC, Prince HM, et al. Panobinostat in patients with relapsed/refractory Hodgkin's lymphoma after autologous stem-cell transplantation: results of a phase II study. J Clin Oncol. 2012;30(18):2197–203. Epub 2012/05/02.
34. Moskowitz AJ, Hamlin Jr PA, Perales MA, Gerecitano J, Horwitz SM, Matasar MJ, et al. Phase II study of bendamustine in relapsed and refractory Hodgkin lymphoma. J Clin Oncol. 2013;31(4):456–60. Epub 2012/12/19.
35. Katz J, Janik JE, Younes A. Brentuximab Vedotin (SGN-35). Clin Cancer Res. 2011;17(20): 6428–36. Epub 2011/10/18.
36. Buglio D, Georgakis GV, Hanabuchi S, Arima K, Khaskhely NM, Liu YJ, et al. Vorinostat inhibits STAT6-mediated TH2 cytokine and TARC production and induces cell death in Hodgkin lymphoma cell lines. Blood. 2008;112(4):1424–33. Epub 2008/06/11.
37. Martin WG, Ristow KM, Habermann TM, Colgan JP, Witzig TE, Ansell SM. Bleomycin pulmonary toxicity has a negative impact on the outcome of patients with Hodgkin's lymphoma. J Clin Oncol. 2005;23(30):7614–20. Epub 2005/09/28.

Chapter 11
Diffuse Large B-Cell Non-Hodgkin's Lymphoma (DLBCL- NHL)

Nils Winkelmann and Ulrich Wedding

Epidemiology

Diffuse large B-Cell Lymphoma (DLBCL) is the most common subtype of maligant lymphoma (ML). The incidence rate is about 10–15 of 100,000 people in the US and in Europe per year. Men are more frequently affected than women [1]. The incidence of DLBCL in people over the age of 65 years is rapidly rising. In the elderly (75 years or older), rates of diffuse large B-cell lymphoma (DLBCL) and follicular lymphoma increased 1.4 %. According to the SEER cancer statistics review 2000–2011, 9 per 100,000 of those younger than 65 years develop the disease, compared to 90 per 100,000 in those aged older than 65 years. The 5-years relative survival rates decreases from 78 % in those younger than 65 years to 62 % in those older than 65 years. The occurrence of all Non-Hodgkin's Lymphomas (NHL) has been rising from 10 to over 20 newly diagnosed patients per 100,000 from 1975 to 2010. For patients over 75 years of age, incidence rates have doubled (50–100 per 100,000) since 1975. Thus DLBCL is predominantly a disease of older individuals, with a median age of diagnosis at approximately 70 years of age. As demographic changes result in an increasing number of older people the occurrence of NHL in this older patient population will pose an increasing problem [2].

Classification

Diffuse large B-cell lymphoma is a heterogeneous group of Non-Hodgkin's Lymphoma (NHL). They are classified based on the WHO-classification based on

N. Winkelmann, MD (✉)
Department of Internal Medicine II, Department of Hematology and Medical Oncology, Jena University Hospital, Erlanger Allee 101, Jena 07747, Germany
e-mail: nils.winkelmann@med.uni-jena.de

U. Wedding, MD
Department of Palliative Care, University Hospital Jena, Erlanger Allee 101, Jena 07747, Thüringen, Germany
e-mail: ulrich.wedding@med.uni-jena.de

U. Wedding, R.A. Audisio (eds.), *Management of Hematological Cancer in Older People*, DOI 10.1007/978-1-4471-2837-3_11

Table 11.1 Classification of DLBCL

(a) Diffuse large B-cell lymphoma (DLBCL), NOS
T-cell/histiocyte rich large B-cell lymphoma (T/HRBCL)
EBV + DLBCL of the "elderly"
(b) DLBCL with a predominant extranodal location
Primary mediastinal (thymic) large B cell lymphoma (PMBL)
Intravascular large B-cell lymphoma (IVLBCL)
Primary cutaneous DLBCL, leg type (PCLBCL, leg type)
Primary DLBCL of CNS
Lymphomatoid granulomatosis
(c) Large-cell lymphomas of terminally differentiated B-cells
ALK positive large B-cell lymphoma
Plasmablastic lymphoma (PBL)
Primary effusion lymphoma (PEL)
DLBCL associated with chronic inflammation
(d) B-cell neoplasms with features intermediated between DLBCL and other lymphoid tumours
B-cell lymphoma, unclassifiable, with features intermediate between diffuse and large B-cell lymphoma and Burkitt lymphoma
B-cell lymphoma, unclassifiable, with features intermediate between diffuse and large B-cell lymphoma and classical Hodgkin lymphoma

clinical data, morphology, phenotype, cytogenetics, and molecular characteristics [3]. Table 11.1 reports the classification of DLBCL.

Aetiology

Often the aetiology remains unclear. Most of the DLBCL develop as a new disease, so called primary DLBCL, others can transform from other lymphatic neoplasia, so called secondary DLBCL. Prior exposure to agents causing DNA-damage and primary and secondary immunodeficiencies are associated with an increased risk of the development of a DLBCL. Certain chronic virus infections are associated with the occurrence of DLBCL, such as HCV, HIV and EBV. In elderly patients secondary lymphoma are more common than in younger ones. The EBV positive DLBCL in elderly patients should be classified as own entity and are associated with a worse prognosis than the EBV negative one [4].

Biology

The origins of DLBCL are not well understood. Usually, it evolves from normal B cells, but it can also result from malignant transformation of other types of malignant lymphatic neoplasia.

In general DLBCL encompasses a biologically and clinically diverse group of diseases, many of which cannot be separated from one another by well-defined and widely accepted criteria. Therefore new methods of genetic analysis are used for further characterization. DLBCL, NOS can be separate in germinal centre B-like DLBCL (GCB), activated B-like (ACB) DLBCL [5]. Lymphoma cells in the germinal centre B-cell-like subgroup resemble normal B cells in the germinal centre closely, and are generally associated with a favourable prognosis. Activated B-cell-like tumour cells are named from studies showing the constant activation of physiologic B-cell- antigen pathways. They are associated with a poorer prognosis [6]. One of the important pathways involved is the NF-κB pathway, which normally helps transforming B cells into plasma cells [7]. ACB subtype is more common in older patients, but compared to other molecular changes, which loose their prognostic importance when age was added as factor, age and ACB subtype independently contributed to poor prognosis [8].

In addition, gene expression studies found out more about cells and microscopic structures that are spreading within the malignant B- cells and form the tumour microenvironment. In particular, gene expression signatures that are linked with macrophages, T cells, and remodelling of the extracellular matrix seems to be associated with an improved prognosis and better overall survival [9]. On the other hand, the expression of genes involved in enhanced angiogenesis is associated with poorer survival [7].

Only a few genetic aberrations constituted valuable prognostic factors so far. Of these, the translocation of the MYC- oncogene has been associated with inferior survival. An additional translocation in BCL2 leads to an even worse prognosis and are named "double hit lymphomas") [10].

With the help of the above diagnostic criteria derived from primary lymphoma tissue, one can distinguish few important subtypes: the T cell/histiocyte rich large B-cell lymphoma and the Primary cutaneous DLBCL, leg type and the Epstein-Barr virus (EBV) DLBCL of the elderly for which data on modern genetic testing come up as well [11, 12]. Other additional subtypes of large- B-cell lymphomas that are diagnosed and treated in the same way are, such as primary mediastinal (thymic) large B-cell lymphoma, intravascular large B-cell lymphoma, ALK+large B-cell lymphoma, plasmoblastic lymphoma and follicular Lymphoma Grade 3B. The DLBCL of the central nervous system displays great differences concerning disease biology and treatment and will thus not be discussed here.

Data on age associated differences in biology of DLBCL are still limited. Patterns of gene expression are not routinely determined in clinical practice but will gain importance. However, as new therapeutic options might help to overcome negative prognostic molecular changes, the tests will become part of routine [13].

Symptoms

DLBCL is cancer of rapid growth which can occur in any part of the body. Typical first signs of this disease are fast growing masses of lymphatic tissue. Others may present as a tumour of unknown origin, with histology revealing a lymphoma instead of a carcinoma. Age associated changes in presentation have not been reported so far. Elderly patients more often present with extranodal disease [14].

In one third of the patients systemic symptoms are present at diagnosis, such as concomitant fever (>38 °C for at least 3 consecutive days), weight loss (>10 % during the 6 months prior to diagnosis), and night sweats, called B-symptoms [15].

Examination

Examination serves (a) the diagnosis of the disease, (b) the extend of the disease and (c) the judgment of the patients fitness for treatment.

The diagnosis is based on a histological examination of a biopsy, preferable from palpable lymph nodes, when ever possible as excisional biopsy. Core needle biopsy should be restricted to cases where no other surgical access is possible, without major surgery.

The procedures to diagnose the extend of the disease are listed in the following Table 11.2. They do not differ between younger and older patients.

The stage of the disease is classified according to the Ann-Arbor-Classification, see Table 11.3. No differences in staging system between younger and older patients exist.

Systemic Symptoms as fever, weight loss or night sweats are also included in the staging process: "A" means these symptoms are not present and "B" means they are.

Table 11.2 Diagnostic procedures in patients with DLBCL

History and physical exam (including evaluation of all lymph node enlargement, recording site and size of all abnormal lymph nodes, inspection of Waldeyer's ring, evaluation of the presence or absence of hepatosplenomegaly, inspection of the skin, and detection of palpable masses)
Performance status according to the Eastern-Cooperative-Oncology-Group (ECOG) and geriatric assessment
Blood tests (full blood count, Lactate Dehydrogenase (LDH), liver and renal function test including creatine-clearance, uric acid, electrolytes, HIV, HBV- and HCV-, EBV-serology, CMV-serology)
Bone marrow aspiration and biopsy
CT scan or PET/CT scan
Lumbal puncture for liquor cytology and brain MRI in patients with high risk for ZNS-involvement or recurrence
In patients with involvement of extranodal sites, further specific investigations might be necessary

Table 11.3 Ann-Arbor classification of stage [16, 17]

Stage I — Only one lymph node region is involved, only one lymph structure is involved, or only one extranodal site (IE) is involved.
Stage II — Two or more lymph node regions or lymph node structures on the same side of the diaphragm are involved.
Stage III — Lymph node regions or structures on both sides of the diaphragm are involved
Stage IV — There is widespread involvement of a number of organs or tissues other than lymph node regions or structures, such as the liver, lung, or bone marrow.

The judgment of a patients fitness for treatment includes cardic, renal and pulmonary function test. In addition a structured geriatric assessment (GA) is recommended at least for patients aged 70 years and older [18]. A screening tool is less specific but might be an approach in a busy clinic [19]. Results of GA are associated with survival in patients with malignant lymphoma [20, 21].

A geriatric assessment was better in judging the patients prognosis than physicians. Tucci et al. included patients with newly diagnoses DLBCL in a prospective cohort trial. All patients received a geriatric assessment. The treating physician was blinded for the results of the geriatric assessment when deciding on patients´ fitness for treatment. Most of the patients were considered fit for an R-CHOP regimen, others not, they received attenuated dose regimens, corticosteroids or single agent Rituximab. The geriatric assessment classified more patients as not fit for R-CHOP. The prognosis of patients classified by physicians as fit but by assessment as unfit was identical to the prognosis of those classified as unfit by the physicians and the assessment [22].

Patients' fitness for treatment should be assessed at the time of diagnosis and after a prophase treatment (see below) [15].

Prognostic Factors

Prognostic factors predicting overall survival can be related to the disease (stage, LDH, extranodal involvement) and to the patients (age, performance-status) and the treatment, as response after treatment is a highly predictive factor for survival.

The following factors have been identified as independently associated with survival and thus are included in the International Prognostic Index (IPI) scoring system. In addition an age-adapted version (aaIPI), was established, see Tables 11.4 and 11.5 [23].

As the prognostic classification according to the IPI and aaIPI was established based on data, prior to the inclusion of Rituximab into the treatment, the scores were re-evaluated based on data of patients treated with Rituximab containing regimes. The data are reported in Table 11.6. Sehn et al. suggest based on their data analysing population based data, to use three instead of four prognostic categories: very good, good, and poor; and renamed the IPI to a revised IPI [24]. The former distribution

Table 11.4 Categories of the IPI and aaIPI [23]

Age younger and older than 60 (0 vs. 1)[a]
LDH level normal or higher than normal (0 vs. 1)
General health status (ECOG performance status score 0–1 or 2 and greater) (0 vs. 1)
Stage I – II or III – IV disease (0 vs. 1)
Involvement of more than one extranodal site present or not (0 vs. 1)[a]

[a]Not included in the age adjusted International Prognostic Index (aaIPI)

Table 11.5 IPI risk groups and 5 years survival rate according to age [15, 23]

Risk group	Number of risk factors in IPI	Number of risk factors in aaIPI	5 years survival rate (all patients)	5 years survival rate (patients >60 years)	3 years survival rate (patients aged >60 years from RICOVER-trial)
Low	0–1	0	73	56	88
Low-intermediate	2	1	51	44	79
High-intermediate	3	2	43	37	68
High	4–5	3	26	21	58

Table 11.6 Revised IPI [24]

Risk group	No of IPI factors	4 years OS
Very good	0	94
Good	1.2	79
Poor	3–5	55

had separated only two different prognostic groups, factors 0–2 and factors 3–4. The median age of the included patients was 61 years. Ziepert et al. analysed treatment results of clinical trials including patients aged 60 years and older with DLBCL. They confirmed the prognostic value of the aaIPI regarding PFS, EFS and OS [25]. As age above 60 years is a factor of IPI, older patients per se can not be in a very good risk group.

Treatment

None or delayed treatment leads to death within weeks to few months. Treatment decision should into account the stage of the disease and the IPI in addition to patients´ fitness. Chemotherapy with CHOP is the backbone of treatment in patients with DLBCL. It was established in 1976. The initial trial included patients with a median age of 53 years [26].

As the IPI identified age, below and above the age of 60 years, as major prognostic factor, as treatment toxicity increases with age, and as in younger patients, strategies to increase dose of chemotherapy, with the hope of increased remission and survival rate, trials often used age limit of 60 years as definition of elderly patients.

1st line Treatment for Fit Patients Aged 60–80 Years

The addition of Rituximab, a chimeric CD 20 antibody, added to CHOP improved treatment results substantially, as demonstrated in different trials. Coiffer et al. were the first to show that the addition Rituximab was able to improve response rate, event-free and overall survival in patient aged 60–80 years [27]. Maintenance therapy with Rituximab following the R-CHOP regime seemed demonstrated no further improvement in outcome [28]. The RICOVER-60 trial compared different dosing intervals and numbers of therapy cycles, R-CHOP given every 14 days (R-CHOP-14) proved most effective in maximizing event free and overall survival for the same patient group [29]. The shorter interval includes obligatory application of G-CSF as part of the dose-dense protocol.

However, there is an ongoing discussion whether this data apply to patients prognostic risk groups in the age adjusted IPI. Furthermore, the application of R-CHOP-14 in this age group resulted in more frequent grade 3 and 4 neutropenia and increased number of transfusions [30, 31]. Table 11.7 summarizes the results of 1st line regimens containing R-CHOP as a treatment arm.

All in all 6–8 cycles of R-CHOP-14 or R-CHOP-21 should be the current standard of care for fit patients and according to these pivotal trials for patients aged younger than 80 years.

Prior to the start of the R-CHOP regimen a prophase treatment is recommended, consisting of a single intravenous injection of vinristin 1 mg day 1 and oral prednisolone for 7 days. Besides not being tested in a randomized fashion, toxicity in the 1st cycle reduced substantially [15].

1st Line Treatment Alternatives and Options for Patients with Comorbidities, Medically Non-Fit, or Patients or Aged More Than 80 Years

All in all data for very elderly patients, especially those aged 80 years and older are limited. Bellera at al. analysed the specific barriers to include elderly patients with malignant lymphoma (not especially patients with DLBCL) in RCTs and identified restrictive inclusion criteria, poor performance status, impaired liver and kidney function and presence of comorbidities as major reasons [32]. Therefore, data especially for these groups of patients are very limited. In addition to data from RCTs, data from cohort trials in phase II trials have to be included in the recommendations for treatment decision, as they better reflect the typical elderly patients seen in clinics or hospitals.

There is no generally agreed definition, which patient is suitable for a classical R-CHOP regimen. Age is one factor associated with increased toxicity. With the increase in age, treatment related toxicity and mortality increases. Predictors of toxicity are analysed by Ziepert et al. [33]. They separately analysed data for patients aged up to 60 years and above 60 years. Low body weight, female gender, poor PS, high LDH, and initial cytopenia where associated with increased hematological toxicity. According to the results of the RICOVER-60 trial, treatment related death rate was 4 % was patients aged 60–65 years, 6.4 % for those aged 66–70 years, 7.0 % for those aged 70–75 years, and 20.1 % for those aged 76–80 years.

A physicians' judgement, that the patient is not suitable for a standard R-CHOP regimen can be based on different criteria. Tucci et al. identified, that a geriatric

Table 11.7 RCTs on 1st line treatment of patients with DLBCL aged 60 years and older

1st author and year	Treatment	N=/Age group/ median	% of patients ECOG-PS-2	% of patients aged 80+	Primary endpoint results	Overall survival
Coffier et al. *NEJM* (2002) [27]	8×CHOP-21 vs. 8×R-CHOP-21	339/60–80/69	20	0	EFS: 2 years-EFS 38 vs. 57 %; p<0.01	2 years-OS 57 vs. 70 %; p<0.01
Pfreundschuh et al. *Lancet Oncol* (2008) [29]	(1) CHOP-14 vs. R-CHOP-14+(2) 6 vs. 8 cycles	1,222/61–80/68	14	0	EFS: 3 years-EFS 47.2 vs. 53.0 % for 6 vs. 8 CHOP and 66.5 vs. 63.1 % for 6 vs. 8 R-CHOP	OS: 3 years-OS 67.7 vs. 66.0 % for 6 vs. 8 CHOP and 78.1 vs. 72.5 % for 6 vs. 8 R-CHOP
Habermann et al. *JCO* (2006) [28]	(1) CHOP 21 vs. R-CHOP+(2) NIL vs. R Maintenance	632/60–92/69	15	8	FFS: 3 years-FFS 46 vs. 53 %; p=0.04	OS: 3 years-OS 58 vs. 67 %;
Delarue et al. *Lancet Oncol* (2013) [30]	8×R-CHOP-21 vs. 8×R-CHOP-14	602/60–80/70	22	0	EFS: 3 years-EFS 56 vs. 60 % p=0.7614 (NS)	OS: 3 years-OS 72 vs. 69 % (NS)
Cunningham et al. *Lancet* (2013) [31]	8×R-CHOP-21 vs. 8×R-CHOP-14	1,080/19–88/61	13	n.r.	OS: 2-years-OS 80.8 vs. 82.7; p=NS	See primary end point

assessment is better to identify patients as fit for treatment than physicians´ judgement [22].

Main strategies followed in the over 80 year old patients and in those unfit for standard R-CHOP treatment are to reduce toxicity of R-CHOP by dose reduction or to use other less toxic drugs.

A variety of studies mainly in the last decade of the last century compared different regimens to CHOP, to find a less toxic protocol. One of the most extensively studies substance, was Mitoxantrone as substitute for Doxorubicin, resulting in CNOP instead of CHOP regimen. In a meta-analysis comparing results of 9 studies, CHOP remained the superior regime regarding efficacy and CNOP was not less toxic. The studies were not restricted to elderly patients, but included a considerable number of older adults [34]. As Rituximab is a very active and less toxic agent, trials using R-Non-CHOP regimens are analysed and reported in Table 11.8.

The dose-reduced R-Mini-CHOP regime is a pragmatic alternative that has shown progression free survival rates by 47 % after 2 years [21, 39].

Most of the previously mentioned trials analysed a liposomal anthracycline. The International Society for Geriatric Oncology (SIOG) provides recommendations for the use of liposomal anthracyclines, beside other tumours in lymphoma patients by which treatment can be delivered more safely [40].

R- Bendamustine is a valuable alternative for anthracycline free treatment in patients that are ineligible for R-CHOP [41].

Patients Aged 80+

As rarely patients aged 80 years and older are included in prospective clinical trials, especially RCTs, cohort trials are an additional method to gain knowledge on treatments used, results obtained, and the value of variables of a comprehensive geriatric assessment (CGA) as prognostic tools [42, 43]. Table 11.9 summarizes articles reporting treatment results in cohorts of patients aged 80 and older.

In patients aged 80 and older, the treatment decision is mainly based on the patients fitness for treatment. A structured geriatric assessment shall help to identify patients fit for standard treatment with R-CHOP and those who should be treated with alternative protocols, when severe comorbidity, e.g. cardiac failure are present, or when the pre-existing performance-status / functional status is poor.

Trials Integrating Comprehensive Geriatric Assessment (CGA)

Only few trials are available reporting the inclusion of CGA in the care for elderly patients with DLBCL. Results of a systematic literature research are listed in Table 11.10.

Table 11.8 Phase II trials of R-Non-CHOP regimen in 1st line treatment

1st author and year	Treatment	N=/Age group/median	% of patients ECOG-PS ≥2	% of patients aged 80+	Primary endpoint results	Reasons against CHOP	Assessment
Visani et al. (2008) [35] [35]	R-COMP-21	20/61–82/73	45	n.r.	CR 63 %,	Frailty	Frail patients
Corazzelli et al. (2011) *BJH* [36]	R-COMP-14	41/62–82/73	32	12	4 years OS 67 %	Cardiomyopathy	aaCCI predicted outcome
Peyrade et al. (2011) *Lancet Oncol* [21]	R-mini-CHOP-21	149/80–95/83	34	100	OS 29 months 2 years-OS: 59 %	Age 80+	IADL Score with prognostic value
Musolino et al. (2011) *Cancer* [37]	DA-POCH-R	23/70–90/77	74	43	RR 83 %, CR 52 % 2nd 3 years OS 56 %	n.r.	Age >80 adverse prognostic factor.
Hainsworth et al. (2010) *Clin Lymphoma Myeloma Leuk* [38]	R-CNOP or R-CVP	51/…/78	37	43	2 years OS 72 %	Age and poor PS	n.r.

ECOG-PS Eastern Cooperative Oncology Group Performance Status, *n.r.* not reported, *aaCCI* age adjusted Charlson Comorbidity Index, *IADL* Instrumental Activities of Daily Living, *RR* response rate, *CR* complete remission, *OS* overall survival

Table 11.9 Cohort trials in patients with DLBCL aged 80+

1st author and year	Treatments	N=/Age group/median	% of patients ECOG-PS-2	Frequency of DLBCL patients	Use of R-CHOP/other regimens	Assessment
Thieblemont et al. (2008) *Ann Oncol* [42]	different protocols	205/80–101/83	36	n=81 (39 %)	8 (12 %)	Not performed
Bairey et al. (2006) *Ann Oncol* [43]	different protocols	104/80–95/84	38	n=66 (61 %)	37 (34 %) CHOP 3 (3 %) R-CHOP	CIRS-G
Italiano et al. (2005) *Haematologica* [39]	R-mini-CHOP	22/80+/n.r.	42	n=19	15	Not performed

Table 11.10 Trials in elderly patients with DLBCL including CGA

Author	Type of study	Endpoint	Data on CGA	Patients
Bairey et al. (2013) [44]	Retrospective	Early death = 4 months survival	Not reported, but postulated	90 with early death
Spina et al. (2012) [45]	Prospective cohort, no RCT	5-years DFS, OS, cause-specific survival, toxicity	CGA as base for classification as fit, unfit and frail	DLBCL, aged 70+, 1st line, 2000–2006, n = 100
Olivieri et al. (2012) [46]	Prospective cohort, no RCT	Survival in CR (follow-up 57 months)	I = fit -> R-CHOP-21 (54)	DLBCL, 1st line, n = 91
		I 57 %	II = comorbid -> R-CDOP-21 (22) lip. Dox.	
		II 32 %	III = frail = dose reduced mini-CHOP (15)	
		III 20 %		
Merli et al. (2012) [47]	Prospective RCT R-CHOP n = 110 R-CEOP n = 114	Survival: data see Table 11.2	Included to define fit patients. 21 % had limitations in IADL-Score, 13 % a CIRS-Score of 3 in at least one organ system. CGA results did not define prognostic groups.	n = 224, aged 65+, DLBCL, fit, 1st line, R-CHOP vs. R-mini-CEOP
Merli et al. (2014) [59]	Prospective cohort	OS associated with age adjusted IPI and comorbidity	Of 334 patients 99 were classified as frail by CGA, fit are included in [47]. Frail: 80 years and older, ADL limitation, comorbidity grad 4 comorbidity or 3 or more grad 3 comorbidities in CIRS, presence of geriatric syndromes	n = 334, 65+ years, DLBCL untreated
Tucci et al. (2009) *Cancer* [22]	Prospective cohort, no RCT	2 years OS 77.6 % in fit, 23.8 % in un-fit	Fit = criteria: age < 80, no ADL dependence, no grad 4 comorbidity in CIRS, less than 3 grad 3 comorbidities, no presence of geriatric syndromes	n = 84 aged 65, DLBCL, 1st line, curative or non-curative
Winkelmann et al. (2011) *JCRCO* [20]	Prospective cohort, no RCT	Prognostic factors for OS age, IADL, comorbidity	ADL limitations 18 %, IADL limitation 21 %, CIRS-G level 3–4 56 %	n = 143, 18–86 years, lymphoma, non only DLBCL, 1st line treatment
Lin et al. *Ann Hematol* (2012) [48]	Retrospective cohort	Treatment intensity and overall survival	Charlson-Comorbidity-Score (CCI) was not associated with treatment intensity but with overall survival	n = 333, 60+ years, median 73 years, DLBCL

In summary the trials including CGA demonstrate the prognostic significance of variable of the CGA for survival in elderly patients with DLBCL. This is true for functional scores, especially IADL score, and for comorbidities, where the CIRS-G score is the most widely used score. Randomised trials comparing CGA based treatment decision to clinical judgement are missing so far. Physician´s judgement of fitness of patients for treatment classifies more patients as fit than CGA [49].

Second Line Therapy

In patients with recurrence or resistant disease second line regimens are used. In younger once and those medically fit, high-dose chemotherapy followed by autologeous blood stem cell retransfusion is treatment of choice. It is especially effective in those patients who responded to 1st line therapy, who had an interval of at least 12 months until recurrence and who responded to second line treatment [50]. A maintenance treatment with rituximab is not beneficial [51]. However, most of elderly patients, especially those aged 70 years and older will not be fit for a high-dose regimen. A variety of treatment protocols are effective in inducing a remission, but most of the patients will have a recurrence again or will develop resistance while on treatment. The treatment approach will be non-curative in most of these patients. Main prognostic factor is the time between 1st line treatment and recurrence. A second curative approach might be possible when the interval is more than 12 months. Suggested treatment protocols are R-GemOx [52], R-ESHAP-[53] and R-mini-CHOP-Regime [21] or less toxic but less effective as well the R-bendamustine regmine [54].

Radiotherapy (RT)

Radiotherapy is an effective method in lymphoma treatment. However which role RT has as part of 1st line treatment remains unclear. Most data on involved-field RT in patients with bulky disease or residual disease after induction chemotherapy, are collected prior to the use of rituximab. The topic is discussed in more detail by Martelli et al. [15].

Patients with Special Comorbidities

Cardiac failure: R-CEOP might be a treatment option when the use of antracyclines is not possible [55]. However liposomal agents are available and effective [40].

Renal failure: Some case reports on treatment of elderly patients with end-stage renal failure on dialysis treated with chemotherapy such as R-mini-CHOP or R-bendamustine are available.

Future Perspectives

With the more and more better understanding of lymphoma biology a variety of new agents are available, with some promising results from phase II trials, to overcome the negative biology and resistance to chemotherapy [56–58].

References

1. Morton LM, Wang SS, Devesa SS, Hartge P, Weisenburger DD, Linet MS. Lymphoma incidence patterns by WHO subtype in the United States, 1992–2001. Blood. 2006;107(1):265–76.
2. Smith BD, Smith GL, Hurria A, Hortobagyi GN, Buchholz TA. Future of cancer incidence in the United States: burdens upon an aging, changing nation. J Clin Oncol. 2009;27(17):2758–65.
3. Swerdlow SH, Campo E, Harris NL, Jaffe ES, Pileri SA, Stein H, Thiele J, Vardiman JW. WHO classification of tumors of haematopoietic and lymphoid tissues. Lyon: IARC Press; 2008.
4. Oyama T, Yamamoto K, Asano N, Oshiro A, Suzuki R, Kagami Y, Morishima Y, Takeuchi K, Izumo T, Mori S, Ohshima K, Suzumiya J, Nakamura N, Abe M, Ichimura K, Sato Y, Yoshino T, Naoe T, Shimoyama Y, Kamiya Y, Kinoshita T, Nakamura S. Age-related EBV-associated B-cell lymphoproliferative disorders constitute a distinct clinicopathologic group: a study of 96 patients. Clin Cancer Res. 2007;13(17):5124–32.
5. Alizadeh AA, Eisen MB, Davis RE, Ma C, Lossos IS, Rosenwald A, Boldrick JC, Sabet H, Tran T, Yu X, Powell JI, Yang L, Marti GE, Moore T, Hudson Jr J, Lu L, Lewis DB, Tibshirani R, Sherlock G, Chan WC, Greiner TC, Weisenburger DD, Armitage JO, Warnke R, Levy R, Wilson W, Grever MR, Byrd JC, Botstein D, Brown PO, Staudt LM. Distinct types of diffuse large B-cell lymphoma identified by gene expression profiling. Nature. 2000;403(6769): 503–11.
6. Lenz G, Wright G, Dave SS, Xiao W, Powell J, Zhao H, Xu W, Tan B, Goldschmidt N, Iqbal J, Vose J, Bast M, Fu K, Weisenburger DD, Greiner TC, Armitage JO, Kyle A, May L, Gascoyne RD, Connors JM, Troen G, Holte H, Kvaloy S, Dierickx D, Verhoef G, Delabie J, Smeland EB, Jares P, Martinez A, Lopez-Guillermo A, Montserrat E, Campo E, Braziel RM, Miller TP, Rimsza LM, Cook JR, Pohlman B, Sweetenham J, Tubbs RR, Fisher RI, Hartmann E, Rosenwald A, Ott G, Muller-Hermelink HK, Wrench D, Lister TA, Jaffe ES, Wilson WH, Chan WC, Staudt LM. Stromal gene signatures in large-B-cell lymphomas. N Engl J Med. 2008;359(22):2313–23.
7. Lenz G, Staudt LM. Aggressive lymphomas. N Engl J Med. 2010;362(15):1417–29.
8. Klapper W, Kreuz M, Kohler CW, Burkhardt B, Szczepanowski M, Salaverria I, Hummel M, Loeffler M, Pellissery S, Woessmann W, Schwanen C, Trumper L, Wessendorf S, Spang R, Hasenclever D, Siebert R. Patient age at diagnosis is associated with the molecular characteristics of diffuse large B-cell lymphoma. Blood. 2012;119(8):1882–7.
9. Linderoth J, Eden P, Ehinger M, Valcich J, Jerkeman M, Bendahl PO, Berglund M, Enblad G, Erlanson M, Roos G, Cavallin-Stahl E. Genes associated with the tumour microenvironment are differentially expressed in cured versus primary chemotherapy-refractory diffuse large B-cell lymphoma. Br J Haematol. 2008;141(4):423–32.
10. Niitsu N, Okamoto M, Miura I, Hirano M. Clinical features and prognosis of de novo diffuse large B-cell lymphoma with t(14;18) and 8q24/c-MYC translocations. Leukemia. 2009;23(4):777–83.
11. Ahn JS, Yang DH, Duk Choi Y, Jung SH, Yhim HY, Kwak JY, Sung Park H, Shin MG, Kim YK, Kim HJ, Lee JJ. Clinical outcome of elderly patients with Epstein-Barr virus positive diffuse

large B-cell lymphoma treated with a combination of rituximab and CHOP chemotherapy. Am J Hematol. 2013;88(9):774–9.

12. Pham-Ledard A, Prochazkova-Carlotti M, Andrique L, Cappellen D, Vergier B, Martinez F, Grange F, Petrella T, Beylot-Barry M, Merlio JP. Multiple genetic alterations in primary cutaneous large B-cell lymphoma, leg type support a common lymphomagenesis with activated B-cell-like diffuse large B-cell lymphoma. Mod Pathol. 2014;27(3):402–11.
13. Witzig TE. Origins research in large cell lymphoma-time for action? Lancet Oncol. 2014;15(7):674–5.
14. Kuper-Hommel MJ, van de Schans SA, Vreugdenhil G, van Krieken JH, Coebergh JW. Undertreatment of patients with localized extranodal compared with nodal diffuse large B-cell lymphoma. Leuk Lymphoma. 2013;54(8):1698–705.
15. Martelli M, Ferreri AJ, Agostinelli C, Di Rocco A, Pfreundschuh M, Pileri SA. Diffuse large B-cell lymphoma. Crit Rev Oncol Hematol. 2013;87(2):146–71.
16. Carbone PP, Kaplan HS, Musshoff K, Smithers DW, Tubiana M. Report of the Committee on Hodgkin's Disease Staging Classification. Cancer Res. 1971;31(11):1860–1.
17. Lister TA, Crowther D, Sutcliffe SB, Glatstein E, Canellos GP, Young RC, Rosenberg SA, Coltman CA, Tubiana M. Report of a committee convened to discuss the evaluation and staging of patients with Hodgkin's disease: Cotswolds meeting. J Clin Oncol. 1989;7(11):1630–6.
18. Extermann M, Aapro M, Bernabei R, Cohen HJ, Droz JP, Lichtman S, Mor V, Monfardini S, Repetto L, Sorbye L, Topinkova E, C. G. A. o. t. I. S. o. G. O. Task Force on. Use of comprehensive geriatric assessment in older cancer patients: recommendations from the task force on CGA of the International Society of Geriatric Oncology (SIOG). Crit Rev Oncol Hematol. 2005;55(3):241–52.
19. Decoster, L, Van Puyvelde K, Mohile S, Wedding U, Basso U, Colloca G, Rostoft S, Overcash J, Wildiers H, Steer C, Kimmick G, Kanesvaran R, Luciani A, Terret C, Hurria A, Kenis C, Audisio R, Extermann M (2014). Screening tools for multidimensional health problems warranting a geriatric assessment in older cancer patients: an update on SIOG recommendations. Ann Oncol. Jan 2014 [Epub ahead of print].
20. Winkelmann N, Petersen I, Kiehntopf M, Fricke HJ, Hochhaus A, Wedding U. Results of comprehensive geriatric assessment effect survival in patients with malignant lymphoma. J Cancer Res Clin Oncol. 2011;137(4):733–8.
21. Peyrade F, Jardin F, Thieblemont C, Thyss A, Emile JF, Castaigne S, Coiffier B, Haioun C, Bologna S, Fitoussi O, Lepeu G, Fruchart C, Bordessoule D, Blanc M, Delarue R, Janvier M, Salles B, Andre M, Fournier M, Gaulard P, Tilly H, i. Groupe d'Etude des Lymphomes de l'Adulte. Attenuated immunochemotherapy regimen (R-miniCHOP) in elderly patients older than 80 years with diffuse large B-cell lymphoma: a multicentre, single-arm, phase 2 trial. Lancet Oncol. 2011;12(5):460–8.
22. Tucci A, Ferrari S, Bottelli C, Borlenghi E, Drera M, Rossi G. A comprehensive geriatric assessment is more effective than clinical judgment to identify elderly diffuse large cell lymphoma patients who benefit from aggressive therapy. Cancer. 2009;115(19):4547–53.
23. The International Non-Hodgkin's Lymphoma Prognostic Factors Project. A predictive model for aggressive non-Hodgkin's lymphoma. N Engl J Med. 1993;329(14):987–94.
24. Sehn LH, Berry B, Chhanabhai M, Fitzgerald C, Gill K, Hoskins P, Klasa R, Savage KJ, Shenkier T, Sutherland J, Gascoyne RD, Connors JM. The revised International Prognostic Index (R-IPI) is a better predictor of outcome than the standard IPI for patients with diffuse large B-cell lymphoma treated with R-CHOP. Blood. 2007;109(5):1857–61.
25. Ziepert M, Hasenclever D, Kuhnt E, Glass B, Schmitz N, Pfreundschuh M, Loeffler M. Standard International prognostic index remains a valid predictor of outcome for patients with aggressive CD20+ B-cell lymphoma in the rituximab era. J Clin Oncol. 2010;28(14):2373–80.
26. McKelvey EM, Gottlieb JA, Wilson HE, Haut A, Talley RW, Stephens R, Lane M, Gamble JF, Jones SE, Grozea PN, Gutterman J, Coltman C, Moon TE. Hydroxyldaunomycin (Adriamycin) combination chemotherapy in malignant lymphoma. Cancer. 1976;38(4):1484–93.

27. Coiffier B, Lepage E, Briere J, Herbrecht R, Tilly H, Bouabdallah R, Morel P, Van Den Neste E, Salles G, Gaulard P, Reyes F, Lederlin P, Gisselbrecht C. CHOP chemotherapy plus rituximab compared with CHOP alone in elderly patients with diffuse large-B-cell lymphoma. N Engl J Med. 2002;346(4):235–42.
28. Habermann TM, Weller EA, Morrison VA, Gascoyne RD, Cassileth PA, Cohn JB, Dakhil SR, Woda B, Fisher RI, Peterson BA, Horning SJ. Rituximab-CHOP versus CHOP alone or with maintenance rituximab in older patients with diffuse large B-cell lymphoma. J Clin Oncol. 2006;24(19):3121–7.
29. Pfreundschuh M, Schubert J, Ziepert M, Schmits R, Mohren M, Lengfelder E, Reiser M, Nickenig C, Clemens M, Peter N, Bokemeyer C, Eimermacher H, Ho A, Hoffmann M, Mertelsmann R, Trumper L, Balleisen L, Liersch R, Metzner B, Hartmann F, Glass B, Poeschel V, Schmitz N, Ruebe C, Feller AC, Loeffler M. Six versus eight cycles of bi-weekly CHOP-14 with or without rituximab in elderly patients with aggressive CD20+ B-cell lymphomas: a randomised controlled trial (RICOVER-60). Lancet Oncol. 2008;9(2):105–16.
30. Delarue R, Tilly H, Mounier N, Petrella T, Salles G, Thieblemont C, Bologna S, Ghesquieres H, Hacini M, Fruchart C, Ysebaert L, Ferme C, Casasnovas O, Van Hoof A, Thyss A, Delmer A, Fitoussi O, Molina TJ, Haioun C, Bosly A. Dose-dense rituximab-CHOP compared with standard rituximab-CHOP in elderly patients with diffuse large B-cell lymphoma (the LNH03-6B study): a randomised phase 3 trial. Lancet Oncol. 2013;14(6):525–33.
31. Cunningham D, Hawkes EA, Jack A, Qian W, Smith P, Mouncey P, Pocock C, Ardeshna KM, Radford JA, McMillan A, Davies J, Turner D, Kruger A, Johnson P, Gambell J, Linch D. Rituximab plus cyclophosphamide, doxorubicin, vincristine, and prednisolone in patients with newly diagnosed diffuse large B-cell non-Hodgkin lymphoma: a phase 3 comparison of dose intensification with 14-day versus 21-day cycles. Lancet. 2013;381(9880):1817–26.
32. Bellera C, Praud D, Petit-Moneger A, McKelvie-Sebileau P, Soubeyran P, Mathoulin-Pelissier S. Barriers to inclusion of older adults in randomised controlled clinical trials on Non-Hodgkin's lymphoma: a systematic review. Cancer Treat Rev. 2013;39(7):812–7.
33. Ziepert M, Schmits R, Trumper L, Pfreundschuh M, Loeffler M. Prognostic factors for hematotoxicity of chemotherapy in aggressive non-Hodgkin's lymphoma. Ann Oncol. 2008;19(4):752–62.
34. Osby E, Hagberg H, Kvaloy S, Teerenhovi L, Anderson H, Cavallin-Stahl E, Holte H, Myhre J, Pertovaara H, Bjorkholm M. CHOP is superior to CNOP in elderly patients with aggressive lymphoma while outcome is unaffected by filgrastim treatment: results of a Nordic Lymphoma Group randomized trial. Blood. 2003;101(10):3840–8.
35. Visani G, Ferrara F, Alesiani F, Ronconi S, Catarini M, D'Adamo F, Guiducci B, Bernardi D, Barulli S, Piccaluga P, Rocchi M, Isidori A. R-COMP 21 for frail elderly patients with aggressive B-cell non-Hodgkin lymphoma: a pilot study. Leuk Lymphoma. 2008;49(6):1081–6.
36. Corazzelli G, Frigeri F, Arcamone M, Lucania A, Rosariavilla M, Morelli E, Amore A, Capobianco G, Caronna A, Becchimanzi C, Volzone F, Marcacci G, Russo F, De Filippi R, Mastrullo L, Pinto A. Biweekly rituximab, cyclophosphamide, vincristine, non-pegylated liposome-encapsulated doxorubicin and prednisone (R-COMP-14) in elderly patients with poor-risk diffuse large B-cell lymphoma and moderate to high 'life threat' impact cardiopathy. Br J Haematol. 2011;154(5):579–89.
37. Musolino A, Boggiani D, Panebianco M, Vasini G, Salvagni S, Franciosi V, Ardizzoni A. Activity and safety of dose-adjusted infusional cyclophosphamide, doxorubicin, vincristine, and prednisone chemotherapy with rituximab in very elderly patients with poor-prognostic untreated diffuse large B-cell non-Hodgkin lymphoma. Cancer. 2011;117(5):964–73.
38. Hainsworth JD, Flinn IW, Spigel DR, Clark BL, Griner PL, Vazquez ER, Doss HH, Shipley D, Franco LA, Burris 3rd HA, Greco FA, C. Sarah Cannon Oncology Research. Brief-duration rituximab/chemotherapy followed by maintenance rituximab in patients with diffuse large B-cell lymphoma who are poor candidates for R-CHOP chemotherapy: a phase II trial of the Sarah Cannon Oncology Research Consortium. Clin Lymphoma Myeloma Leuk. 2010;10(1):44–50.

39. Italiano A, Jardin F, Peyrade F, Saudes L, Tilly H, Thyss A. Adapted CHOP plus rituximab in non-Hodgkin's lymphoma in patients over 80 years old. Haematologica. 2005;90(9):1281–3.
40. Aapro M, Bernard-Marty C, Brain EG, Batist G, Erdkamp F, Krzemieniecki K, Leonard R, Lluch A, Monfardini S, Ryberg M, Soubeyran P, Wedding U. Anthracycline cardiotoxicity in the elderly cancer patient: a SIOG expert position paper. Ann Oncol. 2011;22(2):257–67.
41. Weidmann E, Neumann A, Fauth F, Atmaca A, Al-Batran SE, Pauligk C, Jager E. Phase II study of bendamustine in combination with rituximab as first-line treatment in patients 80 years or older with aggressive B-cell lymphomas. Ann Oncol. 2011;22(8):1839–44.
42. Thieblemont C, Grossoeuvre A, Houot R, Broussais-Guillaumont F, Salles G, Traulle C, Espinouse D, Coiffier B. Non-Hodgkin's lymphoma in very elderly patients over 80 years. A descriptive analysis of clinical presentation and outcome. Ann Oncol. 2008;19(4):774–9.
43. Bairey O, Benjamini O, Blickstein D, Elis A, Ruchlemer R. Non-Hodgkin's lymphoma in patients 80 years of age or older. Ann Oncol. 2006;17(6):928–34.
44. Bairey O, Bar-Natan M, Shpilberg O. Early death in patients diagnosed with non-Hodgkin's lymphoma. Ann Hematol. 2013;92(3):345–50.
45. Spina M, Balzarotti M, Uziel L, Ferreri AJ, Fratino L, Magagnoli M, Talamini R, Giacalone A, Ravaioli E, Chimienti E, Berretta M, Lleshi A, Santoro A, Tirelli U. Modulated chemotherapy according to modified comprehensive geriatric assessment in 100 consecutive elderly patients with diffuse large B-cell lymphoma. Oncologist. 2012;17(6):838–46.
46. Olivieri A, Marchetti M, Lemoli R, Tarella C, Lacone A, Lanza F, Rambaldi A, Bosi A, T Italian Group for Stem Cell. Proposed definition of 'poor mobilizer' in lymphoma and multiple myeloma: an analytic hierarchy process by ad hoc working group Gruppo ItalianoTrapianto di Midollo Osseo. Bone Marrow Transplant. 2012;47(3):342–51.
47. Merli F, Luminari S, Rossi G, Mammi C, Marcheselli L, Tucci A, Ilariucci F, Chiappella A, Musso M, Di Rocco A, Stelitano C, Alvarez I, Baldini L, Mazza P, Salvi F, Arcari A, Fragasso A, Gobbi PG, Liberati AM, Federico M. Cyclophosphamide, doxorubicin, vincristine, prednisone and rituximab versus epirubicin, cyclophosphamide, vinblastine, prednisone and rituximab for the initial treatment of elderly "fit" patients with diffuse large B-cell lymphoma: results from the ANZINTER3 trial of the Intergruppo Italiano Linfomi. Leuk Lymphoma. 2012;53(4): 581–8.
48. Lin TL, Kuo MC, Shih LY, Dunn P, Wang PN, Wu JH, Tang TC, Chang H, Hung YS. The impact of age, Charlson comorbidity index, and performance status on treatment of elderly patients with diffuse large B cell lymphoma. Ann Hematol. 2012;91(9):1383–91.
49. Wedding U, Kodding D, Pientka L, Steinmetz HT, Schmitz S. Physicians' judgement and comprehensive geriatric assessment (CGA) select different patients as fit for chemotherapy. Crit Rev Oncol Hematol. 2007;64(1):1–9.
50. Gisselbrecht C, Glass B, Mounier N, Singh Gill D, Linch DC, Trneny M, Bosly A, Ketterer N, Shpilberg O, Hagberg H, Ma D, Briere J, Moskowitz CH, Schmitz N. Salvage regimens with autologous transplantation for relapsed large B-cell lymphoma in the rituximab era. J Clin Oncol. 2010;28(27):4184–90.
51. Gisselbrecht C, Schmitz N, Mounier N, Singh Gill D, Linch DC, Trneny M, Bosly A, Milpied NJ, Radford J, Ketterer N, Shpilberg O, Duhrsen U, Hagberg H, Ma DD, Viardot A, Lowenthal R, Briere J, Salles G, Moskowitz CH, Glass B. Rituximab maintenance therapy after autologous stem-cell transplantation in patients with relapsed CD20(+) diffuse large B-cell lymphoma: final analysis of the collaborative trial in relapsed aggressive lymphoma. J Clin Oncol. 2012;30(36):4462–9.
52. El Gnaoui T, Dupuis J, Belhadj K, Jais JP, Rahmouni A, Copie-Bergman C, Gaillard I, Divine M, Tabah-Fisch I, Reyes F, Haioun C. Rituximab, gemcitabine and oxaliplatin: an effective salvage regimen for patients with relapsed or refractory B-cell lymphoma not candidates for high-dose therapy. Ann Oncol. 2007;18(8):1363–8.
53. Aydin S, Duhrsen U, Nuckel H. Rituximab plus ASHAP for the treatment of patients with relapsed or refractory aggressive non-Hodgkin's lymphoma: a single-centre study of 20 patients. Ann Hematol. 2007;86(4):271–6.

54. Vacirca JL, Acs PI, Tabbara IA, Rosen PJ, Lee P, Lynam E. Bendamustine combined with rituximab for patients with relapsed or refractory diffuse large B cell lymphoma. Ann Hematol. 2014;93(3):403–9.
55. Li Y, Yimamu M, Wang X, Zhang X, Mao M, Fu L, Aisimitula A, Nie Y, Huang Q. Addition of rituximab to a CEOP regimen improved the outcome in the treatment of non-germinal center immunophenotype diffuse large B cell lymphoma cells with high Bcl-2 expression. Int J Hematol. 2014;99(1):79–86.
56. Vitolo U, Chiappella A, Franceschetti S, Carella AM, Baldi I, Inghirami G, Spina M, Pavone V, Ladetto M, Liberati AM, Molinari AL, Zinzani P, Salvi F, Fattori PP, Zaccaria A, Dreyling M, Botto B, Castellino A, Congiu A, Gaudiano M, Zanni M, Ciccone G, Gaidano G, Rossi G, Fondazione Italiana L. Lenalidomide plus R-CHOP21 in elderly patients with untreated diffuse large B-cell lymphoma: results of the REAL07 open-label, multicentre, phase 2 trial. Lancet Oncol. 2014;15(7):730–7.
57. Ruan J, Martin P, Furman RR, Lee SM, Cheung K, Vose JM, Lacasce A, Morrison J, Elstrom R, Ely S, Chadburn A, Cesarman E, Coleman M, Leonard JP. Bortezomib plus CHOP-rituximab for previously untreated diffuse large B-cell lymphoma and mantle cell lymphoma. J Clin Oncol. 2011;29(6):690–7.
58. Morschhauser FA, Cartron G, Thieblemont C, Solal-Celigny P, Haioun C, Bouabdallah R, Feugier P, Bouabdallah K, Asikanius E, Lei G, Wenger M, Wassner-Fritsch E, Salles GA. Obinutuzumab (GA101) monotherapy in relapsed/refractory diffuse large b-cell lymphoma or mantle-cell lymphoma: results from the phase II GAUGUIN study. J Clin Oncol. 2013;31(23):2912–9.
59. Merli F, Luminari S, Rossi G, Mammi C, Marcheselli L, Ferrari A, Spina M, Tucci A, Stelitano C, Capodanno I, Fragasso A, Baldini L, Bottelli C, Montechiarello E, Fogazzi S, Lamorgese C, Cavalli L, Federico M. Fondazione Italiana Linfomi. Outcome of frail elderly patients with diffuse large B-cell lymphoma prospectively identified by Comprehensive Geriatric Assessment: results from a study of the Fondazione Italiana Linfomi. Leuk Lymphoma. 2014;55(1):38–43.

Chapter 12
Multiple Myeloma

Roberto Mina and Antonio Palumbo

Abstract The introduction of novel agents thalidomide, lenalidomide, and the proteasome inhibitor bortezomib, has dramatically improved the outcome of multiple myeloma and today various effective treatment options are available. Both young and elderly patients with multiple myeloma showed to benefit from sequential approaches including novel agents. In young patients, commonly eligible for transplantation, novel combinations as induction before transplantation led to deeper and long-lasting response, and improved survival. Elderly patients or patients with comorbidities would not tolerate high-dose therapy and transplantation, thus gentler approaches are needed. Also in these patients, novel agents have revolutionized the traditional treatment and new effective approaches are now used.

Here we present an overview of the latest strategies including novel agents used to treat both transplant eligible and ineligible patients with multiple myeloma.

Keywords Multiple Myeloma • New drugs • Thalidomide • Lenalidomide • Bortezomib

Epidemiology

Multiple myeloma (MM) is the second most common hematologic malignancy. It accounts for 1 % of all cancers and 13 % of hematologic neoplasm. The median age at diagnosis is 70 years, with 37 % of patients younger than 65 years, 26 % aged 65–74 years, and 37 % older than 75 years [1–3]. The incidence of MM is expected to rise over time because of the increased life-expectancy of the general population.

Disclosure Statement Roberto Mina has no conflicts of interest. Antonio Palumbo has received consultancy fees from Amgen, Bristol-Myers Squibb, Genmab A/S, Celgene, Janssen-Cilag, Millennium Pharmaceuticals Inc., Onyx Pharmaceuticals, and honoraria from Amgen, Array BioPharma, Bristol-Myers Squibb, Genmab A/S, Celgene, Janssen-Cilag, Millennium Pharmaceuticals Inc, Onyx Pharmaceuticals, Sanofi Aventis.

R. Mina, MD • A. Palumbo, MD (✉)
Myeloma Unit, Division of Hematology, University of Torino,
Azienda Ospedaliera Città della Salute e della Scienza di Torino, Torino, Italy
e-mail: appalumbo@yahoo.com

U. Wedding, R.A. Audisio (eds.), *Management of Hematological Cancer in Older People*, DOI 10.1007/978-1-4471-2837-3_12

Diagnosis

The diagnosis of MM is based on the presence of at least 10 % clonal bone marrow plasma cells and serum and/or urinary monoclonal protein [4, 5]. MM can be asymptomatic or symptomatic, with presence of end-organ damage caused by plasma cell proliferation, defined as CRAB features (hypercalcemia, renal failure, anaemia, bone disease) [4, 5]. In addition, free-light chain assay is considered a useful tool for the diagnosis and monitoring of non-secretory MM, when small amounts of monoclonal protein are secreted in the serum and/or urine, and in light chain only myeloma [6, 7]. Symptomatic MM should be treated immediately, while clinical observation is the best approach for asymptomatic disease [8, 9].

The International Staging System (ISS) defines three risk groups on the basis of serum β_2-microglobulin and albumin levels at diagnosis [10]. Chromosomal abnormality detected on standard cytogenetic analysis may be associated with a worse outcome. Among FISH-based abnormalities, patients with isolated del 13 do not have a less favourable outcome, although del 13 with 17p deletion or t(4:14) are associated with poorer outcomes. By FISH, t(4;14) or t(14:16) is associated with poorer outcome; t(11:14) does not have negative outcome; hypderdiploidy is associated with more favourable outcome [11, 12].

Young and Elderly Patients

Patients with MM are commonly classified into young (<65 years of age) and elderly patients (≥65 years of age). Young patients, without severe comorbidities are usually considered eligible for autologous stem cell transplantation (ASCT). Elderly patients, or younger with serious comorbidities, are usually not considered ASCT candidates, thus gentler approaches are needed. However, the biological age may differ from the chronological age. Therefore, beside age, patient's characteristics and comorbidities should be carefully taken into account when determining eligibility for ASCT [13].

The introduction of novel agents, such as the first in-class proteasome inhibitor bortezomib and the immunomodulatory drugs (IMIDs) thalidomide and lenalidomide, has dramatically changed the treatment paradigm of MM [14]. The main goal of treatment is to prolong both progression-free survival (PFS) and overall survival (OS). The achievement of a complete response was recently found to be associated with longer OS in patients eligible for ASCT, and thus is considered an additional major aim of treatment [15]. Of note, novel agents and new effective combinations enabled to achieve a CR in a larger proportion of patients, not only in the young MM but also in elderly subjects. An analysis of 1,175 elderly patients found a significant association between the achievement of CR and long-term outcome, and this supports the use of novel agents to achieve maximal response also in very elderly patients (≥75 years) [16].

This paper will provide an overview of the latest regimens, including novel agents, for the treatment of newly diagnosed patients with MM. Major adverse events associated with the use of novel agents and related actions are summarized in Table 12.1.

Table 12.1 Common adverse events with novel agents and management

Adverse event	Novel agent	Action	Dose-reductions
Neutropenia	Lenalidomide, Bortezomib	G-CSF until neutrophil recovery in case of uncomplicated grade 4 or grade 2–3 complicated by fever or infection.	25–50 % drug reduction
Thrombocytopenia	Bortezomib, Lenalidomide	Platelet transfusion in case of occurrence of grade 4.	25–50 % drug reduction
Anaemia	Bortezomib, Lenalidomide	Erythropoietin or darbepoietin if hemoglobin level is ≤10 g/dL.	25–50 % drug reduction
Infection	All	Trimetoprin-cotrimoxazole for *Pneumocystis carinii* prophylaxis during high-dose dexamethasone. Acyclovir or valacyclovir for HVZ prophylaxis during bortezomib-containing therapy.	25–50 % drug reduction
Neurotoxicity	Bortezomib, Thalidomide	Neurological assessment before and during treatment. Immediate dose reduction is needed	Bortezomib: 25–50 % reduction for grade 1 with pain or grade 2 peripheral neuropathy; dose interruption until resolution to grade 1 or better with restart at 50 % dose reduction for grade 2 with pain or grade 3 peripheral neuropathy; treatment discontinuation for grade 4 peripheral neuropathy.
			Thalidomide: 50 % reduction for grade 2 neuropathy; discontinuation for grade 3; resume Thalidomide at a decreased dose if neuropathy improves to grade 1.
Skin toxicity	Thalidomide, Lenalidomide	Steroids and antihistamines.	Interruption in case of grade 3–4.
			50 % reduction in case of grade 2.
Gastrointestinal toxicity	All	Appropriate diet, laxatives, physical exercise, hydration, antidiarrheics.	Interruption in case of grade 3–4
			50 % reduction in case of grade 2.

(continued)

Table 12.1 (continued)

Adverse event	Novel agent	Action	Dose-reductions
Thrombosis	Thalidomide, Lenalidomide	Aspirin 100–325 mg if no or one individual/myeloma thrombotic risk factor is present. LMWH or full dose warfarin if there are two or more individual/myeloma risk factors and in all patients with thalidomide-related risk factors.	Drug temporary interruption and full anticoagulation, then resume treatment
Renal toxicity	Lenalidomide	Correct precipitant factors (dehydration, hypercalcemia, hyperuricemia, urinary infections, and concomitant use of nephrotoxic drugs).	Reduce dose according to creatinine clearance:
			If 30–60 mL/min: 10 mg/day;
			If < 30 mL/min without dialysis needing: 15 mg every other day;
			If < 30 mL/min with dialysis required: 5 mg/day after dialysis on dialysis day.

G-CSF granulocyte-colony stimulating factors, *HVZ* herpes-varicella-zoster, *LMWH* low-molecular-weight heparin

Young Patients

ASCT is considered the standard of care in younger patients. However, not all the studies that compared ASCT and conventional chemotherapy demonstrated the superiority of the former over the latter one [17–19]. Eventually, a meta-analysis of randomized studies including 2,411 patients treated with ASCT versus conventional chemotherapy, found that ASCT led to longer PFS, although no significant OS improvement was noted as compared with the conventional approach [20].

The choice of single versus double ASCT is still under debate and this issue has been addressed in various studies [11–24]. Despite conflicting results, particularly in terms of OS, all the studies reported a PFS advantage with tandem ASCT. A study confirmed the superiority of double vs a single ASCT after a long-term follow-up [25]. Because depth of response, particularly the achievement of CR, is a prognostic factor of improved survival [26–28], performing a second ASCT should be suggested in those patients who failed to achieve at least very good PR (VGPR) after the first ASCT [21, 22, 24, 28, 29].

Timing of transplantation is a very important question. In a pilot study, despite OS being equivalent with early or delayed ASCT, EFS and quality of life were improved in patients who underwent ASCT as upfront therapy [30]. A Spanish study showed that patients not responding to induction treatment benefited more from early ASCT [31].

Because of the widespread use of the novel agents as upfront therapy in newly diagnosed MM patients (NDMM), the role of early or delayed ASCT needs to be re-evaluated. Recently, a phase 3 study evaluated whether novel agent-containing regimens used as induction, consolidation and maintenance could delay ASCT to the time of first relapse [32]. This study confirmed the superiority of ASCT vs consolidation with lenalidomide in terms of both PFS and OS, showing that ASCT should not be delayed until time of relapse.

Upfront ASCT is typically preceded by a limited number of cycles of induction therapy, whose aim is to reduce tumour cell mass and infiltration before the collection of peripheral blood stem cells. The efficacy shown by novel agents in the relapse/refractory setting, led to the incorporation of such drugs in induction schemas for NDMM patients.

The combination vincristine-doxorubicin-dexamethasone (VAD) was the standard induction treatment for many years. Four to six cycles of VAD would lead to partial response (PR) rate of 52–63 %, with 3–13 % of CR rate [33]. Conventional induction followed by a single or tandem ASCT resulted in a CR rate of 30–40 %.

Novel agents in combination with established anti-myeloma drugs, such as dexamethasone, doxorubicin, or cyclophosphamide, have challenged the role of standard VAD, and new more effective induction regimens are now available.

Thalidomide-Containing Regimens

Various studies showed that the association of thalidomide plus dexamethasone (TD) as induction regimen before ASCT was superior in terms of response, event-free survival (EFS) and OS, if compared with traditional VAD regimen [34, 35]. As a result, TD has been one of the most commonly used induction regimens before ASCT for the past decade. The positive results obtained with TD provided the basis to evaluate the use of this combination with the addition of cytotoxic drugs, such as doxorubicin or cyclophosphamide, for the treatment of transplant-eligible patients. Both doxorubicin [36] and cyclophosphamide [37] plus TD, followed by double ASCT, led to a significantly higher VGPR/ CR rate and longer PFS compared to VAD induction. In the MRC Myeloma IX trial, in the intensive pathway, patients were randomized to receive TD plus cyclophosphamide (CTD) or cyclophosphamide-vincristine-doxorubicin-dexamethasone (CVAD) before transplantation [37]. After induction, CR rate was 13 % with CTD and 8 % with CVAD. Median PFS was 27 months for CTD and 25 months for CVAD, and OS was comparable in the two treatment arms as well (median not reached for CTD and median 63 months for CVAD). Because of its oral administration and the reduced incidence of infection (grade 3: 9 % vs 16 %) and cytopenia (grade 4: 2 % vs 9 %), CTD may be preferred. Peripheral neuropathy and deep vein thrombosis are some of the most important side effects of thalidomide therapy. Thromboprophylaxis, performed with aspirin in low-risk subjects, and warfarin or low molecular weight heparin in high-risk ones, is recommended in patients treated with thalidomide and high-dose dexamethasone or doxorubicin, and should be tailored according to the presence of individual risk factors for thromboembolic events. When thalidomide is used, peripheral neuropathy and deep vein thrombosis (DVT) may quite commonly occur, inducing a high drug-discontinuation rate.

Lenalidomide-Containing Regimen

Considering the good results obtained with TD combination, a phase 3 randomized trial assessed the role of lenalidomide in association with dexamethasone. Lenalidomide plus high-dose dexamethasone (RD) was compared with lenalidomide plus low-dose dexamethasone (Rd) as induction regimen both in myeloma patients eligible and not eligible for ASCT [38]. RD showed to be more effective than Rd with at least VGPR rate of 42 % vs 24 % respectively. However, the high dose regimen was associated with higher toxicity and early mortality rate, and did not result into longer PFS and OS. In a landmark analysis, the 3-year OS was about 92 % in patients who received ASCT after both RD and Rd.

The association of RD with bortezomib (VRD) showed to be effective and safe in a phase 1/2 study [39]. The maximum tolerated dose (MTD) was determined as bortezomib 1.3 mg/m^2, lenalidomide 25 mg, and dexamethasone 20 mg. All of the patients (100 %) achieved at least a PR, including 30 % of CR. Twenty-eight out of sixty-six patients (42 %) proceeded to transplantation. The estimated 1.5-year PFS and OS for the combination treatment with/without transplantation were 75 and 97 %, respectively. Grade 3–4 hematologic toxicities included neutropenia (9 %), and thrombocytopenia (6 %). Most common extra-hematologic toxicities included grade 2–3 sensory neuropathy (80 %) and fatigue (64 %). DVT was less than 10 % and no treatment-related mortalities were observed. To date, no study has confirmed the superiority of VRD over RD.

A phase 2 study has recently combined VRD with cyclophosphamide (VCRD) in previously untreated MM [40]. Responses were higher with VCRD, with at least PR rate of 96 %, and CR rate of 40 %. Longer follow-up is needed to assess a PFS and OS advantage. A phase 2 study by Kumar and colleagues found that, although the four-drug combination was associated with higher rate of VGPR (58 % vs. 51 %) and CR (25 % vs. 24 %), VRD showed to have a better toxicity profile, with a lower rate of discontinuation and treatment-related deaths. Thus VRD may be preferred in the clinical practice. However, further evaluation in a phase 3 study is necessary [41].

Recently, the addition of pegylated liposomal doxorubicin to the 3-drug regimen VRD (VRDD), was explored in a phase 1/2 trial, in which both patients eligible and not eligible for ASCT were enrolled. Patients received 4 to 8 cycles of VRDD and were allowed to undergo ASCT if they had achieved at least a PR after 4 cycles. After the first 4 cycles, the rates of CR/ near CR and ≥ VGPR were 29 and 57 %, respectively. Forty-nine patients underwent ASCT and their response was analysed three months after the transplant: the rates of CR/ near CR and ≥VGPR were 61 and 85 %, respectively. Since the achievement of a deep response (≥VGPR) with induction treatment before ASCT is associated with longer PFS and OS, the 4-drug combination VRDD may be suitable for younger patients willing to proceed to ASCT, although its role must be confirmed in a larger, phase 3 clinical trial [42].

Bortezomib-Containing Regimens

The association of bortezomib and dexamethasone (VD) showed to be an effective and safe frontline approach both in patients eligible and ineligible for ASCT [43]. In two trials [44, 45], VD combination was given as induction before ASCT. At least VGPR rate increased from 30 % before transplantation to 55–60 % after ASCT.

Chemotherapy with VAD has long been a standard induction for transplant eligible patients. A phase 3 study compared VAD regimen with VD as induction therapy before ASCT [46]. VD showed to be superior to VAD in terms of response (≥VGPR 38 % vs 15 % after induction and 68 % vs 47 % after double ASCT) and of median PFS (36 months vs 30 months), although this benefit was not statistically significant.

Cytotoxic drugs like doxorubicin and cyclophosphamide were added to VD as part of 3-drug regimens before ASCT. The randomized phase 3 HOVON-65/ GMMG-HD4 trial compared the association of bortezomib, doxorubicin and dexamethasone (PAD) with the standard induction regimen VAD; the rate of nCR/CR was significantly higher with the bortezomib schedule (34 % versus 49 %, respectively ($P<0.001$)); median PFS and OS were 28 and 55 months for the VAD arm and 35 and 61 months for the PAD arm [47]. In two phase 2 studies, the addition of cyclophosphamide to bortezomib-dexamethasone (VCD or CyBorD) led to a rate of ≥VGPR that varies between 37 and 61 % [40, 48].

Of note, bortezomib-containing regimens seem to overcome the poor prognosis associated with t(4;14), del 17, and other cytogenetic abnormalities [49–52]. A phase 3 trial compared TD vs TD plus bortezomib (VTD) as induction treatment before double ASCT followed by consolidation/maintenance therapy [49]. After induction, the CR rate was 19 and 5 % in the VTD and TD arm respectively (P<0.0001), they increased to 42 and 30 % respectively after the second ASCT (P=0.0004). VTD confirmed to be superior to TD also after consolidation therapy, with 49 % CR rate after VTD consolidation vs 34 % after TD consolidation (P=0.0012). Three-year PFS was longer with VTD (68 % vs 56 % P=0.005) but the 3-year OS was similar between the two treatment groups (86 % vs 84 % respectively). PFS by subgroup analysis showed an advantage with VTD in high-risk patients, such as patients with chromosome abnormalities (del 13, t(4;14) with or without del 17) advanced ISS and older age. Most common toxicities included skin rash, peripheral neuropathy, infection and DVT, although none of them had an incidence higher than 10 %. The positive results achieved in this study provided the basis for the European Medication Agency to approve VTD combination as induction regimen in transplant-eligible patients.

According to risk-stratification provided by the Mayo Clinic group [53], VRD is suggested for high-risk patients, whereas VCD can be used for intermediate-risk patients before ASCT. Whether a more aggressive strategy should be adopted mainly depends on the importance of achieving a high CR rate and of prolonging OS. In low-risk patients, the achievement of CR seems not to be related to longer OS. In these patients, a lenalidomide-containing regimen such as Rd is suggested before ASCT, subsequently lenalidomide maintenance may be administered as well.

Elderly Patients

Patients older than 65 years, or subject with significant comorbidities, are usually considered ineligible for standard melphalan 200 mg/m^2 followed by ASCT. For these patients gentler approaches, and, if necessary, age-adjusted dose modifications are required (Table 12.2).

Thalidomide-Based Regimens

The combination melphalan and prednisone (MP) has been considered, until recently, the standard of care in patients not eligible for transplantation.

The two-drug combination TD has been assessed in elderly patients. Although TD was more effective than standard MP, TD was also associated with a higher

Table 12.2 Recommended dose reductions based on patient age

Drug	Age 65–75 years	Age ≥75 years
Dexamethasone	40 mg weekly	20 mg weekly
Melphalan	0.25 mg/kg days 1–4 every 6 weeks	0.18 mg/kg days 1–4 every 6 weeks or 0.13 mg/kg days 1–4 every 4 weeks
Thalidomide	100 or 200 mg/day continuously	50 or 100 mg/day continuously
Lenalidomide[a]	15–25 mg/day days 1–21 every 4 weeks	10–25 mg/day days 1–21 every 4 weeks
Bortezomib	1.3 mg/m^2 days 1, 4, 8, 11 every 3 weeks or days 1, 8, 15, 22 every 5 weeks	1.0–1.3 mg/m^2 days 1, 8, 15, 22 every 5 weeks

[a]Based on creatinine clearance

incidence of adverse events, treatment discontinuations, and non-disease-related mortality, mainly due to infections [54].

Six randomized studies have validated the role of thalidomide plus MP (MPT) in this setting [55–60]. The two French studies found both a PFS and an OS advantage with MPT compared to MP [55, 56] while the PFS benefit detected in the Italian study did not translate into a survival advantage [60]. The Dutch/Belgian study found differences in PFS and OS between MPT and MP [59]. No significant PFS and OS differences were reported between MPT and MP in the Nordic study, although MPT patients had improved response during the first year of treatment [58]. Grade 3–4 neutropenia (16–48 %) was the most common toxicity with MPT, and was mainly due to melphalan. Peripheral neuropathy (6–23 %) and venous thromboembolism (3–12 %) were quite frequent and they were associated with thalidomide administration. Importantly, anti-thrombotic prophylaxis is recommended when administering thalidomide [61].

Recently, an efficacy meta-analysis pooling together data from 1,685 patients enrolled in the six MPT was performed, and found that median survival was 32.7 months with MP vs 39.3 months with MPT [62]. Early deaths were more frequent with MPT during the first year of treatment, and the advantage of MPT over MP was evident with longer follow-up: the 2-year PFS was 42.5 % with MPT and 28.4 % with MP. Responses were higher in MPT patients, with at least VGPR rate of 25 % for MPT and 9 % for MP. Although this meta-analysis confirmed that MPT improved PFS and OS in previously untreated MM patients, no particular advantage was seen in patients with poor performance status or renal impairment. However, considering the positive results, MPT is today considered one of the new standards of care for elderly patients with MM.

The role of thalidomide has been also assessed in combination with cyclophosphamide and dexamethasone (CTD) [63]. Responses were improved with CTD, with an overall response rate of 32.6 % with MP vs 63.8 % with CTD ($P<0.001$). The median PFS was similar between the two arms (12.4 months with MP vs 13 months with CTD) and so was also the median OS (30.6 months with MP vs 33.2 months with CTD). Of note, CTD showed to be particularly beneficial in subjects with a good cytogenetic profile by FISH. Constipation (41 %), infection (32 %), sensory neuropathy (24 %), and DVT (16 %) were common with CTD. Although thromboprophylaxis was not initially planned in this trial, it was subsequently used for patients receiving thalidomide. This dramatically decreased the rate of thromboembolic events. CTD showed to be a possible approach for selected elderly newly diagnosed MM patients, and is most beneficial in standard-risk patients by FISH analysis.

Lenalidomide-Based Regimens

The RD vs Rd trial previously mentioned included not only young patients but also elderly patients [38]. RD was associated with a higher rate of side effects than Rd, such as DVT or pulmonary embolism (26 % vs 12 %), and infections (16 % vs 9 %), particularly in patients ≥65 years. Considering the better safety profile, Rd is now to be preferred, especially in the elderly setting. Nevertheless, the use of high-dose dexamethasone is still beneficial for patients with renal failure, hypercalcemia, pain and spinal cord compression, at diagnosis.

Recently, a phase 3 trial compared the combination melphalan-prednisone-lenaldiomide followed by lenalidomide maintenance (MPR-R), with MPR and MP [64]. MPR-R prolonged the median PFS in comparison to MPR and MP (31 vs 14 vs 13 months; P<0.001). However, in patients older than 75 years of age, MPR induction did not improve PFS as compared with MP. This may be due to the higher rate of adverse events with MPR and the need for more frequent dose modifications in older patients than in younger patients. The 3-year OS was similar between the three treatment arms (70 % vs 62 % vs 66 %). Grade 4 neutropenia was reported in 35 % of MPR-R patients and 32 % of MPR patients. Despite the recent concerns about lenalidomide-related occurrence of second primary malignancies (SPMs: the 3-year rate was 7 % with both MPR-R and MPR, and 3 % with MP), the benefits associated with MPR-R outweigh the increased risk of SPMs. Similarly to thalidomide, antithrombotic prophylaxis is recommended when patients receive a lenalidomide-containing regimen [61].

Lenalidomide combined with another alkylant agent, cyclophosphamide, plus dexamethasone (CRD) showed to be effective in a phase 2 study including both young and elderly patients [65]. Of note, CRD led to at least VGPR rate of 30 %. The most common hematologic adverse event was neutropenia, and it was manageable with cyclophosphamide dose reductions. Fatigue was the more frequent non-hematologic adverse event. No thromboprophylaxis was planned in the protocol, but it was recommended for high-risk patients, and DVT occurred in 15 % of the patients enrolled. The 2-year PFS rate was 57 % and the 2-year OS rate was 87 %.

A three-arm randomized phase 3 trial is currently ongoing to compare Rd vs MPR vs CPR in elderly MM patients [66]. The major aim is to evaluate the impact of adding an alkylator to Rd, and which one between melphalan and cyclophosphamide is the is the best. Results are still preliminary, but to date no particular advantage in PFS and OS of the triplets over the doublet has been noted.

Bortezomib-Based Regimens

The combination VD showed to be a valid option for both young and elderly patients [43]. A phase 2 trial reported at least PR rate of 90 %, with at least VGPR rate of 42, and 19 % patients in CR/ near CR after VD. In patients who did not receive ASCT, median PFS was 21 months and the median OS was not reached. Adverse events were quite limited, with few cases of grade 3–4 neutropenia and peripheral neuropathy, and no DVT, although no thromboprophylaxis was given.

Bortezomib plus MP (VMP) has been validated as a new standard of care in the phase 3 Velcade as Initial Standard Therapy (VISTA) study [67, 68]. VMP showed longer median TTP 24 months vs 17 months) and 3-year OS (69 % vs 54 %) in comparison with MP. The incidence of grade 3–4 adverse events was higher with VMP than MP, grades 3–4 peripheral sensory neuropathy rate was 14 % with VMP versus 0 % with MP. Gastrointestinal complications were more frequent in the VMP group (19 % vs 5 %). Treatment-related deaths were similar in both groups (2 %).

The Spanish group compared VMP with bortezomib-thalidomide-prednisone (VTP) as induction therapy, using the weekly bortezomib schedule [69]. Response and OS were similar between VMP and VTP, but the latter was associated with more adverse events: grade 3–4 cardiac toxicity rate was 0 % vs 8.5 % (P=0.001) thromboembolism 1 % vs 2 % (P=0.5), and peripheral neuropathy 5 % vs 9 %, (P=0.6), with VTP and VMP, respectively. However, VMP led to higher incidence of neutropenia (39 % vs 22 %, P=0.008), thrombocytopenia (27 % vs 12 %, P=0.0001) and infections (7 % vs 1 %, P=0.01). Discontinuation rate (12 % vs 17 %, P=0.03) and serious adverse events (15 % vs 31 %, P=0.01) were higher with VTP.

The Italian group assessed the role of a more intense approach including four drugs as induction therapy: VMP plus thalidomide induction followed by bortezomib-thalidomide (VMPT-VT). Response rates and PFS were better with VMPT-VT as compared with VMP, VMPT-VT patients reported more grade 3–4 neutropenia (38 % vs 28 %, P=0.02), cardiac complications (10 % vs 5 %, P=0.04) and thromboembolic events (5 % vs 2 %, P=0.08) [70, 71]. The protocol was amended and bortezomib schedule was reduced from twice-weekly to once-weekly administration in both arms. This strategy reduced peripheral neuropathy without affecting efficacy [72, 73]. In addition, a recent analysis found that VMPT-VT was also associated with an OS advantage (5-year: 61% vs 51%, P=0.01). VMP-VT is a valid therapeutic approach for elderly patients, especially for those aged 65–75 years.

Conclusions

Thanks to the availability of new drugs, namely thalidomide, lenalidomide and bortezomib, physicians may choose among a wide variety of treatment options for both young and elderly patients with MM. This also enables to tailor and better personalize therapies according to patients' characteristics. Patients younger than 65 years are usually suitable for ASCT. Induction treatment with new drugs is the most suitable preparatory regimen before transplant. The three-drug combinations VTD and PAD showed to be more effective than two-drug combinations, and seem to have replaced the old standard VAD. Other combinations such as VRD are under evaluation.

Patients over 65 years do not usually tolerate ASCT, and therefore gentler approaches are needed. Today, MPT and VMP proved to be more effective than the traditional MP and therefore, they can be considered the new standards of care for patients ineligible for ASCT. Recently, MPR-R proved to be a valid strategy in this setting. The more intense combination VMPT-VT recently showed to be more effective than VMP. Reducing bortezomib-schedule further improved outcome, by decreasing treatment-related toxicity, without negatively affecting efficacy.

Future trials will evaluate the role of newer compounds, such as carfilzomib, pomalidomide, elotuzumab and bendamustine.

Acknowledgment The authors thank the editorial assistant Giorgio Schirripa

Conflicts of Interest Antonio Palumbo has received consultancy fees from Amgen, Bristol-Myers Squibb, Genmab A/S, Celgene, Janssen-Cilag, Millennium Pharmaceuticals Inc., Onyx Pharmaceuticals, and honoraria from Amgen, Array BioPharma, Bristol-Myers Squibb, Genmab A/S, Celgene, Janssen-Cilag, Millennium Pharmaceuticals Inc, Onyx Pharmaceuticals, Sanofi Aventis.

References

1. Jemal A, Siegel R, Xu J, Ward E. Cancer statistics, 2010. CA Cancer J Clin. 2010;60(5):277–300.
2. Brenner H, Gondos A, Pulte D. Recent major improvement in long-term survival of younger patients with multiple myeloma. Blood. 2008;111:2521–6.
3. Kumar SK, Rajkumar SV, Dispenzieri A, Lacy MQ, Hayman SR, Buadi FK, Zeldenrust SR, Dingli D, Russell SJ, Lust JA, Greipp PR, Kyle RA, Gertz MA. Improved survival in multiple myeloma and the impact of novel therapies. Blood. 2008;111:2516–20.
4. Durie BG, Kyle RA, Belch A, Bensinger W, Blade J, Boccadoro M, Child JA, Comenzo R, Djulbegovic B, Fantl D, Gahrton G, Harousseau JL, Hungria V, Joshua D, Ludwig H, Mehta J, Morales AR, Morgan G, Nouel A, Oken M, Powles R, Roodman D, San Miguel J, Shimizu K, Singhal S, Sirohi B, Sonneveld P, Tricot G, Van Ness B, Scientific Advisors of the International Myeloma Foundation. Myeloma management guidelines: a consensus report from the Scientific Advisors of the International Myeloma Foundation. Hematol J. 2003;4(6):379–98.
5. Kyle RA, Rajkumar SV. Criteria for diagnosis, staging, risk stratification and response assessment of multiple myeloma. Leukemia. 2009;23:3–9.
6. Kyle RA, Remstein ED, Therneau TM, Dispenzieri A, Kurtin PJ, Hodnefield JM, Larson DR, Plevak MF, Jelinek DF, Fonseca R, Melton 3rd LJ, Rajkumar SV. Clinical course and prognosis of smoldering (asymptomatic) multiple myeloma. N Engl J Med. 2007;356(25):2582–90.
7. Kyle RA, Durie BG, Rajkumar SV, Landgren O, Blade J, Merlini G, Kröger N, Einsele H, Vesole DH, Dimopoulos M, San Miguel J, Avet-Loiseau H, Hajek R, Chen WM, Anderson KC, Ludwig H, Sonneveld P, Pavlovsky S, Palumbo A, Richardson PG, Barlogie B, Greipp P, Vescio R, Turesson I, Westin J, Boccadoro M, International Myeloma Working Group. Monoclonal gammopathy of undetermined significance (MGUS) and smoldering (asymptomatic) multiple myeloma: IMWG consensus perspectives risk factors for progression and guidelines for monitoring and management. Leukemia. 2010;24(6):1121–7.

8. Bradwell AR, Carr-Smith HD, Mead GP, Harvey TC, Drayson MT. Serum test for assessment of patients with Bence Jones myeloma. Lancet. 2003;361(9356):489–91.
9. Dispenzieri A, Katzmann JA, Kyle RA, Larson DR, Melton 3rd LJ, Colby CL, et al. Prevalence and risk of progression of light-chain monoclonal gammopathy of undetermined significance: a retrospective population-based cohort study. Lancet. 2010;375(9727):1721–8.
10. Greipp PR, San Miguel J, Durie BG, Crowley JJ, Barlogie B, Bladé J, Boccadoro M, Child JA, Avet-Loiseau H, Kyle RA, Lahuerta JJ, Ludwig H, Morgan G, Powles R, Shimizu K, Shustik C, Sonneveld P, Tosi P, Turesson I, Westin J. International staging system for multiple myeloma. J Clin Oncol. 2005;23(15):3412–20.
11. Fonseca R, Barlogie B, Bataille R, Bastard C, Bergsagel PL, Chesi M, Davies FE, Drach J, Greipp PR, Kirsch IR, Kuehl WM, Hernandez JM, Minvielle S, Pilarski LM, Shaughnessy Jr JD, Stewart AK, Avet-Loiseau H. Genetics and cytogenetics of multiple myeloma: a workshop report. Cancer Res. 2004;64(4):1546–58.
12. Dewald GW, Therneau T, Larson D, Lee YK, Fink S, Smoley S, Paternoster S, Adeyinka A, Ketterling R, Van Dyke DL, Fonseca R, Kyle R. Relationship of patient survival and chromosome anomalies detected in metaphase and/or interphase cells at diagnosis of myeloma. Blood. 2005;106(10):3553–8.
13. Ferlay J, Bray F, Pisani P, Parkin DM. GLOBOCAN 2002: cancer incidence. Mortality and prevalence worldwide. IARC CancerBase No. 5, version 2.0. Lyon: IARC Press; 2004.
14. Palumbo A, Anderson K. Multiple myeloma. N Engl J Med. 2011;364(11):1046–60.
15. Harousseau JL, Avet-Loiseau H, Attal M, et al. Achievement of at least very good partial response is a simple and robust prognostic factor in patients with multiple myeloma treated with high-dose therapy: long-term analysis of the IFM 99–02 and 99–04 Trials. J Clin Oncol. 2009;27(34):5720–6.
16. Gay F, Larocca A, Wijermans P, Cavallo F, Rossi D, Schaafsma R, Genuardi M, Romano A, Liberati AM, Siniscalchi A, Petrucci MT, Nozzoli C, Patriarca F, Offidani M, Ria R, Omedè P, Bruno B, Passera R, Musto P, Boccadoro M, Sonneveld P, Palumbo A. Complete response correlates with long-term progression-free and overall survivals in elderly myeloma treated with novel agents: analysis of 1175 patients. Blood. 2011;117(11):3025–31.
17. Blade J, Rosinol L, Sureda A, et al. High-dose therapy intensification compared with continued standard chemotherapy in multiple myeloma patients responding to the initial chemotherapy: long-term results from a prospective randomized trial from the Spanish cooperative group PETHEMA. Blood. 2005;106(12):3755–9.
18. Fermand JP, Katsahian S, Divine M, et al. High dose therapy and autologous blood stem-cell transplantation compared with conventional treatment in myeloma patients aged 55 to 65 years: long-term results of a randomized control trial from the Group Myelome-Autogreffe. J Clin Oncol. 2005;23(36):9227–33.
19. Barlogie B, Kyle RA, Anderson KC, et al. Standard chemotherapy compared with high-dose chemoradiotherapy for multiple myeloma: final results of phase III US Intergroup Trial S9321. J Clin Oncol. 2006;24(6):929–36.
20. Koreth J, Cutler CS, Djulbegovic B, Behl R, Schlossman RL, Munshi NC, Richardson PG, Anderson KC, Soiffer RJ, Alyea 3rd EP. High-dose therapy with single autologous transplantation versus chemotherapy for newly diagnosed multiple myeloma: a systematic review and meta-analysis of randomized controlled trials. Biol Blood Marrow Transplant. 2007;13(2):183–96.
21. Attal M, Harousseau JL, Facon T, et al. Single versus double autologous stem-cell transplantation for multiple myeloma. N Engl J Med. 2003;349(26):2495–502.
22. Cavo M, Tosi P, Zamagni E, et al. Prospective, randomized study of single compared with double autologous stem-cell transplantation for multiple myeloma: Bologna 96 clinical study. J Clin Oncol. 2007;25(17):2434–41.
23. Segeren CM, Sonneveld P, van der Holt B, et al. Overall and event-free survival are not improved by the use of myeloablative therapy following intensified chemotherapy in previously untreated patients with multiple myeloma: a prospective randomized phase 3 study. Blood. 2003;101(6):2144–51.

24. Goldschmidt H. Single vs. double high-dose therapy in multiple myeloma: second analysis of the GMMG-HD2 trial. Haematologica. 2005;90(1):Abstract 38.
25. Barlogie B, Attal M, Crowley J, et al. Long-term follow-up of autotransplantation trials for multiple myeloma: update of protocols conducted by the Intergroupe Francophone du Myelome, Southwest Oncology Group, and the University of Arkansas for Medical Sciences. J Clin Oncol. 2010;28(7):1209–14.
26. Harousseau JL, Attal M, Avet-Loiseau H. The role of complete response in multiple myeloma. Blood. 2009;114(15):3139–46.
27. Chanan-Khan GS. Importance of achieving a complete response in multiple myeloma, and the impact of novel agents. J Clin Oncol. 2010;28(15):2612–24.
28. Ladetto M, Pagliano G, Ferrero S, et al. Major tumor shrinking and persistent molecular remissions after consolidation with bortezomib, thalidomide, and dexamethasone in patients with autografted myeloma. J Clin Oncol. 2010;28(12):2077–84.
29. Fermand JP, Alberti C, Marolleau JP. Single versus tandem high dose therapy (HDT) supported with autologous blood stem cell (ABSC) transplantation using unselected or CD34-enriched ABSC: Results of a two by two designed randomized trial in 230 young patients with multiple myeloma (MM). Hematol J. 2003;4(1):S59.
30. Fermand JP, Ravaud P, Chevret S, et al. High dose therapy and autologous peripheral blood stem cell transplantation in multiple myeloma: up-front or rescue treatment? Results of a multicenter sequential randomized clinical trial. Blood. 1998;92(9):3131–6.
31. Blade J, Sureda A, Ribera JM, et al. High-dose therapy autotransplantation/intensification versus continued conventional chemotherapy in multiple myeloma patients responding to initial chemotherapy. Definitive results from PETHEMA after a median follow-up of 66 months. Blood. 2003;102:Abstract 42.
32. Palumbo A, Cavallo F, Gay F, et al. Autologous transplantation and maintenance therapy in multiple myeloma. N Engl J Med. 2014;371(10):895–905.
33. Alexanian R, Barlogie B, Tucker S. VAD-based regimens as primary treatment for multiple myeloma. Am J Hematol. 1990;33(2):86–9.
34. Cavo M, Zamagni E, Tosi P, et al. Superiority of thalidomide and dexamethasone over vincristinedoxorubicin dexamethasone (VAD) as primary therapy in preparation for autologous transplantation for multiple myeloma. Blood. 2005;106(1):35–9.
35. Rajkumar SV, Blood E, Vesole D, et al. Phase III clinical trial of thalidomide plus dexamethasone compared with dexamethasone alone in newly diagnosed multiple myeloma: a clinical trial coordinated by the Eastern Cooperative Oncology Group. J Clin Oncol. 2006;24(3):431–6.
36. Lokhorst HM, van der Holt B, Zweegman S, et al. A randomized phase 3 study on the effect of thalidomide combined with adriamycin, dexamethasone, and high-dose melphalan, followed by thalidomide maintenance in patients with multiple myeloma. Blood. 2010;115(6):1113–20.
37. Morgan GJ, Davies FE, Gregory WM, Bell SE, Szubert AJ, Navarro Coy N, et al. Cyclophosphamide, thalidomide, and dexamethasone as induction therapy for newly diagnosed multiple myeloma patients destined for autologous stem-cell transplantation: MRC myeloma IX randomized trial results. Haematologica. 2012;97(3):442–50.
38. Rajkumar SV, Jacobus S, Callander NS, Fonseca R, Vesole DH, Williams ME, Abonour R, Siegel DS, Katz M, Greipp PR. Lenalidomide plus high-dose dexamethasone versus lenalidomide plus low-dose dexamethasone as initial therapy for newly diagnosed multiple myeloma: an open-label randomised controlled trial. Lancet Oncol. 2010;11:29–37.
39. Richardson PG, Weller E, Lonial S, et al. Lenalidomide, bortezomib, and dexamethasone combination therapy in patients with newly diagnosed multiple myeloma. Blood. 2010;116(5):679–86.
40. Kumar S, Flinn I, Richardson PG, et al. Randomized, multicenter, phase 2 study (EVOLUTION) of combinations of bortezomib, dexamethasone, cyclophosphamide, and lenalidomide in previously untreated multiple myeloma. Blood. 2012;119(19):4375–82.
41. Kumar S, Flinn I, Noga SJ, et al. Bortezomib, dexamethasone, cyclophosphamide and lenalidomide combination for newly diagnosed multiple myeloma: phase I results from the multicenter EVOLUTION study. Leukemia. 2010;24(7):1350–6.

42. Jakubowiak AJ, Griffith KA, Reece DE, et al. Lenalidomide, bortezomib, pegylated liposomal doxorubicin, and dexamethasone in newly diagnosed multiple myeloma: a phase 1/2 Multiple Myeloma Research Consortium trial. Blood. 2011;118(3):535–43.
43. Jagannath S, Durie BG, Wolf JL, et al. Extended follow-up of a phase 2 trial of bortezomib alone and in combination with dexamethasone for the frontline treatment of multiple myeloma. Br J Haematol. 2009;146(6):619–26.
44. Harousseau JL, Attal M, Leleu X, et al. Bortezomib plus dexamethasone as induction treatment prior to autologous stem cell transplantation in patients with newly diagnosed multiple myeloma: results of an IFM phase II study. Haematologica. 2006;91(11):1498–505.
45. Rosinol L, Oriol A, Mateos MV, et al. Phase II PETHEMA trial of alternating bortezomib and dexamethasone as induction regimen before autologous stem-cell transplantation in younger patients with multiple myeloma: efficacy and clinical implications of tumor response kinetics. J Clin Oncol. 2007;25(28):4452–8.
46. Harousseau J-L, Attal M, Avet-Loiseau H, et al. Bortezomib plus dexamethasone is superior to vincristine plus doxorubicin plus dexamethasone as induction treatment prior to autologous stem cell transplantation in newly diagnosed multiple myeloma: results of the IFM 2005–01 phase III trial. J Clin Oncol. 2010;28(30):4621–9.
47. Sonneveld P, Schmidt-Wolf IG, van der Holt B, et al. Bortezomib induction and maintenance treatment in patients with newly diagnosed multiple myeloma: results of the randomized phase III HOVON-65/ GMMG-HD4 trial. J Clin Oncol. 2012;30(24):2946–55.
48. Reeder CB, Reece DE, Kukreti V, et al. Cyclophosphamide, bortezomib and dexamethasone induction for newly diagnosed multiple myeloma: High response rates in a phase II clinical trial. Leukemia. 2009;23:1337–41.
49. Cavo M, Tacchetti P, Patriarca F, et al. Bortezomib with thalidomide plus dexamethasone compared with thalidomide plus dexamethasone as induction therapy before, and consolidation therapy after, double autologous stem cell transplantation in newly diagnosed multiple myeloma: a randomised phase 3 study. Lancet. 2010;376:2075–85.
50. Barlogie B, Anaissie E, van Rhee F, et al. Incorporating bortezomib into upfront treatment for multiple myeloma: early results of total therapy 3. Br J Haematol. 2007;138:176–85.
51. van Rhee F, Szymonifka J, Anaissie E, et al. Total therapy 3 for multiple myeloma: Prognostic implications of cumulative dosing and premature discontinuation of VTD maintenance components, bortezomib, thalidomide and dexamethasone, relevant to all phases of therapy. Blood. 2010;116:1220–7.
52. Nair B, van Rhee F, Shaughnessy Jr JD, et al. Superior results of total therapy 3 (2003–33) in gene expression profiling-defined low-risk multiple myeloma confirmed in subsequent trial 2006–66 with VRD maintenance. Blood. 2010;115:4168–73.
53. Rajkumar SV. Multiple myeloma: 2012 update on diagnosis, risk-stratification, and management. Am J Hematol. 2012;87(1):78–88.
54. Ludwig H, Hajek R, Tóthová E, et al. Thalidomide-dexamethasone compared with melphalan-prednisolone in elderly patients with multiple myeloma. Blood. 2009;113:3435–42.
55. Facon T, Mary JY, Hulin C, et al. Melphalan and prednisone plus thalidomide versus melphalan and prednisone alone or reduced-intensity autologous stem cell transplantation in elderly patients with multiple myeloma (IFM 99–06): a randomised trial. Lancet. 2007;370:1209–18.
56. Hulin C, Facon T, Rodon P, et al. Efficacy of melphalan and prednisone plus thalidomide in patients older than 75 years with newly diagnosed multiple myeloma: IFM 01/01 trial. J Clin Oncol. 2009;27:3664–70.
57. Beksac M, Haznedar R, Firatli-Tuglular T, et al. Addition of thalidomide to oral melphalan/prednisone in patients with multiple myeloma not eligible for transplantation: results of a randomized trial from the Turkish Myeloma Study Group. Eur J Haematol. 2011;86:16–22.
58. Waage A, Gimsing P, Fayers P, et al. Melphalan and prednisone plus thalidomide or placebo in elderly patients with multiple myeloma. Blood. 2010;116:1405–12.
59. Wijermans P, Schaafsma M, Termorshuizen F, et al. Phase III study of the value of thalidomide added to melphalan plus prednisone in elderly patients with newly diagnosed multiple myeloma: the HOVON 49 Study. J Clin Oncol. 2010;28:3160–6.

60. Palumbo A, Bringhen S, Liberati AM, et al. Oral melphalan, prednisone, and thalidomide in elderly patients with multiple myeloma: updated results of a randomized controlled trial. Blood. 2008;112:3107–31014.
61. Palumbo A, Rajkumar SV, Dimopoulos MA, et al. Prevention of thalidomide- and lenalidomide-associated thrombosis in myeloma. Leukemia. 2008;22:414–23.
62. Fayers PM, Palumbo A, Hulin C, et al. Thalidomide for previously untreated elderly patients with multiple myeloma: meta-analysis of 1685 individual patient data from 6 randomized clinical trials. Blood. 2011;118:1239–47.
63. Morgan GJ, Davies FE, Gregory WM, et al. Cyclophosphamide, thalidomide, and dexamethasone (CTD) as initial therapy for patients with multiple myeloma unsuitable for autologous transplantation. Blood. 2011;118:1231–8.
64. Palumbo A, Hajek R, Delforge M, Kropff M, Petrucci MT, Catalano J, et al. Continuous lenalidomide treatment for newly diagnosed multiple myeloma. N Engl J Med. 2012;366(19): 1759–69.
65. Kumar SK, Lacy MQ, Hayman SR, et al. Lenalidomide, cyclophosphamide and dexamethasone (CRd) for newly diagnosed multiple myeloma: Results from a phase 2 trial. Am J Hematol. 2011;86:640–5.
66. Palumbo A, Magarotto V, Bringhen S, et al. A Randomized Phase 3 Trial Of Melphalan-Lenalidomide-Prednisone (MPR) Or Cyclophosphamide-Prednisone-Lenalidomide (CPR) Vs Lenalidomide Plus Dexamethsone (Rd) In Elderly Newly Diagnosed Multiple Myeloma Patients. Blood. 2013;122(21): Abstract 536.
67. San Miguel JF, Schlag R, Khuageva NK, et al. Bortezomib plus melphalan and prednisone for initial treatment of multiple myeloma. N Engl J Med. 2008;359:906–17.
68. Mateos MV, Richardson PG, Schlag R, et al. Bortezomib plus melphalan and prednisone compared with melphalan and prednisone in previously untreated multiple myeloma: updated follow-up and impact of subsequent therapy in the phase III VISTA trial. J Clin Oncol. 2010;28(13):2259–66.
69. Mateos MV, Oriol A, Martínez-López J, et al. Bortezomib, melphalan, and prednisone versus bortezomib, thalidomide, and prednisone as induction therapy followed by maintenance treatment with bortezomib and thalidomide versus bortezomib and prednisone in elderly patients with untreated multiple myeloma: a randomised trial. Lancet Oncol. 2010;11: 934–41.
70. Palumbo A, Bringhen S, Rossi D, et al. Bortezomib-melphalan-prednisone-thalidomide followed by maintenance with bortezomib-thalidomide compared with bortezomib-melphalan-prednisone for initial treatment of multiple myeloma: a randomized controlled trial. J Clin Oncol. 2010;28:5101–9.
71. Palumbo A, Bringhen S, Cavalli M, et al. Bortezomib, Melphalan, Prednisone and Thalidomide Followed by Maintenance with Bortezomib and Thalidomide (VMPT-VT) for Initial Treatment of Elderly Multiple Myeloma Patients: Updated Follow-up and Impact of Prognostic Factors. Blood. 2010;116(21):Abstract 620.
72. Bringhen S, Larocca A, Rossi D, et al. Efficacy and safety of once-weekly bortezomib in multiple myeloma patients. Blood. 2010;116:4745–53.
73. Palumbo A, Bringhen S, Larocca A, et al. Bortezomib-melphalan-prednisone-thalidomide followed by maintenance with bortezomib-thalidomide compared with bortezomib-melphalan-prednisone for initial treatment of multiple myeloma: updated follow-up and improved survival. J Clin Oncol. 2014;32(7):634–40.

Chapter 13
Geriatric Assessment

Martine Extermann

Abstract The majority of hematologic malignancies occur in patients aged more than 65 years. Such patients have very variable health status, comorbidity levels, and geriatric syndromes prevalence Kamalakannan, Munuswamy. It is important to identify who would be a candidate for standard treatment schemes, and who would be a candidate for modified therapeutic approaches. Accurate assessment of patient fitness and comorbidities is key when planning therapy for this group as such factors will affect prognosis. In this paper, we review the published literature on a comprehensive geriatric assessment in patients with hematologic malignancies and its correlation with outcomes. Results are accumulating rapidly. The most explored disease setting had been high-grade non-Hodgkin's lymphoma. Many authors appear to converge on a definition of frailty based on severe comorbidity by CIRS-G, altered Activities of Daily Living, and geriatric syndromes. Two general models have also been constructed to predict tolerance to chemotherapy. Future trials should integrate and compare these assessments as correlates or stratification tools in order to build on the early results already available.

Keywords Comorbidity • CGA • Predictive scores • Charlson • CIRS-G • Sorror index • ADL • IADL • Geriatric syndromes • Frailty • Leukemia • Lymphoma • MDS • Myeloma • CLL

Introduction

The majority of patients with hematologic malignancies are over the age of 65. In the US, the median age at diagnosis is 65 years for chronic myelogenous leukemia (CML), 67 years for acute myelogenous leukemia (AML) and non-Hodgkin's lymphoma (NHL), 69 years for multiple myeloma, and 72 years for chronic lymphocytic leukemia (CLL). Hodgkin's disease remains diagnosed mostly in young people, with a median age of 38 years. Acute lymphoblastic leukemia (ALL) has a bimodal distribution with an incidence peak in early childhood and another one in

M. Extermann
Moffitt Cancer Center, University of South Florida,
12902 Magnolia Drive, Tampa, FL 33612, USA
e-mail: martine.extermann@moffitt.org

U. Wedding, R.A. Audisio (eds.), *Management of Hematological Cancer in Older People*, DOI 10.1007/978-1-4471-2837-3_13

the elderly (http://seer.cancer.gov/). Older patients have a significant amount of comorbidity, functional decline, and geriatric syndromes that might impact the treatment selection and outcome of their hematologic malignancy. Whereas healthy older patients can receive treatment similar to younger ones for most hematologic malignancies, at the cost of some increased toxicity, patients with a heavy comorbidity burden have more limited benefits and increased toxicity and might benefit from alternate treatment options. Comorbidity and geriatric assessment have been extensively studied, but most studies and reviews have focused either exclusively on solid tumors, or on a general sample with a minority of hematologic malignancies. Yet hematologic malignancies have some unique features: e.g. frequent bone marrow involvement; rapid response to chemotherapy, which might lead to dramatic functional improvement; and even in advanced stages, treatments offering good chances of cure or long-term remissions. The purpose of this chapter is to review the evidence on the potential role of a CGA in assessing these patients and selecting their treatment.

Assessment of Patient Fitness

Comprehensive Geriatric Assessment (CGA)

Accurate and consistent assessment of patient fitness is of paramount importance for administering effective and safe treatment to elderly cancer patients. Evidence demonstrates that chronological age alone is not a good predictor of life expectancy, functional reserve, or likelihood of treatment-related complications, and therefore guidelines such as those of the NCCN or the SIOG recommend a CGA of older cancer patients [1, 2].

The specific components of a full CGA are not standardized and are often chosen at the discretion of the physician, sometimes dependent on resources. Elements of the CGA commonly include an estimate of life expectancy [3, 4] in addition to assessments of function, comorbidity, nutrition, polypharmacy, emotional and cognitive function, geriatric conditions, and socioeconomic issues (Table 13.1). A full CGA is feasible by a dedicated multidisciplinary team. Klepin et al. explored the feasibility of a CGA in cohort of hospitalized AML patients [10]. Almost all (92.6 %) of the patients were able to complete the whole assessment. Patients with an ECOG PS 0 or 1 had a significant proportion of geriatric problems, suggesting additional assessment value. However, its conduct in the outpatient setting is more challenging due to time, staff and space constraints. Therefore a two-step approach is recommended in oncology, with first a short screening assessment and then a CGA in the patients who screen positive (about half of an older outpatient oncology population). Several screening instruments are available and the interested reader is invited to refer to a recent review of the data [11]. CGA and geriatric interventions have been demonstrated to correlate with cancer prognosis, treatments outcomes

Table 13.1 Common elements of the CGA and examples of evaluation methods

Component	Reason for assessment	Elements for assessment	Method of evaluation
Function	Functional status measures how independent a patient is and is a key factor for determining treatment success or failure	Activities of daily living (ADL)	Patient questions and then if relevant follow up
		Instrumental activities of daily living (IADL)	Katz ADL scale [5]
		Performance status (PS)	Lawton IADL scale
			PS assessed using
			Karnofsky Index
			Eastern Cooperative Oncology Group (ECOG) [6]
Comorbidity	Serious medical conditions that are not directly related to the cancer should be evaluated and treated accordingly to maximise the benefits of therapy	Seriousness of comorbid conditions	Charlson Score [7]
		Number of comorbid conditions	Cumulative Illness Rating Scale – Geriatric (CIRS-G) [8]
Socioeconomic factors	Socioeconomic issues may negatively affect compliance and thus treatment outcome	Living conditions	Social worker
		Care support	General questions
		Income and availability of financial counsel	Discussion with patient/ caregiver
		Access to transportation	
Emotional and cognitive function	Cognitive impairment can jeopardize treatment safety and lead to worse prognosis. Special precautions should be taken to ensure participation and safety of these patients	Assessment of mental state (memory, orientation, comprehension, and logical thinking)	Orientation and counting tests Folstein Mini-Mental Status
	Depression is a condition common in both geriatric and oncology populations and can adversely affect treatment outcome	Evaluation of depressive state	Geriatric depression scale

(continued)

Table 13.1 (continued)

Component	Reason for assessment	Elements for assessment	Method of evaluation
Geriatric conditions	Geriatric problems should be identified and addressed to ensure maximum treatment benefits are achieved	Dementia, delirium, depression, falls, neglect	Geriatric depression scale
			General questions
Nutrition	Malnutrition impacts on immune function and treatment tolerability	Weight and height	General questions
		Weight loss	Nutritional risk: Mini-Nutritional Assessment
Polypharmacy	Potential drug–drug interactions could impact on patient well-being or treatment outcome; unnecessary drugs can be discontinued	Drug–drug interactions	General questions
		Number of medications	Pharmacy assessment (collect all medicines)
		Avoidance of inappropriate drugs	

Adapted with permission from Extermann and Wedding [9]

and treatment modifications [7, 12–17]. Below, we will first analyze the prognostic impact of individual parameters from the CGA, namely comorbidity, functional status, nutrition, cognition and depression, and geriatric syndromes. We will then review how these parameters have been used to identify frail patients, and finally review attempts at using those criteria to select treatment.

Comorbidity

Comorbidity has long been studied for its association with outcome in several malignancies. The most frequently used instruments are the Charlson comorbidity index (hereafter "Charlson") and the CIRS-G [8, 18]. The properties of those instruments, as well as their advantages over ad hoc lists of diseases, has been discussed elsewhere [19]. Most of the studies included either all types of cancers confounded or solid tumors only. Some studies, however, have focused partially or entirely on hematologic malignancies. The presence of comorbidity has been analyzed as a prognostic factor for different end points, such as overall survival, in-hospital mortality, hospitalization, occurrence of toxicity, quality of life, and treatment allocation. One should note that some diseases have received more attention than others, without direct correlation with their relative prevalence.

Overall Survival

In a prospective cohort trial including patients with solid tumors (44.5 %) and hematological neoplasia (55.5 %), Wedding et al. identified comorbidity as an independent prognostic factor of survival (HR = 1.424; 95 % CI, 1.012–2.003) in addition to age (HR = 1.019; 95 % CI, 1.007–1.032), tumor type (HR = 1.832; 95 % CI, 1.314–2.554), and performance status (HR = 1.455; 95 % CI, 1.059–2.000) [20].

Acute Leukaemia

In a small retrospective series of acute leukemia patients (both AML and ALL), a New York team reported that patients with a comorbid condition involving a major organ had a worse median survival: 49 weeks for the group without comorbidity versus 20 weeks for the group with comorbidities. In patients above the age of 70, the figures were 32 weeks versus 4 weeks [21]. Etienne et al. retrospectively analyzed the treatment outcomes of 133 patients aged 70 years and older with AML treated with an intensive regimen. In a multivariate analysis, four adverse prognostic factors for CR and overall survival were identified: unfavorable karyotype, leukocytosis ≥30 g/L, CD34 expression on leukemic cells, and Charlson score >1 [22]. On the other hand, a retrospective analysis of treatment results in 92 patients aged 80 years and older diagnosed with AML found no significant correlation with 3-month survival of comorbidity, measured with either the Charlson index or the Sorror index [23, 24]. A recent study in 102 patient aged 60 and older found that in patients with favorable or intermediate cytogenetics, age <65, normal LDH, and an HCT-CI score of <3 were good prognostic factors for survival [25]. The authors created a simple prognostic index that still needs external validation.

Myelodysplastic Syndrome (MDS)

In a retrospective analysis of 419 patients with de novo MDS (median age 71 years), Sperr et al. compared two different comorbidity scores, the Hematopoietic Cell Transplant-Comorbidity Index (HCT-CI) and the Charlson index, for their association with overall and event-free survival (OS, EFS). The HCT-CI was associated with OS and with EFS, whereas Charlson was only associated with OS [26]. None of the indices was associated with transformation to AML. In multivariate analyses, comorbidity remained an independent prognostic factor of EFS and OS in patients with low or Int-1 MDS.

Hodgkin's Disease

The SHIELD study enrolled 175 patients aged 60 and older (median 73) [27]. Patients were assessed with a modified ACE-27 comorbidity instrument. Patients having >3 G3 comorbidities or 1 grade 4/5 comorbidity were considered frail and did not receive the main study regimen: VEPEMB. They received treatment at the choice of the physician. Function was assessed with ADL, IADL, and ECOG PS. The VEPEMB treated patients had 74 % CR for early stage and 61 % CR for advanced stage. OS and PFS at 3 years were 62 % and 53 %. Among patients treated with curative intent (VEPEMB, ABVD, or CLVPP) none of the patients deemed frail achieved CR and all died with a median OS of 7 months.

Non-Hodgkin's Lymphoma

Winkelmann et al. prospectively analyzed the prognostic value of CGA items in patients with malignant lymphoma. They identified the presence of severe comorbidity, assessed via the CIRS-G score, and IADL, as independent prognostic variables for survival [28]. In a cohort study by Lin et al., comorbidity by Charlson was not associated with the ability to receive complete treatment for DLCBL, but was associated with a decreased PFS and OS [29]. In a phase II study of DLCBL patients with moderate to high-risk cardiac disease treated with a CHOP-R regimen modified to replace doxorubicin with its non-pegylated liposomal form, patients with an age-adjusted Charlson score >7 had a shorter time to treatment failure [30].

CLL

A Mayo clinic team reviewed their CLL database for the influence of comorbidity on outcome [31]. The list of comorbidities was an ad hoc design, with six comorbidities defined as major. Data on ADL capacity were also available. The median age of the 373 patients was 67.6 years; 89 % of the patients had a comorbidity, and 46 % a major comorbidity; 8.9 % of patients had difficulty with their ADLs. On univariate analysis, the presence of a major comorbidity was associated with worse survival ($P=.042$). However, this effect was outweighed by Rai stage and age in the multivariate analysis. An interesting finding of this study was that 25 % of the patients would have been ineligible for a clinical trial based on typical eligibility criteria, but were treated nevertheless for their disease at similar times.

Intensive Care Unit (ICU) and Hospital Mortality

A study of patients admitted to the ICU for hematologic and solid tumors (mostly lymphomas and leukemias) identified Charlson score as an independent predictor of ICU and hospital mortality [32].

Febrile Neutropenia

Comorbidity was also associated with hospitalizations for neutropenia in older NHL patients. In the Iowa SEER/Medicare database, 21.7 % of patients aged 66 and older treated with chemotherapy had a hospitalization for febrile neutropenia; 41 % were hospitalized during the first cycle and 22 % during the second cycle. A positive Charlson score was an independent predictor with an associated adjusted hazard ratio of 1.50 (95 % CI, 1.03–2.17) [33]. A study in 1,355 community-treated patients of all ages treated with CHOP identified liver comorbity as a risk factor for hospitalization for febrile neutropenia, along with age >65, albumin <3.5, baseline absolute neutrophil count <1,500, planned dose intensity ≥80 % standard, and no early use of G-CSF [34]. A review of the 1992–2002 SEER data for the impact of prophylactic growth factors in 13,283 patients aged 65 and older (median 74.9) receiving chemotherapy for non-Hodgkin's lymphoma recorded comorbidity according to the Klabunde index [35]. On multivariate analysis, comorbidity was associated with an increased risk of febrile neutropenia and documented infection, and a worse OS. The odds ratio (OR) was 1.23 (1.11–1.31) for a score of 1 and 1.15 (1.01–1.31) for a score of 2 or more for febrile neutropenia; 1.27 (1.16–1.39) for a score of 1 and 1.67 (1.50–1.86) for a score of 2 or more for infection. The OR of death was 1.28 (1.21–1.34) for a score of 1, and 1.75 (1.65–1.86) for a score of 2 or more. A retrospective study analyzed NHL and prostate patients treated at Moffitt for the impact of hyperglycemia on toxicity from chemotherapy [36]. The subgroup of 162 NHL patients were all treated with CHOP-rituximab (CHOP-R). Comorbidity, as measured with the CIRS-G, did not impact the occurrence of severe toxicity, whereas in prostate cancer patients the total CIRS-G score was associated with grade 3–4 nonhematologic toxicity. In NHL patients, grade 3–4 nonhematologic toxicity was associated with hyperglycemia, both at baseline and during treatment.

Quality of Life

An international study assessed the impact of comorbidity on the quality of life (QOL) of CLL patients: 1,482 patients answered a web questionnaire that included an evaluation of their Charlson score [37]. Overall, CLL patients had a similar QOL to that of the general population, but their emotional wellbeing scores were dramatically lower. Factors associated with lower overall QOL on multivariate analysis were older age, greater fatigue, severity of comorbid illnesses, and undergoing current treatment for CLL. Wedding et al. identified that elderly cancer patients with severe comorbidities (CIRS-G grade 3 or 4) had a worse quality of life, independently from functional status [38]. Forty-six percent of these patients had hematologic malignancies.

Treatment Allocation

An epidemiologic study by the Eindhoven cancer registry was conducted in Hodgkin's and NHL patients aged 60 and older. It identified a prevalence of comorbidity by Charlson score of 58 % for NHL and 62 % for Hodgkin's patients. This was associated with a decline in administration of chemotherapy and a 10–20 % decline in 5-year survival [39]..

Hematopoietic Cell Transplantation

Although transplant strategies are mostly offered to younger patients, transplantation is increasingly used in the fit elderly. Autologous transplant for multiple myeloma is a case in point. Fit patients in their lower seventies with high-risk disease are sometimes offered autologous or reduced intensity conditioning (RIC) allogeneic transplant. Wildes et al. compared patients aged 60 and over with younger patients for outcome of autologous stem cell transplant for relapsed NHL. They identified that comorbidity rated by Charlson score, rather than age, predicted transplant-related mortality and OS [40]. Labonté et al. compared the performance of the Charlson score, the HCT-CI [23], and the modified pretransplantation assessment of mortality (mPAM) in patients receiving autologous transplant for multiple myeloma [41]. All indexes performed similarly in being associated with serious organ toxicity and length of stay. Artz et al. compared the performance of Charlson and the Kaplan-Feinstein score (KFS) in patients receiving RIC for NHL (median age 52, range 17–70) [42]. The KFS was more sensitive and more strongly associated with transplant-related mortality. When combining the KFS and ECOG performance status (PS), a high-risk category could be identified. The patients with a KFS >2, and ECOG PS >1, or an alteration on both scores, had 4.1 times the risk of transplant-related mortality compared to the low risk group (50 % at 6 months vs 15 %). OS was also significantly reduced in older patients. Pollack et al. reviewed the impact of comorbidity measured by HCT-CI in NHL patients receiving RIC [43]. The median age was 53 years (range 32–74). Patients with 3+ comorbidities had more transplant-related mortality (26.3 % vs 4.5 % at 100 days, and 36.8 vs 13.6 % at 1 year). There was no association with disease-related mortality. Farina et al. similarly reviewed the association of HCT-CI with outcome in patients receiving RIC for lymphoma or myeloma [44]. HCT-CI was an independent determinant of OS ($P<.001$), PFS ($P=.002$), and non-relapse mortality ($P=.03$). Karnofsky PS was the other independent predictor for OS and non-relapse mortality. The effect was similar for lymphomas and myeloma.

Functional Status

ECOG performance status is a strong predictor of outcome in older AML patients. A large study from the Swedish Acute Leukemia Registry demonstrated several aspects of that relationship [45]. Older patients with a low PS score had more early deaths than those with good PS, no matter what their age. However, within each age and PS category, the patients who did receive intensive treatment had lower early death rates than the others (Table 13.2). Although they may represent selection bias, these results are consistent with those of a randomized EORTC study of immediate intensive chemotherapy versus observation followed by low-dose Ara-C [47]. Another study reviewed the safety of phase 1/2 clinical trials among AML patients older versus younger than 60 years [48]. Among 121 patients, there was no difference with age. However, ECOG PS was associated with both short-term and long-term survival. Patients with an ECOG PS of 0–1 had 97.5 % 30 days' survival and 21 % 1 year survival, whereas patients with an ECOG PS of 2 or 3 had survivals of 79 and 9.5 % respectively. In NHL, ECOG PS has a well-established prognostic value as a component of the International Prognostic Index, with a score ≥2 being an adverse prognostic factor [49].

A number of studies in the oncology literature have demonstrated an additional value of geriatric functional scales, such as (instrumental) activities of daily living (ADL, IADL), beyond traditional oncologic instruments such as ECOG and Karnofsky PS. Some studies are specific to hematologic malignancies. In a prospective series of 63 adult patients with AML, their age, cytogenetics, Karnofsky PS, and IADL were associated with survival [50]. In multivariate analysis, IADL, Karnofsky PS, and cytogenetics remained as independent predictors. In the series mentioned above, Winkelmann identified severe comorbidity and IADL as

Table 13.2 Early death rates of acute leukemia patients in the Swedish Acute Leukemia Registry [45]

	Therapy								
	All			Intensive			Palliative		
Age, years	ED	Total	%ED	ED	Total	%ED	ED	Total	%ED
<50	15	342	4	14	336	4	1	6	7
50–54	14	160	9	12	155	8	2	5	40
55–59	25	181	14	17	165	10	8	16	50
60–64	27	242	11	20	223	9	7	19	37
65–69	43	308	14	20	246	8	23	61	38
70–74	83	419	20	35	281	12	47	137	34
75–79	98	448	22	30	202	15	67	244	27
80–84	125	411	30	25	96	26	100	312	32
85+	103	256	40	1	11	9	101	244	41
All groups	533	2,767	19	174	1,715	10	356	1,044	34
WHO/ECOG PS 0-II									
16–55				21	491	4	3	12	25
56–65				22	344	6	6	22	27
66–75				35	435	8	27	131	21
76–89				29	211	14	67	397	17
WHO/ECOG PS III–IV									
16–55				10	38	26	2	4	50
56–65				12	43	28	12	19	63
66–75				21	62	34	50	92	54
76–89				20	56	36	142	271	52

Early death (ED) rates (number of death within 30 days from diagnosis/total number/percentage) according to age and type of therapy, and according to WHO/ECOG performance status

independent predictors of survival in lymphoma patients [28]. In the SHIELD study in Hodgkin's patients, ADL, IADL, and ECOG PS were associated with the achievement of CR [27].

Nutrition

Most of the literature on nutrition in hematologic malignancies comes from studies from developing countries in pediatric ALL [51] Undernutrition is associated with more infections, longer hospital stay, and poorer survival. Although we could not find literature on the independent effect of nutrition in the elderly, nutritional status is an independent predictor of severe toxicity from chemotherapy in recently developed indices (see below).

Other Geriatric Syndromes

This definition usually encompasses multifactorial clinical syndromes such as dementia, incontinence, falls, neglect and abuse, delirium, failure to thrive, etc. We did not find specific literature on other geriatric syndromes and the outcome of hematologic malignancies. In a general cancer cohort including some lymphoma patients, the presence of cognitive impairment was associated with a reduction of survival by half for both early stage and advanced tumors [52].

Frailty Definitions in Hematologic Clinical Trials

Several lymphoma/leukemia studies have used empirical definitions of frailty based on a CGA to either assess prognosis or design adapted regimens:

Frailty and Prognosis

In a very interesting series of 84 patients with diffuse large cell lymphoma (DLCL), aged 65 years and older, Tucci et al. analyzed the performance of a comprehensive geriatric assessment in predicting treatment outcomes [53]. Treatment was chosen by the clinicians on clinical judgment and 62 patients received full-dose curative intent therapy. By CGA, 42 patients were considered fit (<3 CIRS-G grade 3 comorbidities, no grade 4 comorbidity, no geriatric syndrome, and independence in ADL). Whereas all geriatrically fit patients had been treated with curative intent and had a better survival, it is interesting to note that for unfit patients, the receipt of curative intent chemotherapy did not affect median survival (8 months vs 7 months, $P = \text{NS}$). A retrospective study in NHL patients (all types) aged 80 and older used the same frailty criteria [54]. Although frailty was not associated with outcome, impaired ADLs were associated with worse PFS and OS.

Frailty as a Selection Criterion

The EORTC 20992 study defined a frail patient as one aged 70 years or older and having either severe comorbidities (by CIRS-G), WHO performance status of 3 or 4, cardiac contraindication to anthracyclines, creatinine clearance <50 mL/min, baseline neutropenia, or thrombopenia [55]. These criteria were chosen as predictors of inability to receive CHOP for large cell lymphoma, and the patients were treated with CVP. The authors also conducted a CGA on these 32 patients. They turned out to have a high prevalence of impairments: 47 % had a severe comorbidity; 94 % were scoring positive on the geriatric depression scale; 81 % were dependent in at least 1 in 8 instrumental activities of daily living; 37.5 % of patients showed scores at 24 or lower on the Mini-Mental Status. Although a subgroup of patients benefited from chemotherapy, four experienced severe toxicities (febrile neutropenia or toxic death), and there were eight early deaths, five of them unrelated to the lymphoma or treatment toxicity. Therefore, this definition truly captured frail patients. Dr Soubeyran and the Goelams group are now conducting a follow-up study adding rituximab and excluding ECOG four patients. Monfardini et al., in a phase 2 intermediate-/high-grade NHL study, defined a frail patient as: (1) Age ≥80, or (2) Age 70–80 and either 3 grade 3 or 1 grade 4 comorbidities (CIRS-G), or dependence in ADL, or a geriatric syndrome [56]. Such patients were treated with a regimen of vinorelbine and prednisone. The median duration of CR was 29 months, and PR 1 month. The median OS was 10 months. Three of thirty patients died of heart failure within 28 days of therapy, and 1 patient died of rapid lymphoma progression. This definition of frailty is close to that of Balducci [57]. The same definition was also used in Tucci et al's study [53].

Monfardini's criteria were used recently to select patients enrolled in a randomized multicentric study comparing R-CHOP and R-miniCEOP [58]. Within that selected fit cohort, IADLs and lesser degrees of comorbidity did not have further prognostic impact, confirming that older patients deemed fit by these criteria can receive standard curative intent chemotherapy.

Those criteria (without the geriatric syndromes) were also used in a study of low-dose Ara-C and valproic acid for elderly patients with AML/RAEB deemed unfit for standard chemotherapy [5]. These 31 patients had a 35 % response rate. There was no significant difference between frail and non-frail patients, but the power is very low.

Olivieri et al. in a multicentric study [6] stratified chemotherapy for DLCBL according to three levels of frailty as follows: Patients were defined as frail if they had one of the following: age ≥85; dependence in ADLs; a geriatric syndrome; a severe comorbidity (CIRS-G ≥3) or 3 grade 2+ comorbidities. Intermediate patients had one or two grade 2 comorbidities but no other criteria. The other patients were considered fit. Fit patients were treated with R-CHOP, intermediate patients with pegylated liposomal doxorubicin replacing the doxorubicin, and frail patients with a miniCHOP without rituximab. Treatment side effects were tolerable. Response rates were similar. EFS and OS were better in the fit group but the study does not allow discerning whether this was due to comorbidity or a treatment effect. Frail patients were markedly older.

Spina et al. conducted a study where they used elements of a comprehensive geriatric assessment, namely comorbidity and ADL/IADL to adapt the chemotherapy regimen of patients with diffuse large cell B-cell lymphoma (Fig. 13.1) [46]. The median number of cycles given was 6. CR was achieved in 81 patients, and PR in 6 (87 % response rate). The 5-year OS was 60 %, DFS 82 %, and EFS 52 %. Fit patients (no CIRS-G grade 3 comorbidity or less than 3 grade 2 comorbidities, independent in ADL, and/or independent in 7 or 8 IADL), unfit patients (no grade 3 comorbidity, 3–5 grade 2 comorbidities, 1 ADL dependence, and/or IADL score 5 or 6), and frail patients (lower scores) had a 5 year OS of 76, 53, and 29 % respec-

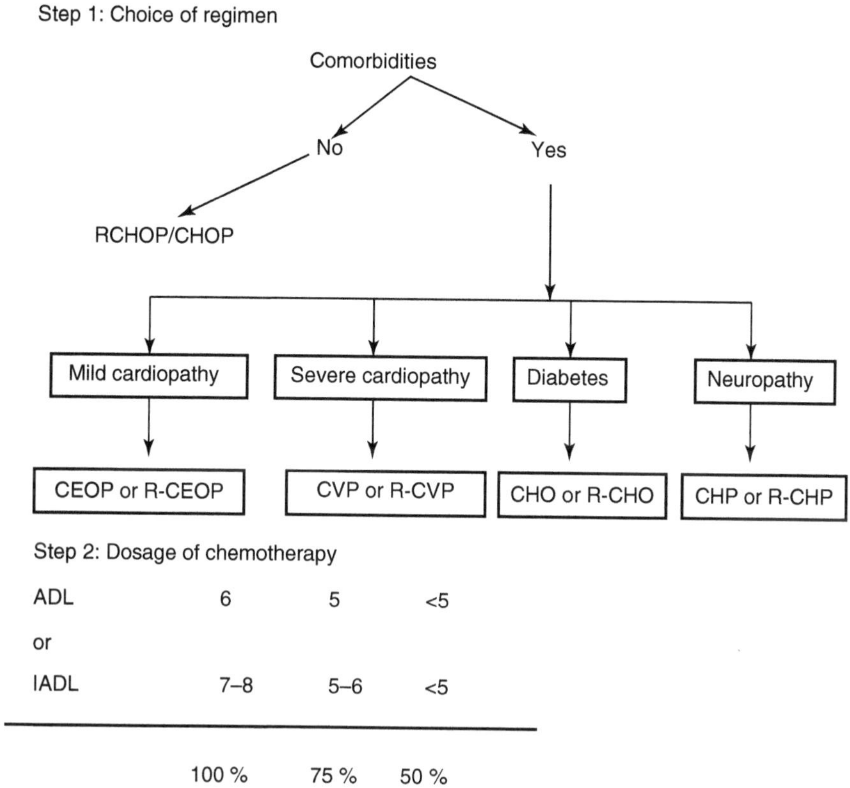

Fig. 13.1 Treatment strategy for diffuse large B-cell lymphoma in Spina et al.'s study (Reproduced with permission from Ref. [46]). Regimen abbreviations: *CEOP* cyclophosphamide, epirubicin, vincristine and prednisone, *CHO* cyclophosphamide, doxorubicin, and vincristine, *CHOP* cyclophosphamide, doxorubicin, vincristine, and prednisone, *CVP* cyclophosphamide, vincristine, and prednisone, *R* rituximab

tively. In multivariate analysis, these geriatric groups and IPI were the elements significantly associated with OS. The toxicity was comparable between groups.

The German CLL Study Group conducted a randomized study of fludarabine and cyclophosphamide with or without rituximab [59]. Since there were concerns about tolerability, they restricted the eligibility to patients with a CIRS-G score of 6 or less. Such patients tolerated equally well both treatments, except for more grade 3–4 neutropenia and leukopenia in the rituximab arm. The same group has an ongoing study to determine the optimal treatment of patients with a higher level of comorbidity.

This half-dozen studies is beginning to provide insights into what might be appropriate criteria to define frailty in lymphoma patients for the purpose of selecting treatment. A combination of comorbidity, function, and geriatric syndromes appears to lead to a reasonable treatment selection. Future work should probably compare such a strategy with alternate models of frailty or treatment toxicity risk and track the trade-offs between effectiveness and toxicity with each model.

Tools Focusing on the Risk of Toxicity from Chemotherapy

Until recently, there were no tools available that could reliably evaluate the individual risk of severe toxicity from different chemotherapy regimens across a range of tumor types. Two new assessment methods that specifically look at the older patient's ability to tolerate chemotherapy were presented at ASCO 2010 and are in the process of further evaluation: The Chemotherapy Risk Assessment Scale for High-age patients (CRASH) and the Cancer and Aging Research Group (CARG) chemotoxicity assessment tools [60, 61].

The CRASH score combines an assessment of the toxicity of the chemotherapy regimen, using the MAX2 index [62], with patient parameters. The score has two subscores: predictors of grade 4 hematologic toxicity, which are lactate dehydrogenase, diastolic blood pressure, IADLs and toxicity of the chemotherapy regimen; and predictors of grade 3–4 nonhematologic toxicity, which are ECOG PS, Mini-Nutritional Assessment, Mini-Mental Status, and toxicity of the regimen. A combined score can be based on the two subscores. The instrument was validated internally and in an independent sample of patients 70 and older. The CARG score has two versions, one with full geriatric instruments, one with individual items, such as age 73 years or over, cancer type, standard dose, poly-chemotherapy, falls in last 6 months, assistance with IADLs, and decreased social activity. It identifies three risk categories for grade 3–5 toxicities in patients 65 and older. Both scores were tested in general populations of older cancer patients and although some patients had hematologic malignancies, they have not been tested specifically in hematologic tumor populations.

In addition, some models focus more specifically on the risk of severe neutropenia or febrile neutropenia. Several were developed in a solid tumor setting but a few are relevant for hematologic malignancies. We mentioned above the model created by Lyman et al. [34] to predict the risk of hospitalization for febrile neutropenia in NHL patients. Intragumtorchai et al., in a population of 145 patients with intermediate-/high-grade NHL treated with CHOP without G-CSF, designed a model based on albumin <3.5 g/dL, LDH above normal range, and bone marrow invasion to identify three risk categories for grade 4 or febrile neutropenia [63]. Blay et al. identified a Day 5 lymphocyte count <700 as a risk factor for febrile neutropenia in a general cancer population. This finding was confirmed in a cohort of lymphoma patients [64]. The same group identified low baseline CD4 count as a risk factor in a general cohort of patients [65]. Although day 1 lymphopenia was also somewhat predictive, it was not as strong a predictor as day 5 lymphopenia [66]. On the other hand, in the CRASH cohort mentioned above, older patients who did not experience any neutropenia during the first cycle and who were receiving a chemotherapy with a MAX2 index <0.20 had only a 4.6 % risk of grade 4 neutropenia and 1.5 % risk of febrile neutropenia during subsequent cycles of treatment [67]. A common characteristic of these neutropenia models, however, is that despite having been created a decade ago, they have failed so far to gain wide interest in their use. They also have not been compared to each other, to our knowledge.

Conclusions and Perspective

A CGA is increasingly used in hematologic malignancies for patient assessment and treatment selection. Italian authors seem to be reaching some convergence around using a definition of frailty derived from Balducci's original proposal [57] that includes at least one of: three or more CIRS-G grade 3 or one grade 4 comorbidity; dependence in basic ADLs; presence of a geriatric syndrome (dementia, delirium, depression, osteoporosis, incontinence, falls, failure to thrive, and neglect/abuse); and sometimes an age threshold at 80 or 85 years old [5, 6, 53, 56, 58]. In solid tumors, similar criteria have been shown to be associated with surgical complications [68] and survival [69].

We also now have two instruments to predict severe toxicity from chemotherapy.

We think it is now time to systematically include these two sets of tools (frailty and predictors of toxicity) into clinical trials for hematologic malignancies in the elderly and correlate them prospectively with complete outcome data and decision strategies.

As the population of patients with hematologic malignancies increases, and as treatment choices become more targeted, there is a clear need to start tailoring the type of treatment we give, not only to the tumor, but to the patient as well.

References

1. Extermann M, Aapro M, Bernabei R, et al. Use of comprehensive geriatric assessment in older cancer patients: recommendations from the task force on CGA of the International Society of Geriatric Oncology (SIOG). Crit Rev Oncol Hematol. 2005;55(3):241–52.
2. NCCN. NCCN Guidelines™. 2011. http://www.nccn.org/professionals/physician_gls/f_guidelines.asp.
3. Walter LC, Covinsky KE. Cancer screening in elderly patients: a framework for individualized decision making. JAMA. 2001;285(21):2750–6.
4. Balducci L, Extermann M. Management of cancer in the older person: a practical approach. Oncologist. 2000;5(3):224–37.
5. Corsetti MT, Salvi F, Perticone S, et al. Hematologic improvement and response in elderly AML/RAEB patients treated with valproic acid and low-dose Ara-C. Leuk Res. 2011;35(8):991–7.
6. Olivieri A, Gini G, Bocci C, et al. Tailored therapy in an unselected population of 91 elderly patients with DLBCL prospectively evaluated using a simplified CGA. Oncologist. 2012;17(5):663–72.
7. Overcash JA, Beckstead J. Predicting falls in older patients using components of a comprehensive geriatric assessment. Clin J Oncol Nurs. 2008;12(6):941–9.
8. Charlson ME, Pompei P, Ales KL, MacKenzie CR. A new method of classifying prognostic comorbidity in longitudinal studies: development and validation. J Chronic Dis. 1987;40(5):373–83.
9. Extermann M, Wedding U. Comorbidity and geriatric assessment for older patients with hematologic malignancies: A review of the evidence. J Geriatr Oncol. 2012;3(1):49–57.
10. Klepin HD, Geiger AM, Tooze JA, et al. The feasibility of inpatient geriatric assessment for older adults receiving induction chemotherapy for acute myelogenous leukemia. J Am Geriatr Soc. 2011;59(10):1837–46.

11. Extermann M. Basic assessment of the older cancer patient. Curr Treat Options Oncol. 2011;12(3):276–85.
12. McCorkle R, Strumpf NE, Nuamah IF, et al. A specialized home care intervention improves survival among older post-surgical cancer patients. J Am Geriatr Soc. 2000;48(12):1707–13.
13. Caillet P, Canoui-Poitrine F, Vouriot J, et al. Comprehensive geriatric assessment in the decision-making process in elderly patients with cancer: ELCAPA study. J Clin Oncol. 2011;29(27):3636–42.
14. Extermann M, Meyer J, McGinnis M, et al. A comprehensive geriatric intervention detects multiple problems in older breast cancer patients. Crit Rev Oncol Hematol. 2004;49(1): 69–75.
15. Audisio RA, Pope D, Ramesh HS, et al. Shall we operate? Preoperative assessment in elderly cancer patients (PACE) can help. A SIOG surgical task force prospective study. Crit Rev Oncol Hematol. 2008;65(2):156–63.
16. Soejono C. The role of comprehensive geriatric assessment (CGA) in the management of stage 3 hepatocellular carcinoma in the elderly. Crit Rev Oncol Hematol. 2006;60(S1):S20.
17. Freyer G, Geay JF, Touzet S, et al. Comprehensive geriatric assessment predicts tolerance to chemotherapy and survival in elderly patients with advanced ovarian carcinoma: a GINECO study. Ann Oncol. 2005;16(11):1795–800.
18. Miller MD, Paradis CF, Houck PR, et al. Rating chronic medical illness burden in geropsychiatric practice and research: application of the Cumulative Illness Rating Scale. Psychiatry Res. 1992;41(3):237–48.
19. Extermann M. Measuring comorbidity in older cancer patients. Eur J Cancer. 2000;36(4): 453–71.
20. Wedding U, Rohrig B, Klippstein A, Pientka L, Hoffken K. Age, severe comorbidity and functional impairment independently contribute to poor survival in cancer patients. J Cancer Res Clin Oncol. 2007;133(12):945–50.
21. Zaheer W, Hashmi A, Lichtman SM, Kolitz J, Cirrone K, Spinek K, Weisman A, Schulman P. Effect of comorbidity and age on survival in 73 patients with de novo acute leukemia. Proc Am Soc Clin Oncol; 1995;13:498.
22. Etienne A, Esterni B, Charbonnier A, et al. Comorbidity is an independent predictor of complete remission in elderly patients receiving induction chemotherapy for acute myeloid leukemia. Cancer. 2007;109(7):1376–83.
23. Sorror ML, Maris MB, Storb R, et al. Hematopoietic cell transplantation (HCT)-specific comorbidity index: a new tool for risk assessment before allogeneic HCT. Blood. 2005;106(8):2912–9.
24. Harb AJ, Tan W, Wilding GE, et al. Treating octogenarian and nonagenarian acute myeloid leukemia patients – predictive prognostic models. Cancer. 2009;115(11):2472–81.
25. Djunic I, Suvajdzic-Vukovic N, Virijevic M, et al. Prognostic risk score for the survival of elderly patients with acute myeloid leukaemia comprising comorbidities. Med Oncol. 2013;30(1):394.
26. Sperr WR, Wimazal F, Kundi M, et al. Comorbidity as prognostic variable in MDS: comparative evaluation of the HCT-CI and CCI in a core dataset of 419 patients of the Austrian MDS Study Group. Ann Oncol. 2010;21(1):114–9.
27. Proctor SJ, Wilkinson J, Jones G, et al. Evaluation of treatment outcome in 175 patients with Hodgkin lymphoma aged 60 years or over: the SHIELD study. Blood. 2012;119(25): 6005–15.
28. Winkelmann N, Petersen I, Kiehntopf M, Fricke HJ, Hochhaus A, Wedding U. Results of comprehensive geriatric assessment effect survival in patients with malignant lymphoma. J Cancer Res Clin Oncol. 2011;137(4):733–8.
29. Lin TL, Kuo MC, Shih LY, et al. The impact of age, Charlson comorbidity index, and performance status on treatment of elderly patients with diffuse large B cell lymphoma. Ann Hematol. 2012;91(9):1383–91.
30. Corazzelli G, Frigeri F, Arcamone M, et al. Biweekly rituximab, cyclophosphamide, vincristine, non-pegylated liposome-encapsulated doxorubicin and prednisone (R-COMP-14) in

elderly patients with poor-risk diffuse large B-cell lymphoma and moderate to high 'life threat' impact cardiopathy. Br J Haematol. 2011;154(5):579–89.
31. Thurmes P, Call T, Slager S, et al. Comorbid conditions and survival in unselected, newly diagnosed patients with chronic lymphocytic leukemia. Leuk Lymphoma. 2008;49(1):49–56.
32. Moran JL, Solomon PJ, Williams PJ. Assessment of outcome over a 10-year period of patients admitted to a multidisciplinary adult intensive care unit with haematological and solid tumours. Anaesth Intensive Care. 2005;33(1):26–35.
33. Chen-Hardee S, Chrischilles EA, Voelker MD, et al. Population-based assessment of hospitalizations for neutropenia from chemotherapy in older adults with non-Hodgkin's lymphoma (United States). Cancer Causes Control. 2006;17(5):647–54.
34. Lyman GH, Delgado DJ. Risk and timing of hospitalization for febrile neutropenia in patients receiving CHOP, CHOP-R, or CNOP chemotherapy for intermediate-grade non-Hodgkin lymphoma. Cancer. 2003;98(11):2402–9.
35. Gruschkus SK, Lairson D, Dunn JK, Risser J, Du XL. Comparative effectiveness of white blood cell growth factors on neutropenia, infection, and survival in older people with non-Hodgkin's lymphoma treated with chemotherapy. J Am Geriatr Soc. 2010;58(10):1885–95.
36. Brunello A, Kapoor R, Extermann M. Hyperglycemia during chemotherapy for hematologic and solid tumors is correlated with increased toxicity. Am J Clin Oncol. 2011;34(3):292–6.
37. Shanafelt TD, Bowen D, Venkat C, et al. Quality of life in chronic lymphocytic leukemia: an international survey of 1482 patients. Br J Haematol. 2007;139(2):255–64.
38. Wedding U, Rohrig B, Klippstein A, Brix C, Pientka L, Hoffken K. Co-morbidity and functional deficits independently contribute to quality of life before chemotherapy in elderly cancer patients. Support Care Cancer. 2007;15(9):1097–104.
39. van Spronsen DJ, Janssen-Heijnen ML, Lemmens VE, Peters WG, Coebergh JW. Independent prognostic effect of co-morbidity in lymphoma patients: results of the population-based Eindhoven Cancer Registry. Eur J Cancer. 2005;41(7):1051–7.
40. Wildes TM, Augustin KM, Sempek D, et al. Comorbidities, not age, impact outcomes in autologous stem cell transplant for relapsed non-Hodgkin lymphoma. Biol Blood Marrow Transplant. 2008;14(7):840–6.
41. Labonte L, Iqbal T, Zaidi MA, et al. Utility of comorbidity assessment in predicting transplantation-related toxicity following autologous hematopoietic stem cell transplantation for multiple myeloma. Biol Blood Marrow Transplant. 2008;14(9):1039–44.
42. Artz AS, Pollyea DA, Kocherginsky M, et al. Performance status and comorbidity predict transplant-related mortality after allogeneic hematopoietic cell transplantation. Biol Blood Marrow Transplant. 2006;12(9):954–64.
43. Pollack SM, Steinberg SM, Odom J, Dean RM, Fowler DH, Bishop MR. Assessment of the hematopoietic cell transplantation comorbidity index in non-Hodgkin lymphoma patients receiving reduced-intensity allogeneic hematopoietic stem cell transplantation. Biol Blood Marrow Transplant. 2009;15(2):223–30.
44. Farina L, Bruno B, Patriarca F, et al. The hematopoietic cell transplantation comorbidity index (HCT-CI) predicts clinical outcomes in lymphoma and myeloma patients after reduced-intensity or non-myeloablative allogeneic stem cell transplantation. Leukemia. 2009;23(6):1131–8.
45. Juliusson G, Antunovic P, Derolf A, et al. Age and acute myeloid leukemia: real world data on decision to treat and outcomes from the Swedish Acute Leukemia Registry. Blood. 2009;113(18):4179–87.
46. Spina M, Balzarotti M, Uziel L, et al. Modulated chemotherapy according to modified comprehensive geriatric assessment in 100 consecutive elderly patients with diffuse large B-cell lymphoma. Oncologist. 2012;17(6):838–46.
47. Lowenberg B, Zittoun R, Kerkhofs H, et al. On the value of intensive remission-induction chemotherapy in elderly patients of 65+ years with acute myeloid leukemia: a randomized phase III study of the European Organization for Research and Treatment of Cancer Leukemia Group. J Clin Oncol. 1989;7(9):1268–74.

48. van Heeckeren W, Fu P, Barr PM, Arfons LM, Kirschbaum MH, Lazarus HM, Cooper BW. Safety and tolerability of phase I/II clinical trials among older and younger patients with acute myelogenous leukemia. J Geriatr Oncol. 2011;2(3):215–21.
49. Anonymous. A predictive model for aggressive non-Hodgkin's lymphoma. The International Non-Hodgkin's Lymphoma Prognostic Factors Project. New Engl J Med. 1993;329(14): 987–94.
50. Wedding U, Rohrig B, Klippstein A, Fricke HJ, Sayer HG, Hoffken K. Impairment in functional status and survival in patients with acute myeloid leukaemia. J Cancer Res Clin Oncol. 2006;132(10):665–71.
51. Lobato-Mendizabal E, Lopez-Martinez B, Ruiz-Arguelles GJ. A critical review of the prognostic value of the nutritional status at diagnosis in the outcome of therapy of children with acute lymphoblastic leukemia. Rev Invest Clin. 2003;55(1):31–5.
52. Robb C, Boulware D, Overcash J, Extermann M. Patterns of care and survival in cancer patients with cognitive impairment. Crit Rev Oncol Hematol. 2010;74(3):218–24.
53. Tucci A, Ferrari S, Bottelli C, Borlenghi E, Drera M, Rossi G. A comprehensive geriatric assessment is more effective than clinical judgment to identify elderly diffuse large cell lymphoma patients who benefit from aggressive therapy. Cancer. 2009;115(19):4547–53.
54. Nabhan C, Smith SM, Helenowski I, et al. Analysis of very elderly (>/=80 years) non-Hodgkin lymphoma: impact of functional status and co-morbidities on outcome. Br J Haematol. 2012;156(2):196–204.
55. Soubeyran P, Khaled H, MacKenzie M, Debois M, Fortpied C, de Bock R, Ceccaldi J, de Jong D, Eghbali H, Rainfray M, Monnereau A, Zulian G, Teodorovic I. Diffuse large B-cell and peripheral T-cell non-Hodgkin's lymphoma in the frail elderly. A phase II EORTC trial with a progressive and cautious treatment emphasizing geriatric assessment. J Geriatr Oncol. 2011;2(1):36–44.
56. Monfardini S, Aversa SM, Zoli V, et al. Vinorelbine and prednisone in frail elderly patients with intermediate-high grade non-Hodgkin's lymphomas. Ann Oncol. 2005;16(8):1352–8.
57. Balducci L, Extermann M, Carreca I. Management of breast cancer in the older woman. Cancer Control. 2001;8(5):431–41.
58. Merli F, Luminari S, Rossi G, et al. Cyclophosphamide, doxorubicin, vincristine, prednisone and rituximab versus epirubicin, cyclophosphamide, vinblastine, prednisone and rituximab for the initial treatment of elderly "fit" patients with diffuse large B-cell lymphoma: results from the ANZINTER3 trial of the Intergruppo Italiano Linfomi. Leuk Lymphoma. 2012;53(4):581–8.
59. Hallek M, Fischer K, Fingerle-Rowson G, et al. Addition of rituximab to fludarabine and cyclophosphamide in patients with chronic lymphocytic leukaemia: a randomised, open-label, phase 3 trial. Lancet. 2010;376(9747):1164–74.
60. Extermann M, Boler I, Reich RR, et al. Predicting the risk of chemotherapy toxicity in older patients: the Chemotherapy Risk Assessment Scale for High-Age Patients (CRASH) score. Cancer. 2012;118(13):3377–86.
61. Hurria A, Togawa K, Mohile SG, et al. Predicting chemotherapy toxicity in older adults with cancer: a prospective multicenter study. J Clin Oncol. 2011;29(25):3457–65.
62. Extermann M, Bonetti M, Sledge GW, O'Dwyer PJ, Bonomi P, Benson 3rd AB. MAX2–a convenient index to estimate the average per patient risk for chemotherapy toxicity; validation in ECOG trials. Eur J Cancer. 2004;40(8):1193–8.
63. Intragumtornchai T, Sutheesophon J, Sutcharitchan P, Swasdikul D. A predictive model for life-threatening neutropenia and febrile neutropenia after the first course of CHOP chemotherapy in patients with aggressive non-Hodgkin's lymphoma. Leuk Lymphoma. 2000;37(3–4):351–60.
64. Blay JY, Chauvin F, Le Cesne A, et al. Early lymphopenia after cytotoxic chemotherapy as a risk factor for febrile neutropenia. J Clin Oncol. 1996;14(2):636–43.

65. Borg C, Ray-Coquard I, Philip I, et al. CD4 lymphopenia as a risk factor for febrile neutropenia and early death after cytotoxic chemotherapy in adult patients with cancer. Cancer. 2004;101(11):2675–80.
66. Ray-Coquard I, Borg C, Bachelot T, et al. Baseline and early lymphopenia predict for the risk of febrile neutropenia after chemotherapy. Br J Cancer. 2003;88(2):181–6.
67. Janssen-Heijnen ML, Extermann M, Boler IE. Can first cycle CBCs predict older patients at very low risk of neutropenia during further chemotherapy? Crit Rev Oncol Hematol. 2011;79(1):43–50.
68. Kristjansson SR, Rønning B, Hurria A, et al. A comparison of two pre-operative frailty measures in older surgical cancer patients. J Geriatr Oncol. 2012;3(1):1–7.
69. Basso U, Falci C, Brunello A, Zafferri V, Fiduccia P, Sergi G, Lonardi S, Lamberti E, Castegnaro E, Solda C, Cossutta F, Chiaron-Sileni V, Monfardini S, Zagonel V. Prognostic value of multidimensional geriatric assessment (MGA) on survival of a prospective cohort of 880 elderly cancer patients (ECP). J Clin Oncol. 2011;29(Suppl):abstr 9065.

Chapter 14
Nursing Issues

Corien M. Eeltink, Angelina Beumer-Grootenhuis, and Carolien Burghout

Abstract It is known that older patients with hematological malignancies can benefit from treatment modalities as long as tailored evaluation of all aspects is used to assess potential problems. Oncology nurses and Nurse Practitioners can play an important role in the collection of information in older patients. However, it is important that the collected information is used for making the right treatment decision and that this decision is taken by a multidisciplinary team.

After the evaluation of all aspects that can be impacted by aging, proactive interventions need to be offered to prevent deterioration. In this chapter we will describe some of the different nursing aspects with regard to the following topics: polypharmacy and medication-adherence, nutritional state, the nursing management of drug related side effects, patient preferences and information needs of older adults. The last paragraph is on caregiving by family and friends and the role of the nurse to support optimal collaboration.

This chapter is intended to focus on the different roles that nurses can have in the care for the older patients, not only by assessing the geriatric assessment or managing the most common side effects of the treatment, but also by educating and the supporting role nurses can have in the care for the older patient and their caregivers.

Keywords Polypharmacy • Medication adherence • Nutritional state • Information needs • Family caregivers • Nursing management

C.M. Eeltink, RN, MA, ANP (✉)
Department of Haematology, VU University Medical Center,
7057, 1007 MB Amsterdam, The Netherlands
e-mail: C.Eeltink@vumc.nl

A. Beumer-Grootenhuis, RN
Department of Oncology, Deventer Ziekenhuis,
Deventer, The Netherlands

C. Burghout, RN, M ANP
Department of Haematology, Jeroen Bosch Hospital,
's-Hertogenbosch, The Netherlands

U. Wedding, R.A. Audisio (eds.), *Management of Hematological Cancer in Older People*, DOI 10.1007/978-1-4471-2837-3_14

Introduction

The diagnosis and treatment of hematological malignancies in older patients is very challenging due to the wide range of potential problems related to the older person's health status which will have to be taken into account.

Prognosis and treatment outcome between older and younger patients do not differ, provided that the intended therapeutic treatment can be given. Therefore, an adequate fitness screening of the elderly patient prior to treatment is important to predict the probability to complete chemotherapy. Screening for comorbidity and loss of function are also important for the severity of the side effects caused by the treatment and the impact this all can have on Quality of Life (QoL). Nurses can have an essential role in the screening and care for the older patients.

Firstly, older persons receive more prescriptions than any other group. Nurses play a major role in identifying people receiving multiple medications and in helping to evaluate their effectiveness. Suggestions for obtaining a complete drug history are presented along with explanations of the role of age-related changes on the effect of those medications on the elderly.

Secondly, malnutrition is becoming increasingly more common among older persons. This is a cause for concern considering malnutrition negatively affects the health of the older adult. Screening to determine malnutrition should be an essential part of the nursing assessment. Giving tips and advice about nutrition in the treatment of cancer is always valuable, also in case of no malnutrition.

Thirdly, to limit severity of the adverse events, early identification and prompt interventions for the most common toxicities are needed. The most common adverse events in older patients with Hematological Malignancies and how to manage these are described.

Fourthly, to increase compliance and decrease anxiety, patient information should be given in a way that the patient and his/her relative clearly understand. Older persons often have a more paternalistic style of making decisions; this may either lead to a lower information need or to a risk for poor communication. Unmet communication needs can occur during psychological and physical health crisis: this may cause non-compliance, and is an important risk factor for the outcome of the medical treatment.

Finally, with the current trends of the increase in home care, more adult children and older partners are becoming involved in caring for their ill relative. The caregiving demands may exist for several months to years. Family caregivers tend to put the needs of their loved ones before their own needs and that they are at increased health risk.

Case Presentation Mr. A, a 78-year-old man, has been diagnosed with a monoclonal gammopathy of undetermined significance (MGUS) since 2006. Recently he has been diagnosed with a Multiple Myeloma on the basis of anemia and lytic lesions. He will be starting treatment with Melphalan, Prednisone and Bortezomib (MPV) [1]. His performance status according to the World Health Organization is 1. His only complaint is mild to moderate fatigue. Mr. A is also known with chronic obstructive pulmonary disease and intermittent claudication since 1998, surgery for aortic aneurysm in 2000, renal disease since 2004.

Mr. A is a widower since 15 years. He lives independently together with his only son, who is 50 years old. Mr. A has had no other relation since his wife died. He enjoys life to the fullest, he is used to travel a lot and he likes to eat preferably in good restaurants.

Physically he is not able to walk long distances, but because they live above a supermarket, he is able to do the shopping. He is dependent on public transportation.

Polypharmacy and Medication Adherence

Comorbidity plays a role in defining the treatment and is in the first place the domain of the physician. Due to the comorbidity, the elderly patient often has a status of polypharmacy. Polypharmacy is promoted by increasing free medication which can be bought without prescription. Some of these may interact with chemotherapy, and some might be considered as potentially inappropriate medications.

To screen for used drugs, the nurse can make enquiry and clarify which medications are used, which are prescribed and which are supplements, and in which doses and for what indications. Most patients do not know what medication they use (in terms of generic name) but they do know exactly what colour and dosage are required. This screening can also be used to identify possible causes for nonadherence. Changes in physical and psychosocial functioning such as difficulty in handling medication containers, diminished sensory abilities, altered cognitive function, reduced self-confidence, depression and social isolation can affect medication behaviour. The following questions can be used to assess patients:

- Do you need help with the use of medications?
- Are you able to read the prescription on the box and can you get the medication out of the blisters?
- Do you ever adapt your medication prescription to physical complaints?
- Do you ever take a drug holiday?
- Do you ever forget to use your medication?

After collecting the information the nurse can propose what interventions for increasing medication adherence can be successful.

- Asking a relative or the local pharmacy to help in case of problems with opening the blisters or reading the information on the package.
- In case of the antitumoral therapy provides supplementary written information with regard to frequency, at what times, when to alarm, and reasons for taking antitumor or co-prescribed medication such as antiemetics, antihistamines, anticoagulants, etc

- Prescribe medication no more than two times a day
- Discuss what times are most convenient for the patient
- Sometimes an extra consultation might be necessary
- Tailoring the therapy to the patients' needs is sometimes necessary

Occasionally, the patient may require a hospital admission during the diagnosis or during the treatment period. At discharge, it is important to go through all medication again: which medication needs to be taken and which medication has been stopped. During admission, medication is not always prolonged, and patients need to be informed about this. Also the drugs taken at home may look different from those used in hospital.

Adherence to the prescribed anti-cancer therapy has become an important issue. According to Medical Subject Headings (MeSH) thesaurus, medication adherence is described as the voluntary cooperation of the patient in taking drugs or medicine as prescribed. This includes the right timing, the right dosage, and the right frequency. Adherence to treatment is a complex issue that can influence the outcomes of therapy. Being adherent to therapy is important because of its close link with effectiveness, as non-adherence can contribute to the patient's worsening due to an absence of drug activity. Non-adherence may also lead to an increased number in physician's visits and unnecessary diagnostic testing, hospitalization or longer in-hospital stays, medication overdose, changes in dose or regimen, and unnecessary medical expenses [2, 3]. A study by Monane et al. [4] measured adherence and related demographic factors in a retrospective cohort of 4,068 elderly outpatients. Good compliance (>or = 80 %) was associated with age of 85 years or older [4]. In most of the published studies age is not an important predictor of medication adherence [3].

Factors that are associated with better adherence to prescribed oral medication in older patients are white race, drug and dosage form, the use of multiple drugs, low costs of medication, insurance coverage, and good physician-patient communication [3]. There are different strategies regarding education, behaviour, and social interventions which can be combined to improve medication adherence [5]. The health of a patient can also affect adherence. For example the patient who is nauseous will have problems to take oral medication.

It is important that the patient knows what he should use and how long for. The prescribed medicine should always be delivered in the same form, and should be easy for the patient to take. All side effects have to be clearly explained. It is important that the medication fits into the patient's lifestyle.

Nursing Role

- At admission or discharge and during outpatient clinic visits: screen and discuss regularly all used medication, prescribed and non-prescribed, and the reasons for non-adherence with your patient.
- To achieve medication adherence, it is very important to educate patients and convince them about the benefits of the regimen.

- Patients should be well informed about the chronic disease and the complications associated with non-adherence.

Nutritional Status

The nursing assessment of the patient's nutrients and fluids intake is to determine functional and dysfunctional patterns. Nutrition is important during hospitalization, but also in the outpatient program. At every intake the nurse has to identify all the risks for malnutrition. The body needs nutrition to produce energy for life functions. It is important for the older patient to prevent weight loss. Weight loss and/or anorexia point towards malnutrition. Malnutrition increases the vulnerability to illness.

However, knowledge about the impact of nutritional intervention on physical and mental function, and on quality of life is still lacking, we do think that there is an association between impaired physical functioning and malnutrition. Some of the causes of malnutrition are reversible, for example depression, physical functioning, biting, chewing and any teeth problems, vision problems, poor appetite, lack of sleep and stress. Furthermore eating is a social activity. When social circumstances change, eating can become less important. To provide sufficient and healthy meals, it is also necessary that the supplies are available.

Providing tips and advice about nutrition in the treatment of cancer is always valuable, even in the case of no malnutrition. To prevent malnutrition or to help your patient stay on weight, there are simple methods such as meals on wheels, meal service by healthcare institute in the surrounding, grocery delivery by the Internet, share meal with family or neighbours once or more times per week, cooking for 2 days at a time. Furthermore nurses can advice patients and their relatives to use whole foods instead of low fat, to use no diet except for specific problems (i.e. kidney damage) and to use multiple small portions of food instead of three large meals per day.

In addition, it is essential to work with validated screening lists in order to determine the nutritional status like the Malnutrition Universal Screening Tool (MUST) or Simplified Nutritional Assessment Questionnaire (SNAQ). In all these screening instruments unintentional weight loss in a short time is a fixed item as a parameter to malnutrition. Nurses can consult the dietician in case of malnutrition.

Nursing Role

- At every intake identify all risk for malnutrition
- To give tips and advice about nutrition in the treatment of cancer is always valuable, also in case of no malnutrition
- To work with validated screening lists in order to determine the nutritional status
- To consult the dietician in case of malnutrition

Management of Side Effects During Antitumoral Therapy

Treatment side effects are frequently more severe among older patients and they also seem to last longer than in adult patients. It is important that the patient is well informed about the expected toxicities and about what patients may do themselves to improve the compliance with chemotherapy. Some treatments may lead to diabetes or complicate the clinical relevance of pre-existing diabetes, iron overload, deep venous thrombosis, osteoporosis, etc. Apart from all the adverse medical events, the disease and/or treatment may also have an effect on the physical, functional, emotional, social, and spiritual wellbeing.

If curative treatment options are available, proactive and competent management of adverse events is essential to allow continuation of treatment in order to obtain optimal response (see Table 14.1). Careful patient observation during treatment allows the nurse to evaluate the physical and psychological condition. The most common adverse events in older patients with Hematological Malignancies and how to manage them are summed up in Table 14.1. It is also important to evaluate psychological problems, in particular, loneliness, abandonment, feelings of being a burden for the family.

To be able to adequately address QoL issues numerous validated QoL questionnaires for cancer patients exist. Older patients can have also other Health Related Quality of Life (HRQOL) concerns than their younger counterparts. Weelwrigt et al. [6] identified 14 specific issues that affect perceived HRQOL in patients older than 70 years with a solid tumor [6]. These 14 items have been grouped into the following conceptually related five scales (mobility, worries about others, future-worries, maintaining purpose and illness burden) and two single items (joint stiffness and family support), and resulted in the EORTC-QLQ-ELD 14 [6].

Nursing Role

- To increase patient's compliance and decrease his/her anxiety, the oncology nurse should discuss all relevant information with the patient and relatives before therapy starts. This information should be delivered in an easily understand way
- Nursing care should also be centred during and after treatment to assist their patients to maintain their QoL.
- To give information on how the chemotherapy affects the disease as well as QoL, and for how long this can be expected before recovery
- Written information on the treatment and the possible adverse events should always be given
- The importance of when to alert the treating physician must be emphasised so that the ongoing treatment can be reassessed as soon as possible

- To adequately address all HRQOL issues which are important to older patients
- To limit the severity of adverse events, their early identification and prompt intervention are needed for the most common ones
- To carefully evaluate psychological problems

Table 14.1 Nursing management of most common adverse events in older patients with hematological malignancies drug related adverse event

	Signs and symptoms	Nursing management
Anaemia	Palpitations	Red blood cell transfusions
	Chest pain	Administration of erythropoietin agents
	Fatigue	
	Dyspnea	
	Dizziness	
	Headaches	
Neutropenia	Fever	Timely recognition of infection
	Cough	Administration of recombinant granulocytic growth factors
	Dysuria	Antimicrobial therapy (prophylactic or for active infections)
	Recurrent/refractory infections	Withhold therapy or dose adjustment
Thrombocytopenia	Petechiae	Timely recognition of risk of bleeding
	Ecchymosis	Platelet transfusion
	Epistaxis	Aminocaproic acid (prophylactic or for active bleeding)
	Hemoptysis	Monitoring medication with anti-platelet effect
	Hematuria	Withhold therapy or dose adjustment
Stomatitis and mucositis	Painful mouth sores	Prevent secondary infection
	Difficulty chewing/swallowing	Provide pain relief
	Reduction of food intake	Maintain dietary intake
	Malnutrition	Motivate routine systematic oral care
	Negative impact on QoL	In case of fungal infection topical or systemic antifungal agents
Nausea and vomiting	Lack of food/fluid intake	Anti-emetics
	Malnutrition	Encourage adequate hydration
	Negative impact on QoL	Check intake, weight,
		Ensure baseline and ongoing renal function

(continued)

Table 14.1 (continued)

	Signs and symptoms	Nursing management
Diarrhoea	Mucositis	Evaluate for infectious aetiology
	Infection	Minimise the complication of dehydration by
	Faecal impaction	Encourage adequate hydration
		Anti-diarrheals
		Dietary consultation
Constipation	Altered bowel elimination	Laxatives
	Nausea	Include foods that have a high fibre content
	Vomiting	Adequate fluid intake
	Abdominal pain	Light exercises
	Malaise	Prevent
		Decreased mobility
		Decreased oral intake
		Use of antiemetics/narcotics
Fatigue	Exhaustion	Rehabilitation should begin with the cancer diagnosis but depends on extent of disease
	Decreased capacity for mental or physical work	Establish a baseline
	Rarely an isolated symptom	Seek information about related factors and offer interventions if possible
		Recent illnesses
		Pain
		Emotional stress
		Medication regimen
		Anaemia
		Sleep disorders
		Altered nutritional status
Malnutrition	Anorexia	Encourage adequate hydration
	Weight loss	Dietary measures/consultation
	Altered and/or loss of taste	Antiemetics
	Reluctance	
	Stomatitis	
	Gastrointestinal toxicity	

Case Presentation (Continued) Mr. A calls the hotline from the hospital. He cannot eat very well. He is feeling nauseous and it feels as if he has a full stomach. When the nurse asks about his bowel elimination, it appears that Mr. A has been constipated since three days. During the nurse's assessment she also asks Mr. A how his fluid intake, diet and physical activity have been. Mr. A admits he has not been out of his chair since the last visit to the hospital. Mr. A is given a prescription for a laxative and the nurse encourages him to walk around more.

She makes a note in the electronic patient's file and also lists him for a recall phone call in a couple of days for reassessment's.

Patient Preferences and Information Needs

Older persons grew up in a culture where decision making was more paternalistic. This may either lead to a lower information need or to a risk for poor communication. Research indicates that patient preferences and information needs differ widely. Patient information should target older patients' needs, in order to prepare them to the prescribed treatment and to help them deal with adverse effects [7].

The majority of older adults must also cope with growing limitations in the physical and cognitive functioning along with age progresses. However cognitive decline due to aging, may limit the understanding and memorization of complex information; this might imply that the need for further information may be inhibited [8]. As a result of this, patients may feel distressed due to the difficulties in understanding what is happening along their clinical course. In the communication with family and friends, stress can also worsen when patients become incapable of understanding the consequences of their decisions [9].

Older patients have unmet communication needs as serious gaps in recalling and understanding may occur during psychological and physical health crisis [9]. A possible explanation for this is that older adults have unique language, cognitive, psychological, and social issues that affect their own health ability to read and write [10]. Unfulfilled information needs may cause non-compliance, and this is an important risk factor for the outcome of the medical treatment.

Patient's coping strategies have been described as influencing their information needs [11]. Each single individual will differ in his/her coping styles (and information needs): this can influence the patient's requests and behaviour. According to Miller et al. [12], individuals can use two main cognitive coping styles in dealing with cancer and other health threats: monitoring (attending to) or blunting (avoiding) potentially threatening information. Individuals may use either coping style at different moments [12]. Patients fare better (psychologically, behaviourally, and physiologically) when the information they receive about their medical condition is tailored to their own coping style: generally those with a monitoring style tend to do better when given more information, and those with a blunting style do better with less information. To explicitly judge patients in advance on their preferences, the following questions may be helpful: 'Do you generally think 'I want to know every detail' or do you tend to say 'I'll will just see what is going to happen'? [13].

Regardless of the monitoring style, patients who are pessimistic about their future or who have uncontrollable medical situations, may require additional emotional support to help them deal with their disease [14].

The meaning of life rests on the belief that life is worth living and suffering can be valuable [15]. Meaning of life refers to the value and purpose of life, important life goals, and for some, spirituality [16]. Meaning enriches life. Several studies show that patients who report more meaning in their life during their cancer diagnosis also report less distress better physical health, better mental health and may be associated with mortality [15–17].

Patients with cancer often experience feelings of reduced QoL, sadness, hopelessness and spiritual distress, such as an evaluation of one's past and problems with finding a new meaning in life while suffering from a sometimes incurable disease. A cancer diagnosis and the associated intensive medical treatment profoundly confront people with the limits of their existence and death. Meaning of life can contribute to effective coping. Research on facilitating meaning-making is still in an early stage. Several studies are presently ongoing.

Nursing Role

- To assist patients to understand their treatment options, to prioritize information needs, and to help them deal with adverse effects.
- To discuss concerns and communicate their care needs.
- To navigate through the healthcare system for symptom management.
- To learn ways of coping with the emotional and existential issues.

Social Support and Caregiving by Family

Most of the older people can function independently. They have successfully managed to adapt to the changed circumstances. This is called 'successful ageing'.

However, as age progresses, social relations and contacts often decrease. Older people lose out a lot. Older people are not employed anymore. Old friends and nearer relatives have also aged; they might also perceive same problems. A reduced mobility can also prevent older patients from going outdoors; friends and near relatives may also become ill or die. When, as a result of comorbidities or of the malignant condition (sudden) functional decline takes place, the social network of the older patient may further decrease. Moreover, the communication with others may become more critical because of problems with hearing, seeing, or cognition. The loss of (in) formal roles and contacts makes the elderly more vulnerable. Because of these above mentioned circumstances the elderly can feel depressed or socially isolated.

Research has shown that the degree in which people receive support from their direct social surroundings relates strongly with perceived health. People with good social contacts have less health problems and can manage sickness better. The lack of social relations has also been correlated to a higher mortality rates and a shorter survival [18]. If the patient is emotionally better supported by his environment, this patient is more likely to adapt better, physically and mentally. This wellbeing plays a role in allowing the patient to remain at home or being admitted to the hospital or nursing home/hospice [19].

Family caregivers are frequently prepared to do everything they can in the best patient's interest. Because of this, their own needs are either ignored or exceeded. Moreover, the daily care of a patient may increase during the course of the illness, not only in its quantity but also in complexity. When the care is provided by the partner of the older patient, who most frequently happens to be an older person him/herself, the reaction to this demanding role is likely to be predicted by age, gender, cultural background, ethnicity, socioeconomic status, educational level, personal health and family dynamics [20].

Case Presentation (Continued) During the visit to the nursing specialist the social network is mapped. Mr. A can only asks his son for help. Because Mr. A can do the shopping and cooking himself, neither the son nor Mr. A. can see any major problems. Mr. A's son is willing to offer informal care to his father in addition to his work as an account manager.

Because the son is not always available to accompany his father to the hospital, Mr. A takes a taxi if his son is not able to accompany him. During each visit to the outpatient clinic the social network and QoL of both the patient and caregiver is a recurring topic of conversation.

Family caregivers of cancer patients often deliver a considerable part of the care themselves. They perform nursing tasks (administer medication, injections or enteral feeding, assist with activities of daily living), domestic tasks, coordinate the needs and give emotional support.

Looking after an ill spouse, a parent or a close relation can give positive feelings such as satisfaction and self-respect, as well as gratitude and love for the other one. The relationship with the patient can be strengthened with activities such as direct communication, psychical contact, laughter, effective problem solving and spending time together.

Providing care to a relative can also be difficult or incriminating. Frequently, the need for care arises suddenly; there is hardly any time to think about the consequences of giving care to a loved one and family caregivers are usually unprepared for such tasks. Decisions must be taken rapidly and sometimes the patient's clinical situation worsens of a sudden. Family caregivers are confronted with high physical and emotional demands: sometimes financial issues, or the disease itself, creates cognitive and emotional disruptions [19, 21]. They themselves are therefore at risk of illness or burn out and can experience physical, mental, and behavioural complaints [19]. Burden on family caregivers is one of the risk factors for the abuse of older persons [22]; a right for support on their own needs should thus be taken into consideration for family carers [19]. When the patient is hospitalised, family carers may experience a far less cooperative approach with the healthcare professionals. This can be explained by the undefined boundaries between formal and informal care, the lack of good information and consultation, or the lack of being involved at the treatment of the patient. Also, family carers have often reported lack of education and skills to deliver their patients' care as well as a lack of social support [21]. All of these can become a burden and strain between the patient and family carers [21].

Quality of Life of Family Caregiver

The experienced QoL of the family carers is affected at an early stage of the disease [23]. Family carers of patients with leukaemia have identified the burden and disruptiveness as their most important concerns for QoL. Key factors for their well-being are expression of feelings, household maintenance and family support [21]. Sometimes, caregivers do not know how to coordinate care [21]. Research has shown that the learning needs of a caregiver were education and information about giving medications, managing side-effects and managing symptoms such as pain, nausea, vomiting and fatigue. Also, communication, getting support, and positive nursing attitudes are important items for the QoL of caregivers [21]. Several instruments have been developed to measure the QoL of caregivers. One of these is the Caregiver Quality of Life Index-Cancer (CQOLC). This self-reporting instrument has a good test-retest reliability (0.95) and an internal consistency (0.91) and also has a sufficient validity [24]. A better mental health status is associated with an improved QoL. The Patient's emotional problems and his deteriorating performance status associate to a worse QoL of the family carrers [25].

There are different types of support, such as everyday emotional support, emotional support with problems, appreciation support, practical support, social companionship and informative support. Everyone needs everyday support in a certain way. The need for the type and the quantity of support depends on the phase of the illness. The quality of life and quality of care of the patient also depends on the wellbeing of the caregiver.

Nursing Role

- To recognize the educational and psychological needs of FCs.
- To provide adequate information, not only about chemotherapy or supportive care, but also about the FCs own health risks.
- To give instruction on how to address common problems.
- To manage the caregiver by offering interventions.
- To give practical support.
- To identify when the FC needs time, every now and then, for himself.
- To prevent physical and mental health problems in caregivers.
- To identify the best person whom the patient can rely for support.
- To encourage the FCs to receive assistance from friends and formal caregivers.
- To monitor and evaluate the caregiver's mental health, emotional distress and QoL.

Case Presentation, Continued Initially the Multiple Myeloma responded very well to the MPV cycles. After 12 months Mr. A renal function worsens due to progressive Multiple Myeloma. Because of the extreme fatigue, and the malaise Mr. A needs more care at home. His son regrets it very much but he is not able to give the care his father needs. After discussing if there is really no assistance to be expected from friends the nurse has to inform Mr. A and his son the possibilities of formal care.

Conclusion

Haematologists, geriatricians, and nurses are involved in the care of older patients. It is important that all disciplines work together and in an harmonised way. Nurses are in a position to assess all aspects that can be impacted by aging, and to monitor the impact of the disease and treatment on patients' and caregivers' QoL. Nurses are also crucially important in supporting and providing interventions to assist patients and (family) caregivers.

References

1. Mateos MV, Richardson PG, Schlag R, Khuageva NK, Dimopoulos MA, Shpilberg O, et al. Bortezomib plus melphalan and prednisone compared with melphalan and prednisone in previously untreated multiple myeloma: updated follow-up and impact of subsequent therapy in the phase III VISTA trial. J Clin Oncol. 2010;28(13):2259–66.
2. Partridge AH, Avorn J, Wang PS, Winer EP. Adherence to therapy with oral antineoplastic agents. J Natl Cancer Inst. 2002;94(9):652–61.
3. Balkrishnan R. Predictors of medication adherence in the elderly. Clin Ther. 1998;20(4):764–71.
4. Monane M, Bohn RL, Gurwitz JH, Glynn RJ, Levin R, Avorn J. Compliance with antihypertensive therapy among elderly Medicaid enrollees: the roles of age, gender, and race. Am J Public Health. 1996;86(12):1805–8.
5. Williams A, Manias E, Walker R. Interventions to improve medication adherence in people with multiple chronic conditions: a systematic review. J Adv Nurs. 2008;63(2):132–43.
6. Wheelwright S, Darlington AS, Fitzsimmons D, Fayers P, Arraras JI, Bonnetain F, Brain E, et al. International validation of the EORTC QLQ-ELD14 questionnaire for assessment of health-related quality of life elderly patients with cancer. Br J Cancer. 2013;109(4):852–8.
7. Jansen J, van Weert J, van Dulmen S, Heeren T, Bensing J. Patient education about treatment in cancer care: an overview of the literature on older patients' needs. Cancer Nurs. 2007; 30(4):251–60.
8. Pinquart M, Duberstein PR. Information needs and decision-making processes in older cancer patients. Crit Rev Oncol Hematol. 2004;51(1):69–80.
9. Rose JH, Radziewicz R, Bowmans KF, O'Toole EE. A coping and communication support intervention tailored to older patients diagnosed with late-stage cancer. Clin Interv Aging. 2008;3(1):77–95.
10. Sparks L, Nussbaum JF. Health literacy and cancer communication with older adults. Patient Educ Couns. 2008;71(3):345–50.
11. Friis LS, Elverdam B, Schmidt KG. The patient's perspective: a qualitative study of acute myeloid leukaemia patients' need for information and their information-seeking behaviour. Support Care Cancer. 2003;11:162–70.
12. Miller SM, Brody DS, Summerton J. Styles of coping with threat: implications for health. J Pers Soc Psychol. 1988;54:142–8.

13. Timmermans LM, van Zuuren FJ, van der Maazen RW, Leer JW, Kraaimaat FW. Monitoring and blunting in palliative and curative radiotherapy consultations. Psychooncology. 2007;16(12):1111–20.
14. Miller SM. Monitoring versus blunting styles of coping with cancer influence the information patients want and need about their disease. Implications for cancer screening and management. Cancer. 1995;76(2):167–77.
15. Jim HS, Richardson SA, Golden-Kreutz DM, Andersen BL. Strategies used in coping with a cancer diagnosis predict meaning in life for survivors. Health Psychol. 2006;25(6):753–61.
16. Vachon ML. Meaning, spirituality, and wellness in cancer survivors. Semin Oncol Nurs. 2008;24(3):218–25.
17. Jim HS, Purnell JQ, Richardson SA, Golden-Kreutz D, Andersen BL. Measuring meaning in life following cancer. Qual Life Res. 2006;15(8):1355–71.
18. Heany CA, Israel BA. Social networks and social support. In: Glanz K, Rimer BK, Lewis FM, editors. Health behavior and health education: theory, research and practice. San Francisco: Jossey-Bass; 2002. p. 185–209.
19. Blum K, Sherman DW. Understanding the experience of caregivers: a focus on transitions. Semin Oncol Nurs. 2010;26:243–58.
20. Hagedoorn M, Buunk BP, Kuijer RG, Wobbes T, Sanderman R. Couples dealing with cancer: role and gender differences regarding psychological distress and quality of life. Psychooncology. 2000;9:232–42.
21. Tamayo GJ, Broxson A, Munsell M, Cohen MZ. Caring for the caregiver. Oncol Nurs Forum. 2010;37:50–7.
22. van der Kruk T, Salentijn C, Schuurmans M. Verpleegkundige zorgverlening aan ouderen. Den Haag: Lemma BV; 2007.
23. Pellegrino R, Formica V, Portarena I, Mariotti S, Grenga I, Del MG, et al. Caregiver distress in the early phases of cancer. Anticancer Res. 2010;30:4657–63.
24. Edwards B, Ung L. Quality of life instruments for caregivers of patients with cancer: a review of their psychometric proportions. Cancer Nurs. 2002;25:342–9.
25. Weitzner MA, Jacobsen PB, Wagner H, Friedland J, Cox C. The Caregiver Quality of Life Index Cancer (CQOLC) scale: development and validation of an instrument to measure quality of life of the family caregiver of patients with cancer. Qual Life Res. 1999;8:55–63.

Chapter 15
General Considerations on Treatment in Older Patients with Hematological Malignancies

Pierre Soubeyran, Camille Chakiba, and Anne-Sophie Michallet

Introduction

Standard treatment relates to disease, not to patients. The question in older patients is consequently most often to adapt standard treatment to the specific situation of the patient through a strict evaluation of risks and benefits since higher risks may consume benefits.

The obvious approach is to propose dose reductions although it will decrease both risks and benefits. In this case, methodological validation will be hampered by the absence of standard treatment since it is, by definition, not feasible. The objective of trials will be mainly the search for the treatment which offers the best risks / benefits ratio. Another alternative – which can be proposed as a second step – is to replace potentially toxic drugs by new, less toxic, compounds – mainly targeted therapies – to maintain benefits while decreasing risks. In this case, it will be necessary to perform phase III trials to compare the new candidate combination to the best adapted standard treatment (at a level which yields low level toxicity).

P. Soubeyran, MD (✉)
Department of Medical Oncology, Institut Bergonié,
229 cours de l'Argonne, 33076 Bordeaux Cedex, France

Site de Recherche Intégrée sur le Cancer, BRIO
(Bordeaux Recherche Intégrée Oncologie), 229 cours de l'Argonne,
33076 Bordeaux Cedex, France

Université Bordeaux Segalen, 146 rue Léo Saignat, 33076
Bordeaux Cedex, France
e-mail: P.Soubeyran@bordeaux.unicancer.fr

C. Chakiba, MD
Department of Medical Oncology, Institut Bergonié,
229 cours de l'Argonne, 33076 Bordeaux Cedex, France

Site de Recherche Intégrée sur le Cancer, BRIO
(Bordeaux Recherche Intégrée Oncologie), 229 cours de l'Argonne,
33076 Bordeaux Cedex, France

A.-S. Michallet, MD
Department of Hematology, Hôpital Lyon-Sud, Hospices Civils de Lyon, Lyon, France

U. Wedding, R.A. Audisio (eds.), *Management of Hematological Cancer in Older People*, DOI 10.1007/978-1-4471-2837-3_15

All along this process, to develop this strategy, we need to control risks and to precisely define endpoints. Major endpoints in the elderly include, beside control of disease, maintenance of quality of life and autonomy and limitation of treatment toxicity to a minimum. All these endpoints should be taken into account to manage older patients but their hierarchical importance will depend on the health status of the individual patient. For fit patients, thanks to a longer life expectancy and lower risks, the primary objective can be to control or even (in a limited number of diseases) cure disease, while in unfit patients, the primary endpoint is to maintain quality of life and autonomy.

The experience of geriatricians can be of major help in this field. Indeed, in a large cohort of 12,480 community-dwelling elders, Mohile et al. [1] showed a higher prevalence of functional impairment, geriatric syndromes and frailty, as defined by Balducci criteria [2] or VES13 questionnaire [3], in patients with a personal history of cancer as compared to respondents without a cancer history. Furthermore, cancer patients had lower self-rated health. However, this evaluation process is time-consuming. Comprehensive geriatric assessment has the necessary capacity to foresee frailties in major geriatric domains such as dependencies, nutrition, mood and falls. Geriatrician's conclusions will allow onco-hematologists to decide how to adapt standard treatment to make it as secure as possible. However, the introduction of this new medical competence in the onco-hematological decision process is not that simple. Decisions cannot be based on thresholds of the score of various questionnaires but should implement the interpretation of the results by an experienced geriatrician, so-called comprehensive geriatric assessment (CGA), a long, time-consuming, process. Consequently, many teams cannot afford this further pre-treatment evaluation. A potential solution is to begin the evaluation by a screening questionnaire which will allow restricting the application of the complete procedure to the only patients who may need it. This approach is now reaching consensus in the Geriatric oncology community [4].

Finally, after the identification of patients at risk and the adaptation of the oncological treatment, geriatricians are able to offer patients interventions to compensate for their inabilities and frailties. Indeed, geriatric management improves outcome in the general population [5]. However, evidence of the effectiveness of this ressource-consuming and thus expensive process is missing in the oncology setting [6] so that it cannot be introduced in the daily practice without previous demonstration of its effects.

Selection Procedure: Search for Factors Predictive of Early Adverse Events

The major objective is to identify, among available baseline data, a limited number of factors which will allow to classify patients according to risks in order to determine which treatment can be reasonably proposed i.e. full dose standard treatment (fit), reduced standard treatment (vulnerable or intermediate) or tailored treatment (frail). Treatment decision will depend on the risk of early events (death, toxicity, functional decline for example) and on the expected life expectancy to be balanced with chances of tumor control (which are disease-specific and will not be analyzed in this chapter).

Classification of patients by either physician's judgment or CGA results, although highly correlated, shows different results with a major underestimation of the frail population by physician's judgment as shown in a prospective series of 200 patients [7] in which the proportion of fit, vulnerable and frail patients were respectively 64.3, 32.4 and 3.2 % by physician's judgment and 25, 25.5 and 49.5 % according to Balducci's classification [2]. Furthermore, some recent data tend to show that the geriatric approach is more valid to identify palliative patients who will not benefit from standard therapy [8]. In a prospective series of 84 consecutive patients with previously untreated diffuse large B-cell lymphomas, patients were classified as fit or unfit either by hematologists, according to standard criteria, or by geriatricians, according to four criteria, age, ADL, CIRS-G and occurrence of geriatric syndromes. Geriatric results were blinded to the hematologists. Proportion of unfit patients was again different (26 % for physicians, 50 % according to geriatric classification). Geriatric criteria appeared more efficient to predict prognosis since patients classified as fit by the physician – and treated accordingly – but frail with geriatric assessment, behaved as patients classified as unfit by the two methods in terms of survival. Another proposal for classification of elderly patients with diffuse large B-cell lymphoma has been proposed by Spina et al. [9] based on the ADL and IADL. However, in a selected population of patients with favorable outcome, no real conclusion can be drawn in the absence of comparison with current daily practice.

Overall, data in hematological malignancies are limited and results observed in other kinds of cancer will be also considered.

Some authors searched for factors to predict survival at various time points in the general population [10, 11]. Based on large series of patients, including validation cohorts, they are robust and discriminate efficiently population with different life expectancy. All include cancer among significant risk factors. Scores of Lee et al. [10] and Schonberg et al. [11] are currently studied in the field of oncology to determine whether they can help in the treatment decision process.

In patients with various types of malignancies, correlations between the severity of comorbid conditions and diverse outcomes have been observed in various types of cancer including colorectal [12] and breast [13] carcinomas. Furthermore, results of geriatric assessment have demonstrated prognostic value on survival. In a series of 83 patients with advanced ovarian cancer, Freyer et al. demonstrated the prognostic value of disease stage but also of geriatric depression scale and of the number of medications [14]. In a series of 364 patients with various types of cancer including one third of lymphomas, the risk of early death (within 6 months of treatment initiation) was predicted by disease extension, sex, mini nutritional assessment and time get up and go [15].

The second important event to predict is certainly toxicity which can depend on treatment intensity on one hand and on patient's health status on the other hand. The only problem is to define the clinically significant threshold that is the one above which the treatment has to be considered either too intense i.e. the endpoint. As often, the analysis of the literature is hampered by the variety of endpoints chosen, from all high grade toxicities to only severe toxicities (with various definitions) and toxic deaths.

Gomez et al. [16] search for predictive factors of treatment-related mortality in a retrospective series of 267 consecutive patients older than 60 with diffuse large B-cell lymphoma treated by CHOP chemotherapy. Geriatric factors were not included and poor performance status was the only independent predictor of treatment-related death. Of note, increased age was not predictive. This result obviously leads to consider that geriatric assessment results which have been demonstrated as superior to performance status assessment should be scrutinized [17]. Many other studies focusing on toxicity predictors were not restricted to hematological cancer. Two major series targeted high grade toxicity. Hurria et al. [18] selected grade 3–5 toxicities as endpoints in a large series of 500 patients. Various factors were identified among which age, biological data (creatinine clearance and hemoglobin level), chemotherapy description (dose intensity, number of drugs) and geriatric status (hearing, falls, medications, walking and social activities). Depending on the risk score, grade 3–5 toxicity rate varied from 25 to 89 %. Of note, performance status was not predictive of toxicity risk. Extermann et al. [19] analyzed separately grade 4 hematological and grade 3–4 non-hematological toxicities in a series of 518 evaluable patients. Factors such as age, diastolic blood pressure, performance status, LDH level, chemotherapy toxicity score were predictive together with IADL, MMS and MNA. The final risk score predicted hematological toxicity risk from 7 to 100 % and non-hematological toxicity rate from 33 to 93 %.

Another approach is to define clinically significant toxicity with different endpoints such as unplanned hospitalization or functional decline during treatment. In a series of 354 evaluable patients older than 70 with various kinds of cancer before chemotherapy, including 110 lymphomas, we defined severe toxicity as unplanned hospitalization during treatment [20]. Forty-seven patients experienced unexpected hospital admission. Patients with low platelet count and low MNA score had a significant higher risk for treatment-related hospitalization (OR 3.763 and 4.194 respectively). Adaptation of chemotherapy schedule and doses by the investigator reduced significantly the risk of hospital admission (OR 0.509). In the same series of patients, we searched for factors predictive of functional decline (defined as a decrease of 0.5 points or more on the ADL scale between baseline and the second cycle of chemotherapy) [21]. With 50 patients experiencing functional decline among 299 evaluable patients, high baseline GDS and low IADL were independently associated with increased risk of functional decline. In a series of 123 patients with colorectal cancer included in a randomized phase III trial, Aparicio et al. [22] searched simultaneously for predictive factors of three different events, grade 3–4 toxicity, dose-intensity reduction and unexpected hospitalization. Predictive factors for grade 3–4 toxicity were experimental arm, MMSE and IADL scores while experimental arm and abnormal alkaline phosphatases were identified for dose-intensity reduction and MMSE and GDS for unexpected hospitalization. Freyer et al. [14] considered severe toxicity to be at least one event among febrile neutropenia, grade 4 neutropenia, early treatment withdrawal or re-hospitalization for more than 7 days because of grade 3/4 toxicity. In their series of 83 patients older than 70 with advanced ovarian cancer, they demonstrate that depression, dependence and poor performance status were predictive of severe toxicity.

Comparison of the different series is somewhat difficult since they did not use the same tools and sometimes did not include important dimensions of geriatric assessment which were considered major in other series. Overall, beside expected factors such as type and dose of chemotherapy or performance status, geriatric assessment data appear to add useful information. Functional impairment (IADL) but also nutrition (MNA), mood (GDS) and cognitive status (MMSE) may be of crucial importance.

Beside a global approach of toxicity risk, specific toxicities may be considered in the elderly. This includes cardiac toxicity and neurological toxicity. Overall data are limited but deserve consideration. It appears that risk of congestive heart failure was related, as expected to anthracycline treatment, but also to other co-factors among which hypertension, diabetes, coronary artery disease or age [23–25]. Furthermore, in a series of 109 patients treated with various types of chemotherapy, Tofthagen et al. [26] analyzed factors predictive of falls and found that number of cycles and loss of balance were independent predictors.

Among possible predictors of crucial events during treatment of elderly with cancer, biological factors can be of importance.

C-reactive protein (CRP) has been found predictive of survival in various kinds of cancer including colorectal [27], gastric [28] and prostate cancer [29]. IL6 level also appeared to have prognostic value in gastric [28] and prostate cancer [29]. Combination of CRP and albumin levels, the modified Glasgow prognostic score [30], have been shown to have prognostic value across all types of cancer including hematological cancer (974 cases).

Indeed, nutritional and inflammatory status are known to be associated with severe hematological toxicity but the data from Alexandre et al. [31], from a series of 107 patients, were not focused on elderly patients (median age: 56; range 33–75). The results of Zauderer et al. [32] are thus more specific and also confirm that baseline albumin <3.5 g/dL and anemia were associated with grade 3–5 chemotherapy-associated toxicity.

Finally, data gathered from the literature demonstrate that geriatric assessment adds to other classical factors to predict early death or survival, toxicity, whatever the definition retained, or functional decline. All dimensions of geriatric assessment may have prognostic value although some domains may prevail. Consequently, baseline geriatric evaluation may help physicians better anticipate potential adverse events which may occur during treatment and thus help him take the right decision about treatment intensity and possible interventions. Yet CGA cannot be offered to all elderly cancer patients since it is time-consuming for physicians and nurses which makes it unaffordable for community hospitals and small cancer hospitals while, in France, 68 % of cancer patients are treated in non-academic hospitals. Consequently, search for a tool to identify patients who can benefit from CGA becomes evident and is the current consensus [4].

This has made the development of shortened instruments essential [4, 33]. To be acceptable for the whole community, such instruments should be performed shortly (less than 10 min) by a nurse or physician trained for the tool completion but not necessarily in geriatry. A few instruments have been identified among which VES13 and G8 are the most studied.

Again, the recurrent question is about the methodology of studies and whether they are comparable or not. The major question is the endpoint which has to be clinically meaningful. As for the above mentioned studies, patients to be detected are those who are exposed to high risk of adverse events such as early death, life-threatening toxicity or functional decline during treatment. Yet, for obvious practical reasons, most series use geriatric assessment questionnaires. Furthermore, each series uses its own set of questionnaires and sometimes omit a few dimensions of assessment. Consequently, comparison between series may be somewhat difficult. The next question is about the threshold to classify a patient in the at-risk group. Most of the time, two different thresholds have been proposed i.e. either at least one or two abnormal questionnaires. However, no one did evaluate whether one threshold is superior to the other in terms of outcome. The question remains thus opened. Finally, this approach, which uses questionnaires only, allows for easy and reproducible studies but the absence of relationship with clinical outcome makes possible that the population identified does not appropriately fit to our needs.

VES13 (Table 15.1) was originally designed to predict functional decline or death over a two-year period in community-dwelling elders [3]. It has been validated in a large series of 6,205 Medicare beneficiaries. It has been later proposed to be used as a screening tool for older patients with prostate cancer [34]. In this series of 50 patients, geriatric assessment included ADL (Activities in Daily Living), IADL (Instrumental ADL), SPPB (Short Physical Performance Battery), CALGB adaptation of the Charlson comorbidity index, number of medications, RAND MOS (Medical Outcomes Study) social support scale and Short Portable Mental Status Questionnaire. Abnormal geriatric assessment was defined as at least two abnormal questionnaires. With the usual VES13 threshold of 3 (questionnaire deemed abnormal if score is 3 or above), sensitivity was 72.7 % and specificity 85.7 %. VES13 was then analyzed in a large series of 419 patients by Luciani et al. [35]. With a geriatric assessment including CIRS-G, ADL, IADL, MMSE and MNA but omitting risk of falls and depression, sensitivity and specificity were respectively 87 and 62 % versus CGA. One third of patients were abnormal as regards to CGA while 53 % had abnormal VES13. The ONCODAGE study evaluated two screening questionnaires, G8 and VES13 [36]. 1,688 patients were included and 1,435 were eligible and evaluable. Geriatric assessments included CIRS-G, ADL, IADL, MMSE, GDS15, MNA and Time Get up and go. For VES13, sensitivity and specificity were 68.7 % (95%CI [66.0 %; 71.4 %]) and 74.3 % (95%CI [68.8 %; 69.3 %]) respectively. For G8, sensitivity was higher at 76.5 % (95%CI = 73.9–78.9 %) and specificity lower at 64.4 % (95%CI = 58.6–70.0 %).

Table 15.1 The VES13 questionnaire [3]

1. Age______________________

SCORE : 1 point for age 75 - 84,

3 points for age ≥ 85

2. In general, compared toother people your age, would you say that your health is:

- □ Poor* **(SCORE = 1 point)**
- □ Fair* **(SCORE = 1 point)**
- □ Good
- □ Very good
- □ Excellent

3. How much difficulty, <u>on average</u>, do you have with the following physical activities?

	No difficulty	A little difficulty	Some difficulty	A lot of difficulty	Unable to do
a. Stooping, crouching or kneeling?	□	□	□	□	□
b. lifting or carrying objects as heavy as 10 pounds?	□	□	□	□*	□*
c. reaching or extending arms above shoulder level ?	□	□	□	□*	□*
d. writing or handling and grasping small objects?	□	□	□	□*	□*
e. walking a quarter of mile ?	□	□	□	□*	□*
f. heavy housework ssuch as scrubbing floors or washing windows ?	□	□	□	□*	□*

Score : 1 point for each * response in Q3a to f.. <u>Maximum of 2 points</u>.

4. Because of your health of physical condition, do you have any difficulty...

a. Shopping for personal items (like toilet items of medicines) ?

□ YES → Do you get help with shopping ? □ YES* □ NO

□ NO

□ DON'T DO → Is that because of your health ? □ YES* □ NO

b. Managing money (like keeping track of expenses or paying bills) ?

□ YES → Do you get help with managing money ? □ YES □ NO

□ NO

□ DON'T DO → Is that because of your health? □ YES* □ NO

c. Walking across the room (USE OF CANE OR WALKER IS OK) ?

□ YES → Do you get help with walking? □ YES* □ NO

□ NO

□ DON'T DO → Is that because of your health? □ YES* □ NO

d. Doing light housework (like washing dishes, straightening up, or light cleaning) ?

□ YES → Do you get help with light housework? □ OUI* □ NON

□ NO

□ DON'T DO → Is that because of your health? □ YES* □ NO

e. Bathing or showering ?

□ YES → Do you get help with bathing or showering? □ YES* □ NO

□ NO

□ DON'T DO → Is that because of your health? □ YES* □ NO

SCORE : 4 POINTS for one or more * responses in Q4a through Q4e

In a series of 400 patients older than 70 with cancer, Luciani et al. [37] studied the SOF (Study of Osteoporotic Fractures) index versus geriatric assessment including 7 questionnaires. Geriatric assessment included CIRS-G, number of medications, ADL, IADL, MMSE, social status assessment and MNA thus omitting evaluation of mood. Risk of falls was not included in geriatric assessment (as endpoint) but SOF has been demonstrated to predict risk of falls and fractures. Abnormal gold standard was defined as one or more abnormal domains. The SOF index includes three components (5 % or more weight loss during the preceding year, inability to rise from a chair five times without using the arms, negative answer to the question "Do you feel full of energy?"). The index is considered positive if two or more of the three components are present. Overall, 68.2 % of patients were classified as unfit according to geriatric assessment and 67.8 % according to SOF. Sensitivity and specificity of SOF were respectively 89 % (95 % confidence interval (CI): 84.7–92.5) and 81.1 % (95 % CI: 73.2–87.5).

In a large series of 259 patients older than 70 with mainly breast and digestive tract cancer, Biganzoli et al. [38] tested two tools, VES13 and CHS (Cardiovascular Health Study). CHS includes the study of five parameters: unintentional weight loss in the past year, self-reported exhaustion, weakness (grip strength), slow walking speed and low physical activity. Patients are considered frail if they have three or more abnormalities, pre-frail if they have one or two and fit if all CHS parameters are normal. CGA included CIRS-G, ADL, IADL, MMSE, GDS and MNA. Risk of falls was not studied. The CGA was considered impaired in the presence of abnormal results in ≥1 domain. Finally, 47, 75 and 66 % were considered impaired according to VES13, CHS and CGA respectively. Sensitivity and specificity of CHS were respectively 87 and 49 % versus 62 and 81 % for VES13. Great variability in specificity of CHS was observed within subgroups.

The G8 questionnaire (Table 15.2) has been developed for the purpose of screening for cancer treatment in a prospective series of 364 consecutive patients with various types of cancer including lymphoma (110 patients) [39]. A cut-off value of 14 provided a good sensitivity estimate (85 %) without deteriorating specificity (65 %). To validate this questionnaire, we launched the Oncodage study in 23 geriatric oncology centers in France [36] (see above). Overall, 1,688 patients have been accrued and 1,435 were eligible and evaluable. Sensitivity was 76.5 % and specificity 64.4 %. The reliability of the questionnaire was good with a kappa coefficient of 0.64 (95%CI: 0.61–0.70). The time required to complete the questionnaire was, on average, 4.4 min (±2.8) and 98.7 % completed it in less than 10 min. Multivariate analysis showed that, together with sex, stage and performance status, G8 was predictive of one-year survival. Another study including 937 prospective patients with various types of cancer including hematological malignancies, confirmed the strong prognostic value of the G8 questionnaire [40]. Geriatric assessment included living alone, ADL, IADL, MMSE, GDS-15, MNA score and presence of at least one comorbidity on the Charlson comorbidity index (risk of falls omitted) and abnormality defined as two or more abnormal questionnaires. G8 was evaluated as a screening tool and showed 86.5 % sensitivity and 59.3 % specificity. fTRST (Flemish version of the Triage Risk Screening Tool) was also proposed for

Table 15.2 The G8 questionnaire [39]

	Items	Possible answers (score)
A.	Has food intake declined over the past 3 months due to loss of appetite, digestive problems, chewing or swallowing difficulties?	0: Severe decrease in food intake
		1: Moderate decrease in food intake
		2: No decrease in food intake
B.	Weight loss during the last 3 months	0: Weight loss >3 kg
		1: Does not know
		2: Weight loss between 1 and 3 kg
		3: No weight loss
C.	Mobility	0: Bed or chair bound
		1: Able to get out of bed/chair but does not go out
		2: Goes out
E.	Neuropsychological problems	0: Severe dementia or depression
		1: Mild dementia or depression
		2: No psychological problems
F.	Body Mass Index (BMI (weight in kg)/(height in month [2])	0: BMI < 19
		1: BMI = 19 to BMI <21
		2: BMI = 21 to BMI < 23
		3: BMI = 23 and >23
H	Takes more than 3 medications per day	0: Yes
		1: No
P	In comparison with other people of the same age, how does the patient consider his/her health status?	0: Not as good
		0.5: Does not know
		1: As good
		2: Better
	Age	0: >85
		1: 80–85
		2: <80
	Total score	**0–17**

screening. Sensitivity was 91.3 % and specificity was 41.9 % with a threshold for abnormality defined as ≥1.

Overall, definition of abnormal CGA was based on various combinations of questionnaires and evaluations leading to a proportion of frail patients of 30 [35] to 94 % [39]. Furthermore, all series focused on a number of abnormal questionnaires as a target although outcome measures would be much preferable. Considering the screening test, the proportion of frail patients varied from 47 [38] to 82 % [39]. It appears that these proportions highly depend on the characteristics of the population screened which highly varies from one study to the other.

Additional tools are available, such as the Barber Questionnaire that was developed as a screening procedure for older adults in general practice [41], but results reported for older adults with breast cancer are disappointing [42]. Further geriatric tools have been proposed for screening purposes such as the short CGA [43], the abbreviated (a)CGA [44], and the Groningen Frailty Index (GFI) [45]. However, overall, most of these instruments have only been presented in feasibility or pilot studies [46], and initial results suggest that they miss too many cases of vulnerable patients [47].

A recent systematic review [48] compared all available screening methods to CGA and reported a median sensitivity for the VES-13 of 68 % (range 39–88 %), and median specificity of 78 % (range 62–100 %) while corresponding results for G8 were 87 and 61 %. A task force has been recently launched by the SIOG (International Society of Geriatric Oncology) to systematically review currently available results on screening tools.

Once screened as frail, patients deserve further attention from their hematologist. CGA is the most obvious solution to propose. However, it may not be possible in all cancer centers depending on the availability of geriatricians. Consequently, other solutions should be considered. This includes increased medical attention from the hematologist such as thorough evaluation of comorbidities, precise evaluation of major functions such as renal and hepatic systems, consideration of nutritional, socio-economic, mood and cognitive conditions of the patients through the involvement of the health professionals of the supportive care team. Another proposal can be a two-step process including screening tool performed in the oncology setting, then a second step performed by geriatric teams, which can be the whole CGA or a specific geriatric tool that remains to be developed. This may be also the evaluation of the patient by a geriatrician which may lead to further intervention to correct identified impairments. Yet, the impact of geriatric intervention in cancer patients is not yet demonstrated. One randomized trial showed significant improvement of survival with home care intervention performed by advanced practice nurses [49] but only in an unplanned sub-analysis on patients with advanced stages of cancer. Further trials showed some benefits of interventions (more appropriate management [50], quality of life [51, 52], physical functioning [51, 53–55]) but there was no reported impact on survival. Furthermore, some of these studies were not exclusively focused on older patients [53, 55]. Finally, the validity of geriatric intervention is not demonstrated up to now and our community should perform randomized controlled trials in the near future to solve this question.

Selection Process in Hematological Malignancies

Overall, it is now possible to foresee what should be the selection procedure to identify frail patients before treatment of hematological malignancies. However, the whole procedure has to be adapted to the hematology setting. Indeed, when the disease can be cured, even with attenuated treatment, it is not possible to decide whether treatment will be palliative or curative based on a screening test, whatever its performances. The question is particularly tricky in the unfit elderly. Diffuse large B-cell lymphoma is such a disease. Some series have already proposed to select patients with geriatric assessment. Tucci et al. selected patients with four

Table 15.3 Comparison of unfit patients as selected by two different approaches

	Italian trial [59]	EORTC trial [56]
Number of patients	30	32
Median age (range)	83 (70–96)	78.5 (70–92)
>80 years old	73 %	34.5 %
PS 2–4	60 %	69 %
Geriatric assessment		
Older than 80	73 %	34.3 %
Dependent in one ADL or more	56 %	53 %
Severe comorbidities	43 %	18.7 %
Lymphoma characteristics		
Stage III or IV	56.5 %	50 %
Elevated LDH	46.5 %	66 %
aaIPI 2–3	56.5 %	72 %
International Prognostic Index (IPI)		
Age-adjusted IPI	56.7 %	72 %
Performance status 2–4	60 %	69 %
Stage III or IV	56.6 %	50 %
Elevated LDH	46.7 %	66 %
Treatment results		
Neutropenia grade 3/4	13.3 %	22 %
Toxic deaths	3	3
Overall response rate	40 %	44.5 %
Complete response rate	10 %	18.5 %
Median survival	10 months	10.1 months

parameters: age, ADL, CIRS-G and occurrence of geriatric syndromes in a prospective series of 84 evaluable patients [8]. This procedure was blinded to the physicians who classified patients as fit or unfit on usual criteria. Indeed, geriatric criteria appeared more efficient to predict prognosis than physician evaluation.

A few prospective trials have been proposed in a search for optimal treatment for frail patients. In the EORTC 20992 phase II trial [56], we proposed to vulnerable/frail patients a cautious strategy including the well-known COP regimen with its low toxicity profile, specific chemotherapy dose adaptations and geriatric assessment. Among 32 registered patients, 27 were evaluable for efficacy and toxicity. Main characteristics of the patients are outlined in Table 15.3. As expected, results were poor with quite a low response rate, short median survival, but also, despite all precautions, four severe toxicities (three toxic deaths and one febrile neutropenia) (Table 15.3) leading to early termination of the trial. Yet specific precautions were proposed to reduce toxicity including upfront dose reductions based on baseline blood counts, creatinine clearance and performance status. Furthermore, chemotherapy doses were reduced during treatment (and maintained thereafter as already performed in another elderly-specific trial [57]) according to specific toxicities including, among others, febrile neutropenia, but also significant weight loss and degradation of autonomy. These precautions were efficient since only seven patients experienced grade 3 or 4 neutropenia (22 %). However, as observed in the retrospective series of Thieblemont et al. [58], three of them experienced febrile neutropenia and two died thus highlighting again the real frailty of these patients. Finally, geriatric evaluation data showed the specificity of the selected population with 53 % ADL-dependent, 81 % IADL-dependent, 94 % high GDS15 (≥6), 37.5 % MMS<24.

In a prospective trial of 30 patients, Monfardini proposed a cautious treatment with vinorelbine and prednisone at reduced doses [59]. In a population of patients with adverse features (Table 15.2), again, outcome was poor with 10 % complete response rate and 10 months median overall survival. Although toxicity profile appeared quite favorable with only 13.3 % grade 3 and 4 neutropenia, 3 toxic deaths occurred because of cardiac failure (Table 15.3).

Peyrade et al. selected patients older than 80 as the sole unfit criteria [60] and proposed R-miniCHOP. Although selection was not based on health status, it was a large series of 150 patients with a median age of 83 ranging from 80 to 95. Results were good for such a population with 29 months median survival. An important result of this trial is certainly to show that factors such as albumin level and IADL score have prognostic value which appears to be superior to the International Prognostic Index in the elderly.

These results show that a significant proportion of patients can benefit from adapted chemotherapy and that some patients can even be cured (or at least their tumor controlled until death) with low dose treatment despite adverse prognostic features at baseline.

Finally, it is necessary to stress a point which is particularly accurate in aggressive lymphoma. Indeed, many patients will be classified as unfit because of impaired performance status. This can be related either to lymphoma or, sometimes, to other comorbidities. In the first situation, improvement can be expected if treatment response can be obtained. In the second one, hope for a better status will remain quite limited. A simple way to evaluate this situation is to ask patient or family about the observed performance status three to six months before lymphoma. This factor should be taken into account before any clinical decision.

Conclusion

Management of elderly patients with hematological malignancies remains challenging. Patients' outcome can be improved through better evaluation of patients' health status which results should be combined with complete pre-treatment work-up to adapt treatment strategies. While treatment of fit patients is largely based on standard strategy with specific precautions such as use of growth factors according to guidelines, management of unfit patients should take into account much higher risks of toxicity and poor outcome. However, proposal of geriatric assessment and intervention can be a solution to reverse critical situation. A first screening test followed, for patients screened as frail, by either increased medical attention or geriatric assessment may be efficient solutions although both the selection procedure and the interventions to apply once impairments have been identified remain to be more precisely defined. Yet, tools have been identified with good prognostic value on major outcomes which should be used to optimize patients' management.

References

1. Mohile SG, Xian Y, Dale W, Fisher SG, Rodin M, Morrow GR, et al. Association of a cancer diagnosis with vulnerability and frailty in older Medicare beneficiaries. J Natl Cancer Inst. 2009;101(17):1206–15.
2. Balducci L, Extermann M. Management of cancer in the older person: a practical approach. Oncologist. 2000;5(3):224–37.
3. Saliba D, Elliott M, Rubenstein LZ, Solomon DH, Young RT, Kamberg CJ, et al. The Vulnerable Elders Survey: a tool for identifying vulnerable older people in the community. J Am Geriatr Soc. 2001;49(12):1691–9.
4. McNeil C. Geriatric oncology clinics on the rise. J Natl Cancer Inst. 2013;105(9):585–6.
5. Stuck AE, Siu AL, Wieland GD, Adams J, Rubenstein LZ. Comprehensive geriatric assessment: a meta-analysis of controlled trials. Lancet. 1993;342(8878):1032–6.
6. Soubeyran P. From suboptimal to optimal treatment in older patients with cancer. J Geriatr Oncol. 2013;4:291–3.
7. Wedding U, Ködding D, Pientka L, Steinmetz HT, Schmitz S. Physicians' judgement and comprehensive geriatric assessment (CGA) select different patients as fit for chemotherapy. Crit Rev Oncol Hematol. 2007;64(1):1–9.
8. Tucci A, Ferrari S, Bottelli C, Borlenghi E, Drera M, Rossi G. A comprehensive geriatric assessment is more effective than clinical judgment to identify elderly diffuse large cell lymphoma patients who benefit from aggressive therapy. Cancer. 2009;115(19):4547–53.
9. Spina M, Balzarotti M, Uziel L, Ferreri AJ, Fratino L, Magagnoli M, et al. Modulated chemotherapy according to modified comprehensive geriatric assessment in 100 consecutive elderly patients with diffuse large B-cell lymphoma. Oncologist. 2012;17(6):838–46.
10. Lee SJ, Lindquist K, Segal MR, Covinsky KE. Development and validation of a prognostic index for 4-year mortality in older adults. JAMA. 2006;295(7):801–8.
11. Schonberg MA, Davis RB, McCarthy EP, Marcantonio ER. Index to predict 5-year mortality of community-dwelling adults aged 65 and older using data from the National Health Interview Survey. J Gen Intern Med. 2009;24(10):1115–22.
12. Ouellette JR, Small DG, Termuhlen PM. Evaluation of Charlson-Age Comorbidity Index as predictor of morbidity and mortality in patients with colorectal carcinoma. J Gastrointest Surg. 2004;8(8):1061–7.
13. Louwman WJ, Janssen-Heijnen ML, Houterman S, Voogd AC, van der Sangen MJ, Nieuwenhuijzen GA, et al. Less extensive treatment and inferior prognosis for breast cancer patient with comorbidity: a population-based study. Eur J Cancer. 2005;41(5):779–85.
14. Freyer G, Geay JF, Touzet S, Provencal J, Weber B, Jacquin JP, et al. Comprehensive geriatric assessment predicts tolerance to chemotherapy and survival in elderly patients with advanced ovarian carcinoma: a GINECO study. Ann Oncol. 2005;16(11):1795–800.
15. Soubeyran P, Fonck M, Blanc-Bisson C, Blanc JF, Ceccaldi J, Mertens C, et al. Predictors of early death risk in older patients treated by first-line chemotherapy for cancer. J Clin Oncol. 2012;30(15):1829–34.
16. Gomez H, Hidalgo M, Casanova L, Colomer R, Pen DL, Otero J, et al. Risk factors for treatment-related death in elderly patients with aggressive non-Hodgkin's lymphoma: results of a multivariate analysis. J Clin Oncol. 1998;16(6):2065–9.

17. Repetto L, Fratino L, Audisio RA, Venturino A, Gianni W, Vercelli M, et al. Comprehensive geriatric assessment adds information to Eastern Cooperative Oncology Group performance status in elderly cancer patients: an Italian Group for Geriatric Oncology Study. J Clin Oncol. 2002;20(2):494–502.
18. Hurria A, Togawa K, Mohile SG, Owusu C, Klepin HD, Gross CP, et al. Predicting chemotherapy toxicity in older adults with cancer: a prospective multicenter study. J Clin Oncol. 2011;29(25):3457–65.
19. Extermann M, Boler I, Reich RR, Lyman GH, Brown RH, DeFelice J, et al. Predicting the risk of chemotherapy toxicity in older patients: the Chemotherapy Risk Assessment Scale for High-Age Patients (CRASH) score. Cancer. 2012;118(13):3377–86.
20. Warkus T, Rainfray M, Fonck M, Bellera C, Blanc-Bisson C, Blanc JF, et al. Low MNA score and thrombacytopenia are predictive of unexpected hospital admission during treatment in elderly patients receiving chemotherapy. J Geriatr Oncol. 2011;2 Suppl 1:S46.
21. Hoppe S, Rainfray M, Fonck M, Hoppenreys L, Blanc JF, Ceccaldi J, et al. Functional decline in older patients with cancer receiving first-line chemotherapy. J Clin Oncol. 2013;31(31):3877–82.
22. Aparicio T, Jouve JL, Teillet L, Gargot D, Subtil F, Le Brun-Ly V, et al. Geriatric factors predict chemotherapy feasibility: ancillary results of FFCD 2001–02 phase III study in first-line chemotherapy for metastatic colorectal cancer in elderly patients. J Clin Oncol. 2013;31(11):1464–70.
23. Pinder MC, Duan Z, Goodwin JS, Hortobagyi GN, Giordano SH. Congestive heart failure in older women treated with adjuvant anthracycline chemotherapy for breast cancer. J Clin Oncol. 2007;25(25):3808–15.
24. Hershman DL, McBride RB, Eisenberger A, Tsai WY, Grann VR, Jacobson JS. Doxorubicin, cardiac risk factors, and cardiac toxicity in elderly patients with diffuse B-cell non-Hodgkin's lymphoma. J Clin Oncol. 2008;26(19):3159–65.
25. Aapro M, Bernard-Marty C, Brain EGC, Batist G, Erdkamp F, Krzemieniecki K, et al. Anthracycline cardiotoxicity in the elderly cancer patient: a SIOG expert position paper. Ann Oncol. 2011;22(2):257–67.
26. Tofthagen C, Overcash J, Kip K. Falls in persons with chemotherapy-induced peripheral neuropathy. Support Care Cancer. 2012;20(3):583–9.
27. McMillan DC, Canna K, McArdle CS. Systemic inflammatory response predicts survival following curative resection of colorectal cancer. Br J Surg. 2003;90(2):215–9.
28. Kim DK, Oh SY, Kwon HC, Lee S, Kwon KA, Kim BG, et al. Clinical significances of preoperative serum interleukin-6 and C-reactive protein level in operable gastric cancer. BMC Cancer. 2009;9:155.
29. Stark JR, Li H, Kraft P, Kurth T, Giovannucci EL, Stampfer MJ, et al. Circulating prediagnostic interleukin-6 and C-reactive protein and prostate cancer incidence and mortality. Int J Cancer. 2009;124(11):2683–9.
30. Proctor MJ, Morrison DS, Talwar D, Balmer SM, O'Reilly DS, Foulis AK, et al. An inflammation-based prognostic score (mGPS) predicts cancer survival independent of tumour site: a Glasgow Inflammation Outcome Study. Br J Cancer. 2011;104(4):726–34.
31. Alexandre J, Gross-Goupil M, Falissard B, Nguyen ML, Gornet JM, Misset JL, et al. Evaluation of the nutritional and inflammatory status in cancer patients for the risk assessment of severe haematological toxicity following chemotherapy. Ann Oncol. 2003;14(1):36–41.
32. Zauderer MG, Sima CS, Korc-Grodzicki B, Kris MG, Krug LM. Toxicity of initial chemotherapy in older patients with lung cancers. J Geriatr Oncol. 2013;4(1):64–70.
33. Extermann M, Aapro M, Audisio R, Balducci L, Droz JP, Steer C et al. SIOG 10 priorities. 1-2-2011.
34. Mohile SG, Bylow K, Dale W, Dignam J, Martin K, Petrylak DP, et al. A pilot study of the vulnerable elders survey-13 compared with the comprehensive geriatric assessment for identifying disability in older patients with prostate cancer who receive androgen ablation. Cancer. 2007;109(4):802–10.

35. Luciani A, Ascione G, Bertuzzi C, Marussi D, Codeca C, Di MG, et al. Detecting disabilities in older patients with cancer: comparison between comprehensive geriatric assessment and vulnerable elders survey-13. J Clin Oncol. 2010;28(12):2046–50.
36. Soubeyran P, Bellera C, Goyard J, Heitz D, Curé H, Rousselot H, et al. Validation of the G8 screening tool in geriatric oncology: the *ONCODAGE* project. J Clin Oncol. 2011;29(15S Part I):550 s.
37. Luciani A, Dottorini L, Battisti N, Bertuzzi C, Caldiera S, Floriani I, et al. Screening elderly cancer patients for disabilities: evaluation of study of osteoporotic fractures (SOF) index and comprehensive geriatric assessment (CGA). Ann Oncol. 2013;24(2):469–74.
38. Biganzoli L, Boni L, Becheri D, Zafarana E, Biagioni C, Cappadona S, et al. Evaluation of the cardiovascular health study (CHS) instrument and the Vulnerable Elders Survey-13 (VES-13) in elderly cancer patients. Are we still missing the right screening tool? Ann Oncol. 2013;24(2):494–500.
39. Bellera CA, Rainfray M, Mathoulin-Pelissier S, Mertens C, Delva F, Fonck M, et al. Screening older cancer patients: first evaluation of the G-8 geriatric screening tool. Ann Oncol. 2012;23:2166–72.
40. Kenis C, Decoster L, Vanpuyvelde K, de Greve J, Conings G, Milisen K, et al. Performance of two geriatric screening tools in older cancer patients. Eur J Cancer. 2013;49 Suppl 2:S338.
41. Barber JH, Wallis JB, McKeating E. A postal screening questionnaire in preventive geriatric care. J R Coll Gen Pract. 1980;30(210):49–51.
42. Molina-Garrido MJ, Guillen-Ponce C. Comparison of two frailty screening tools in older women with early breast cancer. Crit Rev Oncol Hematol. 2011;79(1):51–64.
43. Hurria A, Gupta S, Zauderer M, Zuckerman EL, Cohen HJ, Muss H, et al. Developing a cancer-specific geriatric assessment: a feasibility study. Cancer. 2005;104(9):1998–2005.
44. Overcash JA, Beckstead J, Moody L, Extermann M, Cobb S. The abbreviated comprehensive geriatric assessment (aCGA) for use in the older cancer patient as a prescreen: scoring and interpretation. Crit Rev Oncol Hematol. 2006;59(3):205–10.
45. Slaets JP. Vulnerability in the elderly: frailty. Med Clin North Am. 2006;90(4):593–601.
46. Extermann M, Green T, Tiffenberg G, Rich C. Validation of the Senior Adult Oncology Program (SAOP) 2 screening questionnaire. Crit Rev Oncol Hematol. 2009;69(2):183–5.
47. Kellen E, Bulens P, Deckx L, Schouten H, Van Dijk M, Verdonck I, et al. Identifying an accurate pre-screening tool in geriatric oncology. Crit Rev Oncol Hematol. 2010;75(3):243–8.
48. Hamaker ME, Jonker JM, de Rooij SE, Vos AG, Smorenburg CH, van Munster BC. Frailty screening methods for predicting outcome of a comprehensive geriatric assessment in elderly patients with cancer: a systematic review. Lancet Oncol. 2012;13(10):e437–44.
49. McCorkle R, Strumpf NE, Nuamah IF, Adler DC, Cooley ME, Jepson C, et al. A specialized home care intervention improves survival among older post-surgical cancer patients. J Am Geriatr Soc. 2000;48(12):1707–13.
50. Goodwin JS, Satish S, Anderson ET, Nattinger AB, Freeman JL. Effect of nurse case management on the treatment of older women with breast cancer. J Am Geriatr Soc. 2003;51(9): 1252–9.
51. Galvao DA, Taaffe DR, Spry N, Joseph D, Newton RU. Combined resistance and aerobic exercise program reverses muscle loss in men undergoing androgen suppression therapy for prostate cancer without bone metastases: a randomized controlled trial. J Clin Oncol. 2010;28(2):340–7.
52. Rao AV, Hsieh F, Feussner JR, Cohen HJ. Geriatric evaluation and management units in the care of the frail elderly cancer patient. J Gerontol A Biol Sci Med Sci. 2005;60(6):798–803.
53. Courneya KS, Sellar CM, Stevinson C, McNeely ML, Peddle CJ, Friedenreich CM, et al. Randomized controlled trial of the effects of aerobic exercise on physical functioning and quality of life in lymphoma patients. J Clin Oncol. 2009;27(27):4605–12.
54. Morey MC, Snyder DC, Sloane R, Cohen HJ, Peterson B, Hartman TJ, et al. Effects of home-based diet and exercise on functional outcomes among older, overweight long-term cancer survivors: RENEW: a randomized controlled trial. JAMA. 2009;301(18):1883–91.

55. Demark-Wahnefried W, Clipp EC, Lipkus IM, Lobach D, Snyder DC, Sloane R, et al. Main outcomes of the FRESH START trial: a sequentially tailored, diet and exercise mailed print intervention among breast and prostate cancer survivors. J Clin Oncol. 2007;25(19):2709–18.
56. Soubeyran P, Khaled H, MacKenzie M, Debois M, Fortpied C, de Bock R, et al. Diffuse large B-cell and peripheral T-cell non-Hodgkin's lymphoma in the frail elderly: a phase II EORTC trial with a progressive and cautious treatment emphasizing geriatric assessment. J Geriatr Oncol. 2011;2(1):36–44.
57. Tirelli U, Errante D, Van Glabbeke M, Teodorovic I, Kluin-Nelemans JC, Thomas J, et al. CHOP is the standard regimen in patients>or=70 years of age with intermediate-grade and high-grade non-Hodgkin's lymphoma: results of a randomized study of the European Organization for Research and Treatment of Cancer Lymphoma Cooperative Study Group. J Clin Oncol. 1998;16(1):27–34.
58. Thieblemont C, Grossoeuvre A, Houot R, Broussais-Guillaumont F, Salles G, Traulle C, et al. Non-Hodgkin's lymphoma in very elderly patients over 80 years. A descriptive analysis of clinical presentation and outcome. Ann Oncol. 2008;19(4):774–9.
59. Monfardini S, Aversa SM, Zoli V, Salvagno L, Bianco A, Bordonaro R, et al. Vinorelbine and prednisone in frail elderly patients with intermediate-high grade non-Hodgkin's lymphomas. Ann Oncol. 2005;16(8):1352–8.
60. Peyrade F, Jardin F, Thieblemont C, Thyss A, Emile JF, Castaigne S, et al. Attenuated immunochemotherapy regimen (R-miniCHOP) in elderly patients older than 80 years with diffuse large B-cell lymphoma: a multicentre, single-arm, phase 2 trial. Lancet Oncol. 2011;12(5):460–8.

Chapter 16
General Consideration on Radiotherapy in Older Patients with Hematological Malignancies

Youlia M. Kirova

Abstract The highest incidence of non-Hodgkin's lymphoma (NHL) is in the 60–79 year age group. Close to 30 % of patients with Hodgkin's lymphoma (HL) are >60 years old. Multiple myeloma (MM) is also a disease in older patients. Age is a major prognostic factor for MM, HL and NHL and is included in prognostic indices. The effect of age is partly due to the co morbidities seen in most elderly lymphoma patients limiting their ability to tolerate intensive chemotherapy. New highly conformal irradiation modalities have emerged for treatment of hematological malignancies and they are adapted for the treatment of old patients. Helical Tomotherapy (HT) offers both intensity-modulated irradiation and accurate patient positioning and was shown to significantly decrease radiation doses to the critical organs. Here we review some of the most promising applications of helical Tomotherapy in hematological malignancies. By decreasing doses to the heart or lungs, helical Tomotherapy might decrease the risk of cardiac toxicity, which is a major concern in patients receiving chest radiotherapy especially in elderly. However, new safe and highly highly conformal therapies applied to hematological malignancies are available for the treatment of hematological malignancies in elderly.

Keywords Lymphoma • Multiple Myeloma • Helical Tomotherapy • Toxicity • Elderly

Introduction

Treatment of hematological malignancies is based on systemic chemotherapy and on biological agents, particularly Rituximab, lenalidomide, thalidomide and other new agents [1]. Unfortunately, in elderly, some patients can not support the side effects of the systemic treatments [1]. Radiation therapy still plays a major role in the management of hematological malignancies, especially in elderly when the

Y.M. Kirova, MD
Radiation Oncology, Institut Curie, 26, rue d'Ulm, 75005 Paris, France
e-mail: youlia.kirova@curie.net

U. Wedding, R.A. Audisio (eds.), *Management of Hematological Cancer in Older People*, DOI 10.1007/978-1-4471-2837-3_16

disease is localized as well as in case of bad tolerance of the systemic treatment. Its place and modalities for treatment of lymphoma have evolved over recent decades. First, randomized studies supported reduction of field size and dose radiation in treatment programs for Hodgkin disease [2]. These developments were encouraged by reports that mediastinal radiotherapy was associated with cardiac toxicity and second malignancies, particularly when chemotherapy agents were used concomitantly or sequentially. Second, sophisticated imaging technologies and new radiation delivery techniques have become available [3]. With the recent advances in irradiation devices, new intensity modulated irradiation modalities have emerged. Those offer both increased target dose conformality and improved normal tissue avoidance. Helical tomotherapy combines inversely planned intensity modulated radiotherapy (IMRT) with on-board megavoltage imaging devices [4]. In this way, it has become possible to tailor very sharp dose distributions around the target volumes, close to critical organs [5]. It has emerged as one of the most promising techniques for IMRT delivery. These techniques are particularly adapted for old patients because their good tolerance, the sparing of organs at risk (OAR).

Clinical Applications of Less Toxic Techniques in Elderly

For lymphoma irradiation, it is now the standard of care to use involved-field radiotherapy rather than the extended radiation fields of the past [6]. In this setting of volume reduction, implementation of new strategies aimed at further improving target coverage is promising. Helical tomotherapy combines inversely planned IMRT with on-board megavoltage imaging devices [4]. In this way, it has become possible to tailor very sharp dose distributions around the target volumes, close to critical organs. Improving dose conformality around the volumes has become an important end-point for radiation oncologists who are involved in the treatment of old patients. Dosimetric results from planning studies of helical tomotherapy have demonstrated its ability in better sparing critical organs from irradiation, in comparison with more conventional irradiation modalities. Helical tomotherapy was shown to provide similar target coverage, and to improve both dose conformality and dose homogeneity within the target volume. This modern irradiation device allows accurate repositioning and critical organs visualization. Tomita et al. [7] compared radiation treatment plans that used IMRT with helical tomotherapy or three-dimensional conformal radiation therapy for nasal natural killer/T-cell lymphoma. Authors found that IMRT achieved significantly better coverage of the planning target volume (PTV), with more than 99 % of the PTV receiving 90 % of the prescribed dose, whereas 3D-CRT could not provide adequate coverage of the PTV, with only 90.0 % receiving 90 % ($P<0.0001$). These results and others demonstrated that helical tomotherapy could significantly improve target coverage when the PTV was close to critical organs.

Prospective data with long-term follow-up evidenced that heart dose exposure may cause cardiac disease and adversely affect quality of life, particularly in patients with mediastinal radiotherapy for Hodgkin lymphoma [8]. Recent data reported that helical tomotherapy could decrease radiation dose exposure for breasts, lung, heart and thyroid gland in patients treated for advanced Hodgkin's disease [9].

Since radiation-induced cardiovascular pathology is a major concern in patients undergoing therapeutic chest irradiation, helical tomotherapy has been logically investigated for improving heart avoidance. The physiopathology and manifestations of radiation-induced heart disease may considerably vary according to the dose, volume and technique of irradiation, and every effort should be made to avoid irradiating cardiac structures [10]. In this way, it will be possible to substantially decrease the risk of death from ischemic heart disease associated with radiation, which is particularly significant in patients receiving other cardiotoxic agents, such as anthracyclines. Actually, helical tomotherapy also allows treatments that would be difficult for conventional radiotherapy machines to deliver, such as treating mediastinal lymph nodes [11]. Several other promising applications for helical tomotherapy have emerged. These strategies include treatment of patients who are at high risk of radiation-induced toxicity because of individual susceptibility, such as patients with acquired immunodeficiency [12]. Helical tomotherapy could also be used for decreasing the doses to critical structures in patients treated with concurrent targeted agents, which might potentially increase the risk of side effects [13] (Figs. 16.1 and 16.2). Moreover, it permits re-irradiation of relapsed disease, a setting that considerably increases the risk of consequent delayed toxicity. Introducing helical tomotherapy to the field of lymphoma may also provide safer and more accurate radiotherapy to selected patients with bulky residual disease [2]. In other malignancies, our retrospective data in patients with solitary plasmocytoma and multiple myeloma demonstrated that doses to critical organs, including the heart, lungs, or kidneys could be decreased [14]. This may be clinically relevant in heavily pretreated patients who are at risk for subsequent treatment-related cardiac toxicity. High response rates were also reported and encouraged further prospective assessment, and most patients experienced a complete response prior to stem cell transplantation (SCT). In elderly the localized radiotherapy can be used also in case of recurrence after SCT.

Alternative Irradiation Modalities

We have pointed out the potential of helical tomotherapy in the light of our institutional experience. Actually, helical tomotherapy is not the only solution to improve both dose conformality and dose homogeneity within the target volume, and its availability remains rather limited (low number of helical tomotherapy devices) [15]· Other IMRT techniques could also be applied for delivering highly conformal irradiation [16–21]. In 2005, Goodman et al. [18] assessed the feasibility and potential advantages of linear accelerator based IMRT in the treatment of lymphoma involving large mediastinal disease volumes or requiring re-irradiation. Compared to conventional parallel-opposed plans and conformal radiotherapy plans, IMRT could decrease the dose delivered to the lung by 12 and 14 %, respectively. The PTV coverage was also improved, compared with conventional RT [18]. Recent dosimetric data demonstrated that the forward planned IMRT technique could be easily used for improving PTV conformity while sparing normal tissue in Hodgkin's lymphoma [20].

Volumetric modulated arc therapy (VMAT) has also demonstrated its ability in tailoring accurate dose distributions around the target volumes. Weber et al. compared VMAT to conventional fixed beam IMRT in ten patients with early Hodgkin disease [21]. They found no difference in levels of dose homogeneity. However, for involved node radiotherapy, doses to the PTV and OAR were higher and lower with VMAT when compared to IMRT, respectively.

Finally, the dosimetric advantages of proton therapy could also be used for reducing the risk of late radiation-induced toxicity related to low-to-moderate doses in critical organs. Chera et al. [19] compared the dose distribution in Hodgkin's lymphoma patients using conventional radiotherapy, IMRT, and 3D proton therapy in Hodgkin's lymphoma patients with stage II disease. Authors found that 3D proton therapy could reduce the dose to the breast, lung, and total body. However, the availability of proton therapy is very low and only a few patients could benefit from this highly conformal irradiation modality .

Other treatment modalities, as the electron beams can be used in elderly as safe, well tolerated and less toxic treatment, especially for cutaneous and orbital lymphomas, Fig. 16.3 [22].

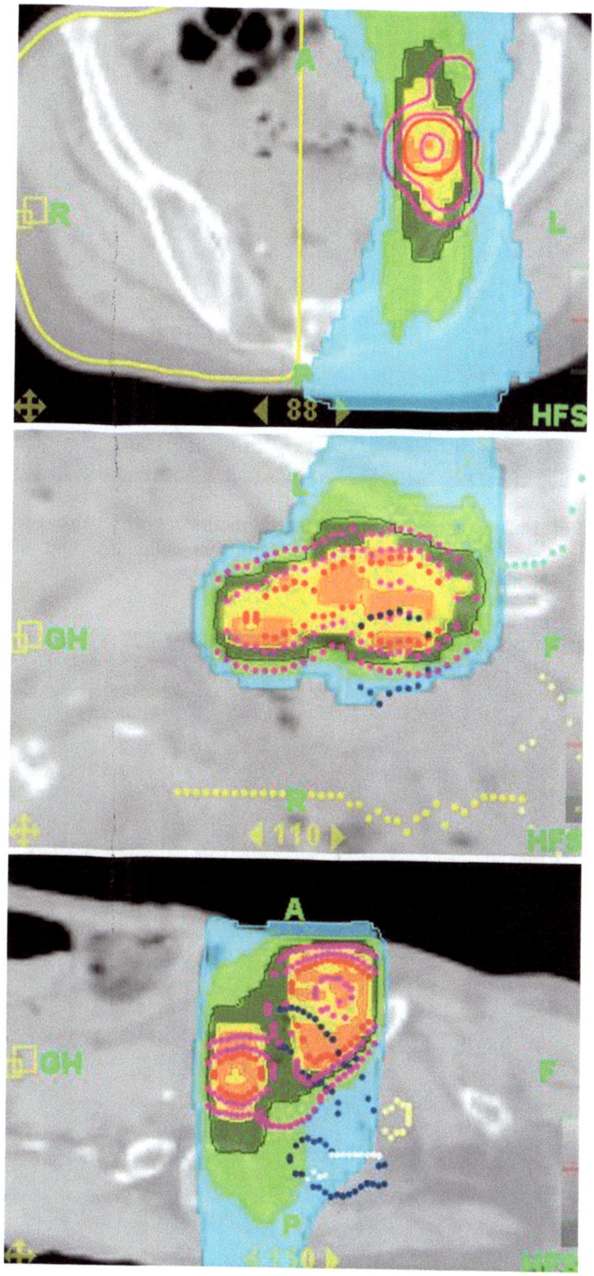

Fig. 16.1 Shows the distribution dose during radiotherapy of an old female patient who was diagnosed with pelvic lesion from high grade lymphoma and who was unable to support the chemotherapy and rituximab treatment (she stopped her treatment after 1 cycle). Dose-volumes histograms evidence accurate sparing of some organs at risk, especially the digestive system

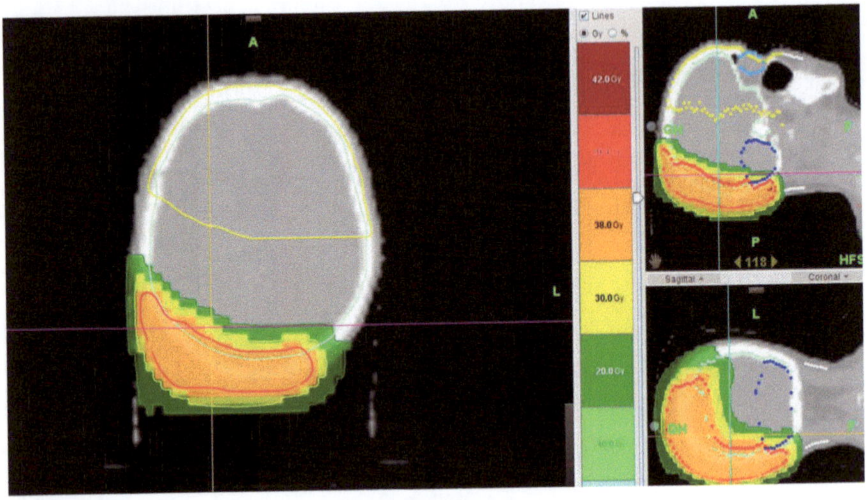

Fig. 16.2 Irradiation using helical tomotherapy of localized recurrence in 75 years old patient treated for multiple myeloma with chemotherapy and stem cell transplantation (dose distribution)

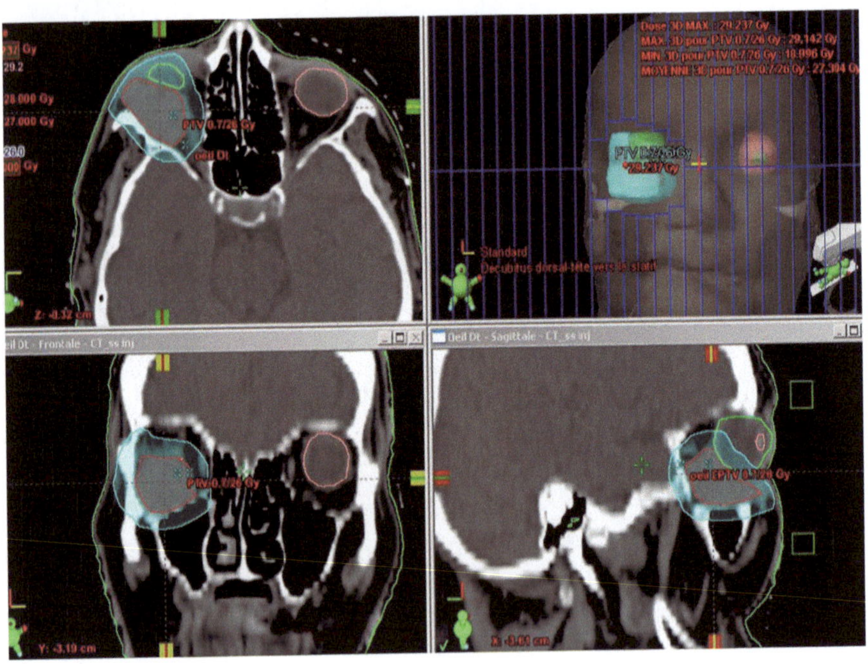

Fig. 16.3 Irradiation of low grade lymphoma in 73 old patient using electron beams

Conclusion

There is growing dosimetric evidence that highly conformal irradiation modalities may improve critical organs sparing, with clinically relevant consequences. Prospective clinical evaluation in needed to confirm the potential benefits of highly conformal therapies applied to hematological malignancies in elderly.

Acknowledgements To Dr. C. Chargary for his precious help

References

1. Westin EH, Longo DL. Lymphoma and myeloma in older patients. Semin Oncol. 2004;31: 19–23.
2. Yahalom J. Transformation in the use of radiation therapy of Hodgkin lymphoma: new concepts and indications lead to modern field design and are assisted by PET imaging and intensity modulated radiation therapy (IMRT). Eur J Haematol Suppl 2005;90–7.
3. Girinsky T, Ghalibafian M. Radiotherapy of Hodgkin lymphoma: indications, new fields, and techniques. Semin Radiat Oncol. 2007;17:206–22.
4. Welsh JS, Patel RR, Ritter MA, Harari PM, Mackie TR, Mehta MP. Helical tomotherapy: an innovative technology and approach to radiation therapy. Technol Cancer Res Treat. 2002;1: 311–6.
5. Beavis AW. Is tomotherapy the future of IMRT? Br J Radiol. 2004;77:285–95.
6. Fermé C, Eghbali H, Meerwaldt JH, et al. Chemotherapy plus involved-field radiation in early-stage Hodgkin's disease. N Engl J Med. 2007;357:1916–27.
7. Tomita N, Kodaira T, Tachibana H, Nakamura T, Nakahara R, Inokuchi H, Mizoguchi N, Takada A. A comparison of radiation treatment plans using IMRT with helical tomotherapy and 3D conformal radiotherapy for nasal natural killer/T-cell lymphoma. Br J Radiol. 2009;82:756–63.
8. Hudson MM, Poquette CA, Lee J, Greenwald CA, Shah A, Luo X, Thompson EI, Wilimas JA, Kun LE, Crist WM. Increased mortality after successful treatment for Hodgkin's disease. J Clin Oncol. 1998;16:3592–600.
9. Prosnitz RG, Chen YH, Marks LB. Cardiac toxicity following thoracic radiation. Semin Oncol. 2005;32:71–80.
10. Vlachaki MT, Kumar S. Helical tomotherapy in the radiotherapy treatment of Hodgkin's disease – a feasibility study. J Appl Clin Med Phys. 2010;11:3042.
11. Gagliardi G, Constine LS, Moiseenko V, Correa C, Pierce LJ, Allen AM, Marks LB. Radiation dose-volume effects in the heart. Int J Radiat Oncol Biol Phys. 2010;76:S77–85.
12. Chargari C, Vernant JP, Tamburini J, Zefkili S, Fayolle M, Campana F, Fourquet A, Kirova YM. Feasibility of Helical Tomotherapy for debulking irradiation prior to stem cells transplantation in malignant lymphoma. Int J Radiat Oncol Biol Phys. 2011;81(4):1184–9.
13. Chargari C, Zefkili S, Kirova YM. Potential of helical tomotherapy for sparing critical organs in a patient with AIDS who was treated for Hodgkin lymphoma. Clin Infect Dis. 2009;48: 687–9.
14. Kirova YM, Chargari C, Amessis M, Vernant JP, Dhedin N. Concurrent involved field radiation therapy and Temsirolimus in refractory mantle cell lymphoma (MCL). Am J Hematol. 2010;85(11):892.

15. Chargari C, Kirova YM, Zefkili S, Caussa L, Amessis M, Dendale R, Campana F, Fourquet A. Solitary plasmocytoma: improvement in critical organs sparing by means of helical tomotherapy. Eur J Haematol. 2009;83:66–71.
16. McCutchen KW, Watkins JM, Eberts P, Terwilliger LE, Ashenafi MS, Jenrette 3rd JM. Helical tomotherapy for total lymphoid irradiation. Radiat Med. 2008;26:622–6.
17. Wong JY, Liu A, Schultheiss T, Popplewell L, Stein A, Rosenthal J, Essensten M, Forman S, Somlo G. Targeted total marrow irradiation using three-dimensional image-guided tomographic intensity-modulated radiation therapy: an alternative to standard total body irradiation. Biol Blood Marrow Transplant. 2006;12:306–15.
18. Goodman KA, Toner S, Hunt M, Wu EJ, Yahalom J. Intensity-modulated radiotherapy for lymphoma involving the mediastinum. Int J Radiat Oncol Biol Phys. 2005;62:198–206.
19. Chera BS, Rodriguez C, Morris CG, Louis D, Yeung D, Li Z, Mendenhall NP. Dosimetric comparison of three different involved nodal irradiation techniques for stage II Hodgkin's lymphoma patients: conventional radiotherapy, intensity-modulated radiotherapy, and three-dimensional proton radiotherapy. Int J Radiat Oncol Biol Phys. 2009;75:1173–80.
20. Cella L, Liuzzi R, Magliulo M, Conson M, Camera L, Salvatore M, Pacelli R. Radiotherapy of large target volumes in Hodgkin's lymphoma: normal tissue sparing capability of forward IMRT versus conventional techniques. Radiat Oncol. 2010;5:33.
21. Weber DC, Peguret N, Dipasquale G, Cozzi L. Involved-node and involved-field volumetric modulated arc vs. fixed beam intensity-modulated radiotherapy for female patients with early-stage supra-diaphragmatic Hodgkin lymphoma: a comparative planning study. Int J Radiat Oncol Biol Phys. 2009;75:1578–86.
22. Gherbi BJ, Kirova YM, Orecchia R. Clinical applications of high-energy electrons. 5th ed. Levitt. 2012.

Chapter 17
Supportive Care in Older Patients with Hematological Malignancies

Karin Jordan, Berit Jordan, Camilla Leithold, and Jörn Rüssel

Abstract The management of hematological neoplasms is particularly difficult in elderly patients, as non-tumor related life expectancy is highly variable and the benefit-to-risk ratio for oncological treatments depends on comorbidities and pharmacological factors. In this patient population an excellent supportive care is of utmost importance to allow the administration of effective treatment. In this chapter the supportive care management strategies with a special focus on myelosuppression, chemotherapy-induced nausea and vomiting, cancer-related fatigue, diarrhoea, mucositis, cardiotoxicity, neurotoxicity and nutrition will be discussed.

Keywords Supportive Care • Elderly patients • Emesis • Fatigue • Myelosuppression • Mucositis • Cardiotoxicity • Diarrhoea • Neurotoxicity • Nutrition

Introduction

Older and younger patients benefit to the same extent from chemotherapy of common neoplasms, but aging is usually associated with increased risk of short- and long-term complications of treatment and of cancer itself. Therefore, the challenges of aging, comorbidities, and polypharmacy require special attention for supportive care in the elderly to address potential side effects.

K. Jordan, MD (✉)
Department of Hematology/Oncology, University Hospital Halle (Saale),
Ernst-Grube-Str. 40, 06120 Halle (Saale), Germany
e-mail: karin.jordan@uk-halle.de

B. Jordan, MD
Department of Neurology, University Hospital Halle (Saale),
Halle (Saale), Germany

C. Leithold, MSc • J. Rüssel, MD
Department of Hematology and Oncology, University Hospital Halle (Saale),
Halle (Saale), Germany

U. Wedding, R.A. Audisio (eds.), *Management of Hematological Cancer in Older People*, DOI 10.1007/978-1-4471-2837-3_17

Chemotherapy-induced Nausea and Vomiting

The goal of each antiemetic therapy is to completely prevent nausea and vomiting. Twenty years ago, nausea and vomiting were common adverse side effects of distinct types of chemotherapy and forced up to 20 % of patients to postpone or refuse potentially curative treatment [1, 2]. Continuous research over the past 25 years has led to steady improvements in the control of chemotherapy-induced nausea and vomiting (CINV).

When evaluating elderly cancer patients for a particular type of chemotherapy, a number of factors have to be considered; these include co-morbidity, poly-pharmacy, compliance, possible decrease in organ function and specific risk factors related to chemotherapy-induced side effects [3].

Classification of CINV

CINV classification is widely agreed upon the antiemetic community. CINV is classified into three categories: acute onset (mostly serotonin related), occurring within 24 h of initial administration of chemotherapy; delayed onset (in part substance P related), occurring 24 h to several days after chemotherapy treatment; and anticipatory nausea and vomiting, observed in patients whose emetic episodes are triggered by taste, odour, sight, thoughts, or anxiety due to a history of poor response to antiemetic agents.

Emetogenicity of Chemotherapeutic Agents

The emetogenic potential of the chemotherapeutic agents used is the main risk factor for the degree of CINV. The emetogenic potential of the chemotherapeutic agents are classified into four emetic risk groups: high (90 %), moderate (30–90 %), low (10–30 %) and minimal (<10 %) (the figures in parentheses represent the percentage of patients having emetic episode/s when no prophylactic antiemetic protection provided) [4]. Therefore, the antiemetic prophylaxis is directed to the emetogenic potential of the chemotherapy (Table 17.1) [5].

Agents such as Lenalidomide, Thalidomide, Nilotinib, Dasatinib and Ruxolitinib are not classified yet.

Patient Related Risk Factors

Age is an important prognostic factor when dealing with chemotherapy-induced nausea and vomiting. Several studies have shown that complete response from nausea and vomiting are significantly more frequent in patients over 65 years of age [3].

Table 17.1 Emetogenic risk of intravenous chemotherapeutic agents

High (emesis risk >90 % without antiemetics)	
Carmustine, BCNU	Lomustine
Cisplatin	Mechlorethamine
Cyclophosphamide (>1,500 mg/m²)	Pentostatin
Dacarbazine, DTIC	Procarbazine
Moderate (emesis risk 30–90 % without antiemetics)	
Azacytidine	Doxorubicin
Alemtuzumab	Imatinib
Cyclophosphamide (<1,500 mg/m²)	Melphalan i.v.
Cytarabine (>1 g/m²)	Mitoxantrone (>12 mg/m²)
Daunorubicin	Oxaliplatin
Low (emesis risk 10–30 % without antiemetics)	
Asparaginase	Methotrexat (>100 mg/m²)
Bortezomib	Mitoxantrone (<12 mg/m²)
Cytarabine (<1 g/m²)	Pegasparaginase
Etoposide i.v.	Teniposide
Gemcitabine	Thiotepa
Minimal (emesis risk <10 % without antiemetics)	
Bleomycin	Melphalan p.o.
Busulfan	Mercaptopurine
Chlorambucil	Methotrexat (<100 mg/m²)
Cladribine	Sorafenib
Cytarabine (<100 mg/m²)	Thioguanine
Fludarabine	Vinblastine
Hydroxyurea	Vincristine
α-, β-, γ- Interferone	Vinorelbine

Adapted from Refs. [5, 11, 16]

Patient risk factors including further female gender, a history of low alcohol intake, experience of emesis during pregnancy, impaired quality of life and previous experience of chemotherapy are known to increase the risk of nausea and vomiting after chemotherapy.

Co-morbidity

Treatment of elderly cancer patients is often complicated by the circumstance that elderly have a higher incidence of concomitant diseases, e.g. hypertension. Heart diseases are seen in approximately 20 % of elderly patients. This should be considered when treating nausea and vomiting with serotonin receptor antagonists. For example some serotonin receptor antagonists have been shown to lead to prolongation of the QTc interval which increases the risk of cardiac arrhythmia. Diabetes (10–15 % in this population) is frequent in elderly cancer patients and leads to increased risk of hyperglycemia with corticosteroids and increased risk of constipation (side effect of serotonin receptor antagonists, 10–15 %) due to autonomic neuropathy [3].

Antiemetics

With modern antiemetics, vomiting can completely be prevented in up to 70–80 % of patients [6, 7].

5-HT3 serotonin receptor antagonists (5-HT3 RAs): The 5-HT3 RAs form the cornerstone of therapy for the control of emesis with chemotherapy agents with moderate to high emetogenic potential. Five 5-HT3-RAs, dolasetron, granisetron, ondansetron, palonosetron and tropisetron are available in Europe. When administering 5-HT3-RAs, several points should be taken into consideration [8–10]:

- The lowest fully effective dose for each agent should be used; higher doses do not enhance any aspect of activity because of the receptor saturation.
- Oral and intravenous route are equally effective.
- No schedule is better than a single dose daily (exception ondansetron) given before chemotherapy.

Neurokinin1 receptor antagonist (NK1 RA): Aprepitant-containing regimens have been shown to significantly reduce acute and delayed emesis in patients receiving highly emetogenic chemotherapy (HEC) and moderately emetogenic chemotherapy (MEC), compared with regimens containing a 5-HT3-RA plus dexamethasone only. Aprepitant is available for oral and as fosaprepitant in the intravenous administration form and should be administered as indicated in Table 17.2. Aprepitant is well tolerated. The most common low grade adverse effects reported during clinical trials include headache, anorexia, fatigue, diarrhoea, hiccups and mild transaminase elevation. Aprepitant is metabolised by cytochrome P450 (CYP) 3A4. It is a moderate inhibitor and an inducer of CYP3A4 [11] and has been shown to cause a twofold increase in the area under the plasma concentration curve (AUC) of dexamethasone, which is a sensitive substrate of CYP3A4. Potential interactions with cytotoxic drugs metabolised by CYP3A4 were intensively studied and did not resulted in clinically significant interactions [12]. However, the potential interactions should be carefully selected when treating elderly patients.

Steroids, dexamethasone: Although not approved as an antiemetic, dexamethasone plays a major role in the prevention of acute and delayed CINV and is an integral component of almost each antiemetic regimen (Table 17.2). Dexamethasone is the most frequently used corticosteroid, although no study reports the superiority of one corticosteroid over another in terms of efficacy. Because of the risk of insomnia, administering corticosteroids in the evening should be avoided. Elderly are often treated with NSAIDs which especially in combination with corticosteroids can lead to gastric bleeding. Elderly patients with a diagnosis of diabetes should be closely monitored, when receiving steroids [3].

Olanzapine: Olanzapine is an atypical neuroleptic drug. By the ASCO (American Society of Clinical Oncology) guidelines olanzapine is recommended

Table 17.2
Dose of antiemetics

$5\text{-}HT_3$-receptorantagonist	Route	Recommended dose (once daily)
Ondansetron	p.o.	8 mg twice daily
	i.v.	8 mg (0.15 mg/kg)
Granisetron	p.o.	2 mg
	i.v.	1 mg (0.01 mg/kg)
Tropisetron	p.o.	5 mg
	i.v.	
Palonosetron	p.o.	0.5 mg
	i.v.	0.25 mg
Steroids		
Dexamethasone	p.o./ i.v.	12 mg (highly emetogenic with aprepitant)
		20 mg w/o aprepitant
		8 mg (moderately emetogenic)
NK_1-receptorantagonist		
Aprepitant	p.o.	125 mg day 1,
		80 mg day 2+3
Fosaprepitant	i.v.	150 mg day 1 only

Adapted from Refs. [5, 11, 16]

as an adjunctive drug and also for patients who experience nausea and vomiting despite optimal antiemetic prophylaxis [5]. This recommendation is supported by the latest study by Navari where olanzapine showed superior efficacy in comparison to metoclopramide in the rescue setting [13].

Dopamine receptor antagonists: Prior to the introduction of $5\text{-}HT_3$ RAs, dopamine-receptor antagonists formed the basis of antiemetic therapy [14]. One of the most frequently used benzamides is metoclopramide. Current guidelines do not recommend metoclopramide for prevention of acute CINV. The current ASCO guidelines recommend that metoclopramide should be reserved for patients intolerant of or refractory to $5\text{-}HT_3$-RAs, dexamethasone and aprepitant [5]. Just recently, the EMA (european medical agency) recommended that metoclopramide should only be prescribed for short-term use (up to 5 days) because of side effects on the nervous system. In addition, the maximum recommended dose in adults has been restricted to 30mg per day.

Benzodiazepines: These drugs can be a useful addition to antiemetic regimens in certain circumstances such as anxiety and risk reduction of anticipatory CINV or in patients with refractory and breakthrough emesis as suggested by all antiemetic guidelines.

Summary of Antiemetic Guideline Based Management of CINV

Three international antiemetic guidelines are available [5, 10, 15]. None of these guidelines have specific recommendations for prophylaxis of CINV in the elderly.

Table 17.3 Antiemetic prevention based on the emesis risk category. Adapted from [5, 11, 16]

Emesis risk	Acute phase (day 1)	Delayed phase (day 2–5)
High	**5-HT_3-RA**	
	Granisetron; 2 mg p.o./1 mg i.v.	
	Ondansetron; 16 mg p.o./8 mg i.v.	
	Palonosetron; 0,5 mg p.o./ 0,25 mg i.v.	
	Tropisetron; 5 mg p.o./i.v.	
	Dolasetron; 100 mg p.o.	
	+	
	Steroid	**Steroid**
	Dexamethasone; 12 mg p.o./i.v.	Dexamethasone; 8 mg p.o./i.v. day 2–3 (4)
	+	+
	NK-1-RA	**NK-1-RA**
	Aprepitant; 125 mg p.o.	Aprepitant; 80 mg p.o. day 2–3
	or	
	Fosaprepitant 150 mg i.v. single-dose	
Moderate	**5-HT_3-RA**, Palonosetron preferred	
	0.50 mg p.o. / 0.25 mg i.v.	
	+	
	Steroid	**Steroid**
	Dexamethasone; 8 mg p.o/ i.v.	Dexamethasone, 8 mg p.o /i.v. day 2–3
Low	**Steroid**	None
	Dexamethasone; 8 mg p.o/i.v.	
Minimal	None	None

HEC; acute CINV: The guidelines suggest unanimously a combination of 5-HT_3 RA, dexamethasone and aprepitant/fosaprepitant within the first 24 h (Table 17.3).

HEC; delayed CINV: All guidelines suggest the combination of dexamethasone and aprepitant. If fosaprepitant was given on day 1, no further application of fosaprepitant is necessary.

MEC; acute CINV: Patients undergoing MEC regimens should be given a combination of a 5-HT3 RA, preferably palonosetron and the corticosteroid dexamethasone. The ASCO guideline stated that the triple combination (5-HT_3 RA, dexamethasone and aprepitant) can be considered in selected patients.

MEC; delayed CINV: Dexamethasone is the preferred agent to use. Nonetheless, when aprepitant was used for the prevention of acute CINV then aprepitant should be used also for the prophylaxis of delayed CINV. 5-HT_3 RA can be used as an alternative. However, if palonosetron was the 5-HT3 RA of choice a repeated application is not useful.

Low emetogenic chemotherapy: In patients receiving chemotherapy of low emetic risk, a single agent, such as a low dose of a corticosteroid, is effective. In principle 5-HT3-RAs are not constituents of the prophylactic armamentarium.

Minimal emetogenic chemotherapy: It is suggested by all guidelines that for patients treated with agents of low emetic risk, no antiemetic drug should be routinely administered before chemotherapy.

Chemotherapy Induced Myelosuppression

Evidence suggests that elderly patients are at greater risk of chemotherapy-related toxicities than younger patients. Myelotoxicity is of particular concern, as the haematopoietic reserves of elderly patients have been found to decrease progressively with time [16]. Age-related haematologic changes are reflected by a decline in bone marrow cellularity, an increased risk of anemia, and a declining adaptive immunity.

Neutropenia

The purpose of G-CSF (Granulocyte-Colony Stimulating Factors) is to enable administration of chemotherapy, regardless of the age of the patient. Prophylactic G-CSF may provide elderly patients with the chance of receiving curative doses of chemotherapy and thus, potentially improve survival rates. Additionally, the value of palliative chemotherapy should also be considered in elderly patients and appropriate growth factor prophylaxis facilitates the administration of such therapy.

In a systematic review and meta-analysis of randomised controlled trials comparing primary prophylactic G-CSF with placebo or untreated controls in adults with solid tumors or lymphomas reported a 40 % reduction in febrile neutropenia with the use of G-CSF in patients older than 65 years [17]. The EORTC (European Organisation for Research and Treatment of Cancer) Guidelines, the NCCN (National Comprehensive Cancer Network) Guidelines for Senior Adult Oncology as well as ASCO recommend the prophylactic use of G-CSF in clinical situations where the risk of neutropenia is greater than 20 %. Age older than 65 years was identified as an important patient characteristic that identified individuals for the receipt of prophylactic growth factor treatment. G-CSF are also recommended in older patients receiving curative therapy in the treatment of non-hodgkin lymphomas where maintenance of dose intensity is essential to achieve a good outcome. The use of G-CSF therapy is also appropriate in this group when the risk of neutropenia from individual regimens is less than 20 %, if other patient-related factors suggest a high risk of morbidity and mortality from neutropenia (Table 17.4). Treatment with G-CSF can be used to reduce the duration of neutropenia and the incidence of hospitalizations in these patients. Prophylactic antibiotic use with or without G-CSF has shown similar beneficial effect in some studies but no clear recommendation has been made about their use in elderly patients for prophylactic or secondary use for chemotherapy-induced neutropenia.

Table 17.4 Prophylactic use of G-CSF in the Elderly

Risk of febrile neutropenia from chemotherapy ≥20 %
Risk of febrile neutropenia from chemotherapy 10–20 % and presence of additional risk factors for infectious complications:
Previous episode of febrile neutropenia
Advanced disease
Heavily pretreated patients
Presence of cytopenias due to bone marrow involvement
Malnutrition
Current infections
Liver or renal dysfunction
Multiple comorbidities
Poor performance status

Adapted from Aapro et al. [43]

The risk of administration of growth factors is minimal, although a slight increase in thrombocytopenia has been reported with the use of GM-CSF (not confirmed for G-CSF).

Anaemia

Please see special Chap. 2 in this book.

Thrombocytopenia

Platelet transfusions are the only effective way to manage thrombocytopenia associated with chemotherapy, besides chemotherapy dose reductions or delay of chemotherapy. The appropriate threshold for platelet transfusion during chemotherapy recommended by the ASCO is a platelet count less than 10×10^9/L [18]. These recommended levels may have to be modified in the elderly population who may have other risk factors for bleeding including the use of anticoagulant drugs for thromboembolic events or cerebrovascular or cardiovascular diseases. The thrombopoetin receptor agonists romiplostim and eltrombopag are still under investigation for management for chemotherapy induced thrombocytopenia.

Fatigue

Fatigue is an attendant and very burdening symptom for patients with chronic diseases. Especially the pathophysiology of cancer-related fatigue (CRF) is not well understood. It can last for several months after having stopped a cytostatic therapy.

CRF is of course a multifactorial disorder and may come from the disease itself or the application of chemotherapy. Personal factors like age, gender, physical conditions, comorbidities, subacute or chronic inflammation and infection and mental health may play an essential role. CRF highly impacts the quality of life and can be associated with a poor adherence to follow the recommended chemotherapy regimen that would be an indirect risk for therapy failure. Therefore the main diagnostic step to become aware of clinically significant fatigue is to keep this symptom in mind. Unfortunately the treatment or prophylactic options against CRF are limited. Because of the possibility of hazardous drug interactions in elderly patients who generally are treated for several comorbidities the use of stimulating antidepressants is only investigated for episodes of real depression which should be ensured by a specialist. It is already known that phytotherapeutics like ginseng may reduce symptoms from CRF. A recent placebo-controlled phase III trial provides data to support that American ginseng that is in some way different from Asian ginseng reduces general and physical CRF over 8 weeks without side effects when given in a dose of 2,000 mg/day [19]. A beneficial therapeutic approach that was shown by a recent published Cochrane Review of clinical trials [20] is aerobic exercise for individuals with CRF during and after cancer therapy. Apart from that the consequent and generous treatment of chronic anaemia is thought to be important to avoid the worsening of CRF although clinical data providing any thresholds for hemoglobin are missing.

Mucositis

Muscositis may be an undesirable effect of any therapy against hematological malignancies such as classical cytostatics and radiation and is defined by a damage of any mucosal region with more or less serious consequences for the whole organism. The pathophysiology is not entirely understood, notably not for the new and smart drugs like kinase inhibitors, immunomodulatos or antibodies. Mucosal injury provides an opportunity for infection to flourish, placing the patient at risk of bacteraemia, sepsis and septicaemia [21]. Whereas severe pain might be the most discomfortable consequence of oral mucositis for patients, diarrhoea is a very common symptom of gastrointestinal mucositis which will be discussed in an extra chapter. In older individuals, mucositis may become rapidly very severe as a result of limited reserve. Mucositis is therefore an area of huge medical need. The grade of severity is not only dependent on the particular drug, drug combination, the field of radiation or dose pattern but also on the individual composition and strength of the mucosal barrier influenced by genetical aspects. Unfortunately, no antidote to mucositis is available. All treatment strategies aimed at improving mouth care are dependent on good assessment as the severity of mucositis spans a wide area of clinical signs and symptoms [22]. Mostly the World Health Organisation (WHO) Oral Toxicity Scale (Table 17.5) is used in practice.

The only generally accepted treatment options for chemotherapy induced mucositis are based on simple symptom control like the use of systemic and topical

Table 17.5 WHO oral toxicity scale

OM grade	Clinical presentation
1	Soreness ± erythema, no ulceration.
2	Erythema, ulcers. Patients can swallow solid diet.
3	Ulcers, extensive erythema. Patients cannot swallow solid diet.
4	OM to the extent that alimentation is not possible.

analgetics, antibiotics in the case of myelosuppression or existent signs of infection and nutritional supplementation in severe cases once incapability of food intake is induced by ulcerations. In contrast to haematopoetic stem cell transplantation protocols which are established for a well-defined population of mostly young and medically fit patients no specific agent for prevention or treatment of oral mucositis in elderly patients treated with standard dose protocols can be recommended [23]. However, in accordance with the latest MASCC mucositis guideline the most important statements are summarized as follow (www.mascc.org):

- "The panel *suggests* that oral care protocols be used to prevent oral mucositis in all age groups and across all cancer treatment modalities (Level of Evidence III)."
- "The panel *suggests* that transdermal fentanyl may be effective to treat pain due to oral mucositis in patients receiving conventional and high-dose chemotherapy, with or without total body irradiation (Level of Evidence III)."
- "The panel *suggests* that 0.5 % doxepin mouthwash may be effective to treat pain due to oral mucositis (Level of Evidence IV)."

Diarrhoea

Diarrhoea is one of the main drawbacks for cancer patients, especially for elderly patients who are commonly at a higher risk of dehydration and infectious complications. Possible etiologies could be classical gastrointestinal mucosal damage by radiotherapy, chemotherapeutic agents or other reasons like decreased physical performance, graft versus host disease and infections. Especially chemotherapy induced diarrhoea (CID) is a common problem in patients with advanced cancer and the incidence of CID has been reported to be as high as 50–80 % of treated patients (≥30 % CTC grade 3–5). Regardless of the molecular targeted approach of tyrosine kinase inhibitors and antibodies, diarrhoea is a common side effect in up to 60 % of patients with up to 10 % severe diarrhoea. Furthermore the pathophysiology is still under investigation [24].

Despite the amount of clinical trials evaluating therapeutic or prophylactic measures in CID, there are just three drugs recommended in current guidelines: loperamide, deodorized tincture of opium and octreotide. There is no approach for any prophylactic treatment.

Guideline Based Drug Recommendation

So far, only loperamide, octreotide and tincture of opium are recommended in the updated treatment guidelines by the consensus conference on the management of CID from Benson et al. due to a lack of efficacy or insufficient evidence level of the other mentioned therapeutical approaches [25].

Opioids: Loperamide is an opioid which functions by decreasing intestinal motility by directly affecting the smooth muscle of the intestine and has no systemic effects due to a minimal absorption. The recommendation in current treatment guidelines [25] is based on an effective reduction in fecal incontinence, frequency of bowel movements and stool weight. The dosage of loperamide is an initial 4 mg dose followed by 2 mg every 2–4 h or after every unformed stool.

Deodorized tincture of opium (DTO) is another widely used antidiarrhoeal agent, despite the absence of literature reports supporting the efficacy for treatment of chemotherapy-induced diarrhoea. DTO contains the equivalent of 10 mg/ml morphine. The recommended dose is 10–15 drops in water every 3–4 h [25]. The camphorated (alcohol-based) tincture is a less concentrated preparation containing the equivalent of 0,4 mg/ml morphine, leading to a dose of 5 ml (one teaspoon) every 3–4 h.

Octreotide: Octreotide, a synthetic somatostatin analog, acts via several mechanisms: decreased secretion of a number of hormones, such as vasoactive intestinal peptide (VIP), prolongation of intestinal transit time and reduced secretion and increased absorption of fluid and electrolytes. It is approved by the US Food and Drug Administration for the treatment of diarrhoea related to VIP-secreting tumors and symptoms due to carcinoid syndrome. Octreotide is beneficial in patients with CID. Although one randomised trial in 41 5-FU-treated patients showed that octreotide was more effective than standard-dose loperamide (90 versus 15 % resolution of diarrhoea by day 3) [26], octreotide is generally reserved as a second-line treatment for patients who are refractory after 48 h, despite a loperamide-escalation because of its high cost. Patients developing a gastrointestinal syndrome including severe diarrhoea, nausea, vomiting, anorexia, and abdominal cramping should receive an aggressive management with i.v. fluids and upfront octreotide. These recommendations by the consensus conference mentioned above reflect the risk of life-threatening complications and the reduced activity of loperamide in case of severe diarrhoea. The optimal dosage of octreotide is not well defined. Current treatment guidelines recommend a starting dose of 100–150 μg subcutaneously (sc) or intravenously (iv) three times a day. Doses could be escalated to 500 μg sc/iv three times a day or by continuous iv infusion 25–50 μg/h three times daily showing a dose-response relationship without significant toxicities. As for oral mucositis the latest MASCC mucositis guideline has provided treatment recommendations and suggestions for gastrointestinal mucositis causing diarrhoea. There is only one important statement for elderly patients treated for hematological malignancies (www.mascc.org):

- "The panel *recommends* that octreotide, at a dose of ≥100 μg subcutaneously twice daily, be used to *treat* diarrhoea induced by standard- or high-dose chemotherapy associated with haematopoetic stem cell transplant, if loperamide is ineffective (Level of evidence II)."

Summary of the consensus recommendations:The commonly used CTC classification divides the grade of severity by the increase of stools over baseline. This is not helpful when searching for specific therapeutic decisions. Rather the volume and duration of diarrhoea and also lifestyle and eating habits that could play a contributory role should be always determined by a comprehensive clinical approach. Other factors that can aggravate CID like intestinal infections, radiation etc. should be always kept in mind. The indication for hospitalization depends on the individual medical assessment of potential life-threatening consequences. Recommendations for the daily clinical practice in an oncology unit come from of a consensus conference on the management of CID and were published in 1998 and updated in 2004. Guidelines for evaluation and management of patients with CID are presented in Fig. **17.1** [25, 27]. The tempo and specific nature of treatment is guided by the classification of the symptom constellation as complicated or uncomplicated. Uncomplicated patients may be managed conservatively in the outpatient setting (at least initially), while those with severe diarrhoea or a potentially exacerbating condition (eg. abdominal cramping, nausea, vomiting, fever, sepsis, neutropenia or bleeding) should be admitted to the hospital and treated aggressively with octreotide, i.v. fluids, antibiotics and a diagnostic workup.

Chemotherapy-induced Cardiotoxicity

Anthracyclines and mitoxantrone have been the anchor drugs of cancer chemotherapy for longer than 60 years. Cardiotoxicity associated with their use has been the most extensively studied non-haematologic complication of chemotherapy and is the most widely recognized cardiac complication of cancer therapy by clinicians. They are known to cause both short- and long-term cardiotoxicity, including potentially fatal congestive heart failure (CHF). Elderly patients are likely to be particularly susceptible to these problems because of comorbidities, such as hypertension and diabetes, and limited cardiac reserve [28].

Anthracyclines: Chronic heart failure following anthracyclines appears to be caused by cumulative damage to myocytes. Data from clinical trials showed that the rate of conventional doxorubicin-related CHF was 5 % at a cumulative dose of 400 mg/m^2, 16 % at a dose of 500 mg/m^2 and 26 % at a dose of 550 mg/m^2 [29]. Age was clearly a risk factor, with a hazard ratio of 2.25 in patients older than 65 years compared with those aged 65 years or younger. In an effort to preserve or increase antitumor efficacy while reducing cardiotoxicity, pegylation or liposomal encapsulation of anthracyclines was developed. It appears that encapsulated doxorubicin/daunorubicin probably has a decreased incidence of cardiotoxicity compared with

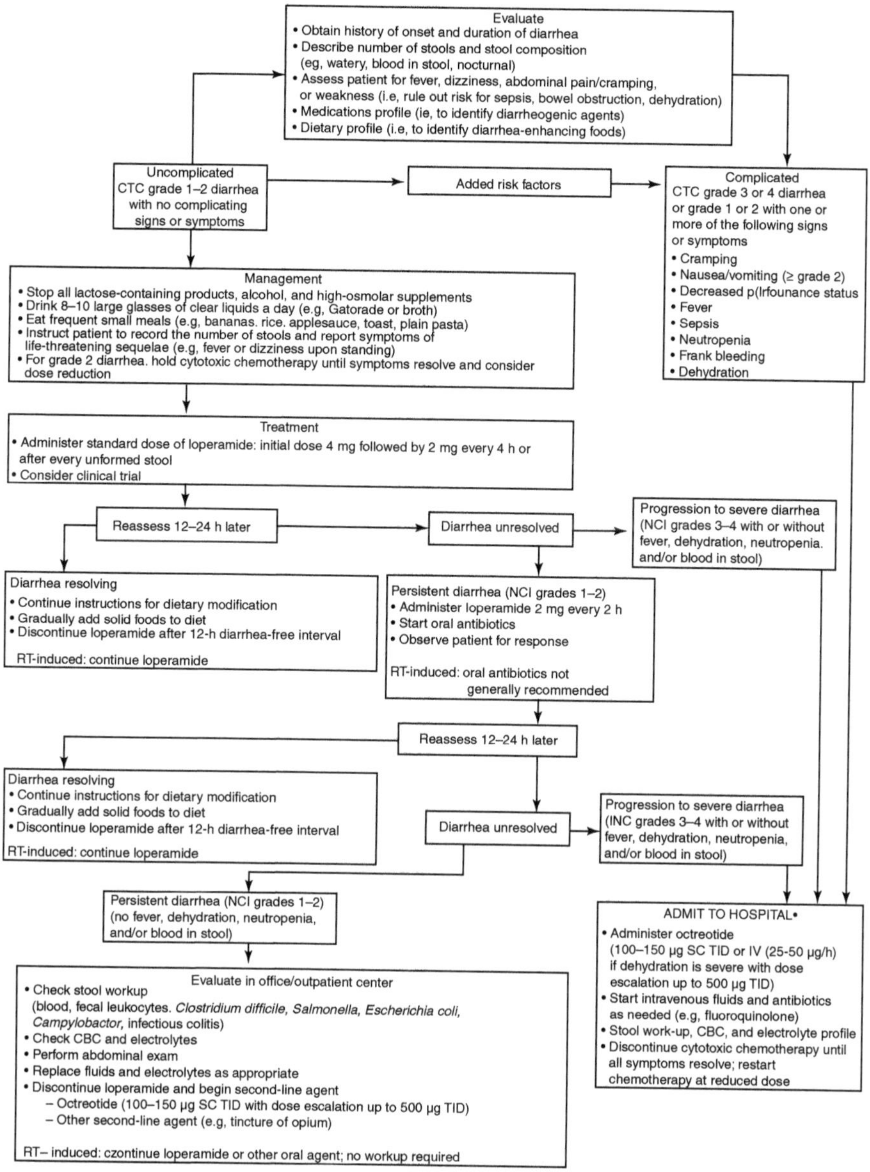

Fig. 17.1 Consensus guideline for the treatment of chemotherapy induced diarrhoea (Benson et al. [26]. Reprinted with permission © 2013 American Society of Clinical Oncology. All rights reserved)

conventional anthracycline administration but their use is limited by their high costs and lacking of a wide body of evidence.

Cyclophosphamide: Unlike the chronic cardiotoxicity associated with anthracyclines that is related to cumulative dosing, the cardiotoxicity associated with cyclophosphamide is related to the magnitude of single dosing, is more often reversible without permanent structural myocardial damage, and lacks the latency for development, with all cases occurring within a week to 10 days of treatment.

Imatinib (and probably other tyrosine kinase inhibitors): In patients with risk factors and/or preexisting cardiovascular disease, the incidence of cardiotoxicity manifested by heart failure with imatinib is in the range of 1–2 %. Non-cardiac oedema is common, and asymptomatic increases in biomarker levels with unknown clinical significance may be detected. In most reported studies, rechallenge with a lower dose of imatanib has been tolerated after resolution of acute heart failure.

Diagnosis

Patients considered for chemotherapy should undergo a baseline electrocardiogram and should be evaluated for conduction block or repolarisation abnormalities. Echocardiography measured left ventricular ejection fraction (LVEF) is one of the most important predictors of prognosis even if there is no clear international opinion on the frequency and method of LVEF assessment. A baseline Doppler echocardiogram with the evaluation of LVEF needs to be obtained particularly in the presence of cardiovascular risk factors, age >60 years, previous cardiovascular disease, prior mediastinal irradiation. Serum biomarkers such as N-terminal-pro-brain natriuretic peptide (NT-proBNP), cardiac troponin or creatinine kinase MB have been assessed as a possible marker of early detection of cardiac dysfunction induced by anthracyclines. However, the results to date are not consistent and therefore the routine use cannot be recommended in general [28].

Prevention and Treatment

Attempts to prevent the myocardial toxicity of chemotherapeutic agents focused on drug formulation and delivery and chemoprotective agents. Semisynthetic formulations of the anthracyclines (e.g. epirubicin) promised to maintain efficacy with reduced cardiotoxicity. However, in equivalent doses for efficacy, cardiotoxicity remains virtually identical to the original preparations. Varying the administration duration from bolus to prolonged infusion has had limited acceptance and has not been widely adopted. The use of standard heart failure therapy [30] in a chemopreventive mode has been reported in several small studies. These include angiotensin receptor blockers, beta blockers and angiotensin-converting enzyme (ACE) inhibitors. Liposomal pegylation may offer reduced cardiotoxicity in exchange for increased acquisition costs of the medication. Chemoprotective agents have also been controversial and cannot be generally recommended. Dexrazoxane, an iron chelator, was originally reported as the first drug to reduce

Table 17.6 SIOG proposals for the managment of anthracyclines cardiotoxicity risk

Recommendations	Proposal
Rigorous screening to exclude patients at unacceptably high cardiac risk (level 1a)	Comprehensive patient history Current signs or history of CHF Cardiovascular comorbidity (i.e. hypertension, diabetes or coronary artery disease) Prior exposure to anthracyclines for this or previous malignancy (level 1a)
Not exceeding the recommended upper cumulative dose (level 1a)	Reduction in maximum cumulative dose (level 5)
Use of less cardiotoxic therapy (level 1a)	Use of continuous infusion (level 1a) Epirubicin (level 1a) Dexrazoxane (level 1b, Elderly level 5) Liposomale anthracycline formulations (level 1b, Elderly: level 5)
Regular monitoring of cardiac function, signs and symptoms (level 1a)	Measure of LVEF by ultrasound (preferred, level 5) or MUGA scan (use the same method trough the follow-up), every two to three cycles of anthracyclines (level 1a) Special attention needed if drop in LVEF exceeds 10 %, even if remaining within normal range (level 5) Long-term follow-up (level 1a)
Cardiovascular risk reduction interventions (level 1a)	Early management of dysfunction (level 1a) Lifestyle modifications (i.e. smoking cessation, regular exercise, weight loss where appropriate) (level 1a) Beta blockers and ACE inhibitors (level 1a) Reduced lipid levels (level 1a)

Adapted from Aapro et al. [29]
CHF congestive heart failure, *MUGA* multiple uptake gated acquisition, *ACE* angiotensin-converting enzyme

cardiotoxicity from anthracyclines. The addition of dexrazoxane is restricted only in adult patients with breast cancer who have received >300 mg/m^2 doxorubicin or >540 mg/m^2 epirubicin according to the Food and Drug Administration and the European Medicines Agency indications [31].

Treatment starts by withdrawal of the causing chemotherapeutic agent, along education about the disease and the effects of diet on its natural history (e.g. salt and fluid restriction, achieving ideal weight); it includes risk factor modification (treatment of hypertension, lipid level reduction, smoking cessation, alcohol abstinence or moderation). Pharmacologic interventions begin with initiation of an ACE inhibitor or an angiotensin receptor blocker or a beta blocker as initial therapy with slow titration to achieve maximally tolerated doses. In contrast loop diuretics should be reserved and used only when fluid overload is evident.

In summary, general recommendations by the International Society of Geriatric Oncology (SIOG) to minimise the myocardial cardiotoxicity of chemotherapy are presented in Table 17.6.

Neurotoxicity

Chemotherapy induced peripheral neuropathy (CIPN) is a common and debilitating side effect associated with a variety of chemotherapeutic agents. Currently, there is a lack of well-proven, effective therapeutic interventions for CIPN including vinca alkaloids, bortezomib i.v. and thalidomide. Due to several possible comorbidities like diabetes in elderly cancer patients CIPN may become rapidly severe. Besides the reduction of quality of life due to CIPN, functional ability and falls has to be considered especially in older cancer patients. It may also result in missed or reduced chemotherapy doses, therefore limiting the efficacy of these therapies.

Prophylaxis of CIPN

In a recently published Cochrane Review none of the potential chemoprotective agents (acetylcysteine, amifostine, gluthatione, Org 2766, oxycarbazepine, diethyldithiocarbamate or Vitamine E) prevent or limit the neurotoxicity [32].

Prophylaxis of oxaliplatin induced CIPN: A clinical trial by Grothey et al. showed a protective effect of a CaMg infusion without loss of efficacy of adjuvant oxaliplatin in colorectal cancer [33]. These data were in accordance to the results of a retrospective analysis [34]. Therefore the use of CaMg as neuroprotectant, although being not very effective were endorsed by the ESMO (European Society for Medical Oncology) Colon Consensus [35]. However, the latest very well designed phase III study presented at ASCO annual meeting 2013 showed no activity of i.v. CaMg as a neuroprotectant against oxaliplatin-induced neurotoxicity [36]. In summary, after these obtained results the use of CaMg to prevent oxaliplatin-induced neurotoxicity is rather discouraged.

Treatment of CIPN

Given limited definitive data in CIPN, extrapolation of a treatment algorithm from the non-CIPN neuropathic pain literature seems to be rational. For individual patients, the choice of agent to try should be influenced by co-morbidities. There are multiple potential therapeutic strategies for treating CIPN, most of which have however little evidence. In view of the latest published trial duloxetine [37] is a favorable treatment option in patients with CIPN (start with 30 mg/day, yielded dose is 60 mg/day), with the similar drug, venlafaxine, being another alternative. However, it is rather difficult to make a definitive recommendation about which of the other potential alternatives, are best to try next, though alpha lipoic acid, topical menthol, or topical baclofen may be a possible treatment option.

It is important to acknowledge that an adequate duration of a therapeutic trial should last 4–6 weeks at target dosing. If the patient has ongoing pain, despite maximal dosing, adding, or substituting, an additional agent with a different mechanism of action can be considered.

Nutrition

Cancer patients are under risk to develop malnutrition over time due to disease and side effects of the therapy. The prevalence of malnutrition is significant higher among hospitalized patients with malignancies than in patients without malignancies [38]. Malnutrition and unintended weight loss are associated with an unfavorable prognosis, reduced quality of life, increased chemotherapy-induced toxicity and a decreased response to therapy [39]. Especially older cancer patients are at an increased risk to develop malnutrition [40]. Table 17.7 lists potential causes of malnutrition.

The nutritional status of older cancer patients can be improved by nutritional interventions such as oral, enteral or parenteral nutrition [41]. It is therefore necessary to identify patients' nutritional status and their individual risk of malnutrition. However, there is neither an uniform and accepted definition of malnutrition, nor a generally accepted method for the assessment of malnutrition in terms of a gold standard. These facts complicate the diagnosis of malnutrition and a timely intervention to counteract the loss of body mass. The European Society for Clinical Nutrition and Metabolism (ESPEN) recommends the use of the Mini Nutritional Assessment (MNA) as a screening tool to evaluate the risk of malnutrition among elderly patients [42]. The MNA includes information about eating behavior, weight loss, mobility, acute illness, psychological stress and neuropsychological problems of the patients.

Furthermore the registration of biochemical markers that reflect the amount of visceral protein, such as albumin, prealbumin and retinol-binding protein could be assessed to identify patients at risk of malnutrition. The interpretation of these values should be made with caution, because diseases of the liver or the kidney as well as acute or chronic inflammation could affect these parameters.

Conclusions

Supportive Care in the elderly patient is based on the same principles as for younger patients. As older patients may have serious problems related to side effects the use of any drug needs special precaution. Age is associated with increased risk of short and long-term complications. The NCCN guidelines and SIOG guidelines for special management strategies for the management of older patients with cancer have been partly endorsed by the EORTC and provide a framework of reference for ameliorating the complications of cancer and cancer treatment and for accommodating emerging information in this rapidly evolving field.

Table 17.7 Causes of malnutrition

Reduced dietary intake	
Physical causes	Stenoses Pain Xerostomia Dysphagia Chronic inflammation Loss of appetite Nausea/Emesis Mucositis Diarrhoea
Mental causes	Anxiety Depression Lonesomeness
Disturbed nutrient use efficiency	Insulin resistance Protein catabolism
Increased basal metabolic rate	Chronic Inflammation Hyperactivity of the sympathetic nervous system

References

1. Herrstedt J. Nausea and emesis: still an unsolved problem in cancer patients? Support Care Cancer. 2002;10(2):85–7.
2. Jordan K, Schmoll HJ, Aapro MS. Comparative activity of antiemetic drugs. Crit Rev Oncol Hematol. 2007;61(2):162–75.
3. Jakobsen JN, Herrstedt J. Prevention of chemotherapy-induced nausea and vomiting in elderly cancer patients. Crit Rev Oncol Hematol. 2009;71(3):214–21.
4. Roila F, Hesketh PJ, Herrstedt J. Prevention of chemotherapy- and radiotherapy-induced emesis: results of the 2004 Perugia International Antiemetic Consensus Conference. Ann Oncol. 2006;17(1):20–8.
5. Basch E, et al. Antiemetics: American Society of Clinical Oncology clinical practice guideline update. J Clin Oncol. 2011;29(31):4189–98.
6. Hesketh PJ, et al. The oral neurokinin-1 antagonist aprepitant for the prevention of chemotherapy-induced nausea and vomiting: a multinational, randomized, double-blind, placebo-controlled trial in patients receiving high-dose cisplatin – the Aprepitant Protocol 052 Study Group. J Clin Oncol. 2003;21(22):4112–9.
7. Poli-Bigelli S, et al. Addition of the neurokinin 1 receptor antagonist aprepitant to standard antiemetic therapy improves control of chemotherapy-induced nausea and vomiting. Results from a randomized, double-blind, placebo-controlled trial in Latin America. Cancer. 2003;97(12):3090–8.
8. Kris MG, et al. Consensus proposals for the prevention of acute and delayed vomiting and nausea following high-emetic-risk chemotherapy. Support Care Cancer. 2005;13(2):85–96.
9. Gralla RJ, et al. Recommendations for the use of antiemetics: evidence-based, clinical practice guidelines. American Society of Clinical Oncology. J Clin Oncol. 1999;17(9):2971–94.
10. Ettinger D, Dwight D, Kris M, editors. National Comprehensive Cancer Network: antiemesis, clinical practice guidelines in oncology. 1st ed. Jenkintown: NCCN; 2013.
11. Shadle CR, et al. Evaluation of potential inductive effects of aprepitant on cytochrome P450 3A4 and 2C9 activity. J Clin Pharmacol. 2004;44(3):215–23.

12. Aapro MS, Walko CM. Aprepitant: drug-drug interactions in perspective. Ann Oncol. 2010;21(12):2316–23.
13. Navari RM, Nagy CK, Gray SE. The use of olanzapine versus metoclopramide for the treatment of breakthrough chemotherapy-induced nausea and vomiting in patients receiving highly emetogenic chemotherapy. Support Care Cancer. 2013;21(6):1655–63.
14. Feyer P, Jordan K. Update and new trends in antiemetic therapy: the continuing need for novel therapies. Ann Oncol. 2011;22(1):30–8.
15. Roila F, et al. Guideline update for MASCC and ESMO in the prevention of chemotherapy- and radiotherapy-induced nausea and vomiting: results of the Perugia consensus conference. Ann Oncol. 2010;21 Suppl 5:v232–43.
16. Repetto L, et al. Use of growth factors in the elderly patient with cancer: a report from the Second International Society for Geriatric Oncology (SIOG) 2001 meeting. Crit Rev Oncol Hematol. 2003;45(2):123–8.
17. Dubois RW, et al. Benefits of GM-CSF versus placebo or G-CSF in reducing chemotherapy-induced complications: a systematic review of the literature. Support Cancer Ther. 2004;2(1): 34–41.
18. Schiffer CA, et al. Platelet transfusion for patients with cancer: clinical practice guidelines of the American Society of Clinical Oncology. J Clin Oncol. 2001;19(5):1519–38.
19. Barton DL, et al. Wisconsin Ginseng (Panax quinquefolius) to improve cancer-related fatigue: a randomized, double-blind trial, N07C2. J Natl Cancer Inst. 2013;105(16):1230–8.
20. Cramp, F and Byron-Daniel J. Exercise for the management of cancer-related fatigue in adults. Cochrane Database Syst Rev. 2012;(11):CD006145.
21. Rubenstein EB, et al. Clinical practice guidelines for the prevention and treatment of cancer therapy-induced oral and gastrointestinal mucositis. Cancer. 2004;100(9 Suppl):2026–46.
22. Sonis ST, et al. Perspectives on cancer therapy-induced mucosal injury: pathogenesis, measurement, epidemiology, and consequences for patients. Cancer. 2004;100(9 Suppl):1995–2025.
23. Elad S, et al. Development of the MASCC/ISOO Clinical Practice Guidelines for Mucositis: considerations underlying the process. Support Care Cancer. 2013;21(1):309–12.
24. Stein A, Voigt W, Jordan K. Chemotherapy-induced diarrhea: pathophysiology, frequency and guideline-based management. Ther Adv Med Oncol. 2010;2(1):51–63.
25. Benson 3rd AB, et al. Recommended guidelines for the treatment of cancer treatment-induced diarrhea. J Clin Oncol. 2004;22(14):2918–26.
26. Cascinu S, et al. Octreotide versus loperamide in the treatment of fluorouracil-induced diarrhea: a randomized trial. J Clin Oncol. 1993;11(1):148–51.
27. Wadler S, et al. Recommended guidelines for the treatment of chemotherapy-induced diarrhea. J Clin Oncol. 1998;16(9):3169–78.
28. Aapro M, et al. Anthracycline cardiotoxicity in the elderly cancer patient: a SIOG expert position paper. Ann Oncol. 2011;22(2):257–67.
29. Swain SM, Whaley FS, Ewer MS. Congestive heart failure in patients treated with doxorubicin: a retrospective analysis of three trials. Cancer. 2003;97(11):2869–79.
30. McMurray JJ, et al. ESC guidelines for the diagnosis and treatment of acute and chronic heart failure 2012: The Task Force for the Diagnosis and Treatment of Acute and Chronic Heart Failure 2012 of the European Society of Cardiology. Developed in collaboration with the Heart Failure Association (HFA) of the ESC. Eur J Heart Fail. 2012;14(8):803–69.
31. Berardi R, et al. State of the art for cardiotoxicity due to chemotherapy and to targeted therapies: a literature review. Crit Rev Oncol Hematol. 2013;88(1):75–86.
32. Albers JW, et al. Interventions for preventing neuropathy caused by cisplatin and related compounds. Cochrane Database Syst Rev. 2011;2, CD005228.
33. Grothey A, et al. Intravenous calcium and magnesium for oxaliplatin-induced sensory neurotoxicity in adjuvant colon cancer: NCCTG N04C7. J Clin Oncol. 2011;29(4):421–7.
34. Gamelin L, et al. Prevention of oxaliplatin-related neurotoxicity by calcium and magnesium infusions: a retrospective study of 161 patients receiving oxaliplatin combined with 5-Fluorouracil and leucovorin for advanced colorectal cancer. Clin Cancer Res. 2004;10 (12 Pt 1):4055–61.

35. Schmoll HJ, et al. ESMO Consensus Guidelines for management of patients with colon and rectal cancer. a personalized approach to clinical decision making. Ann Oncol. 2012;23(10):2479–516.
36. Loprinzi, CL, et al. Phase III randomized, placebo-controlled, double-blind study of intravenous calcium and magnesium to prevent oxaliplatin-induced sensory neurotoxicity (N08CB/Alliance). J Clin Oncol. 2014;32(10):997–1005.
37. Smith EM, et al. Effect of duloxetine on pain, function, and quality of life among patients with chemotherapy-induced painful peripheral neuropathy: a randomized clinical trial. JAMA. 2013;309(13):1359–67.
38. Pirlich M, et al. Prevalence of malnutrition in hospitalized medical patients: impact of underlying disease. Dig Dis. 2003;21(3):245–51.
39. Andreyev HJ, et al. Why do patients with weight loss have a worse outcome when undergoing chemotherapy for gastrointestinal malignancies? Eur J Cancer. 1998;34(4):503–9.
40. Sorbye LW. Cancer in home care: unintended weight loss and ethical challenges. A cross-sectional study of older people at 11 sites in Europe. Arch Gerontol Geriatr. 2011;53(1):64–9.
41. Blanc-Bisson C, et al. Undernutrition in elderly patients with cancer: target for diagnosis and intervention. Crit Rev Oncol Hematol. 2008;67(3):243–54.
42. Kondrup J, et al. ESPEN guidelines for nutrition screening 2002. Clin Nutr. 2003;22(4):415–21.
43. Aapro MS, et al. EORTC guidelines for the use of granulocyte-colony stimulating factor to reduce the incidence of chemotherapy-induced febrile neutropenia in adult patients with lymphomas and solid tumours. Eur J Cancer. 2006;42(15):2433–53.

Chapter 18
Patients Reported Outcome/Quality of Life

Barbara Deschler

Abstract Measures of patient-reported outcomes and quality of life in people with hematological malignancies resemble the subjective and thus highly personal aspects of what impacts life most when facing a malignant disease. They are of importance to both, the patients as well as their treating physicians. Despite this obvious relevance, we have a relatively poor knowledge and understanding of how these outcomes are affected in elderly patients with hematological malignancies.

We are beginning to appreciate the scope of aspects, including the presumably correct measurement of patient-reported outcomes and the various possibilities for utilization (e.g. comparing treatment effectiveness, risk factor assessment, longitudinal analyses of a treatment's impact on functionality, quality of life, or treatment decision-making, etc.). In addition, possibilities of psycho-oncological interventions tailored to patient-reported outcomes are now increasingly utilized.

Still, there is plenty of room for meaningful contribution to the research of these matters of highest individual relevance.

Keywords Patient-reported outcomes • Quality of life • Geriatric hematology • Prognostication • Treatment decision-making

Abbreviations

ADL	Activities of daily living
AML	Acute myeloid leukemia
CML	Chronic myeloid leukemia
HRQOL	Health related quality of life
PRO	Patient-reported outcome
QOL	Quality of life

B. Deschler, MD
Interdisciplinary Clinical Trials Office, Comprehensive Cancer Center Mainfranken, University Hospital Würzburg, Josef-Schneider-Stzr 6, 97080 Würzburg, Germany

Department of Hematology/Oncology, University of Freiburg Medical Center, Freiburg, Germany
e-mail: deschler_b@ukw.de

U. Wedding, R.A. Audisio (eds.), *Management of Hematological Cancer in Older People*, DOI 10.1007/978-1-4471-2837-3_18

Introduction

The easiest task to commence the chapter on Patient-Reported Outcomes (PROs) might be to give a definition: PROs describe parameters that focus on assessing health outcomes from the patient's perspective.

To be more precise: PROs measure various aspects of a given health status and should – whenever possible – come directly from the patient. PROs may measure one specific symptom but can range to multifaceted, multidimensional outcomes. The evaluation of every subjective condition – be it purely symptomatic or complex concepts of reporting physical, mental and social well-being – is a PRO. The documentation and communication of PROs are thus the patients' chance to be heard. Clearly, they are of highest relevance for supporting clinical decision-making. Further, they are used in clinical trials to reflect treatment effectiveness and compatibility. Regulatory agencies now support the consideration of PROs as key outcomes in cancer research.

While all the above seems obvious enough, PROs are far too often forgotten when dealing with other, seemingly more urgent concerns. Communicating PROs importance and motivating an extended use is therefore much more difficult than giving its definition.

Recently, there has been an increase in the availability of questionnaires for obtaining PROs. Scales that measure states of health and illness from the patient's perspective obtain more and more recognition.

So far, however, psycho-social issues remain relatively unstudied in patients with hematological cancer compared with other common types of cancer. Only very few randomized controlled trials in hematology have evaluated PROs prospectively; single studies have studied them in a cross sectional fashion. Even rarer publications have dealt with PROs in the growing subset of older patients with hematological cancer. But those that did indicated, that with rising age, the PROs subjective importance even increased. It appears that in older people the topic becomes even more relevant and they seem less willing to trade off quantity of life against its quality.

High levels of patient distress have been reported for hematological cancer patients. Diagnosis and treatment can have a devastating impact on a vast number of aspects of life and the ability to fulfill roles. Major findings of PRO research in older hematological patients suggest that at diagnosis of – for example – acute leukemia in elderly patients, not only general quality of life (QOL) is compromised. Fatigue is one very prevalent condition with a devastating impact on QOL. Contrary to what one may expect, there is not necessarily a correlation between the physicians' medical assessment of physical function and patient-reported outcomes.

Several PROs provide independent prognostic information for clinical outcomes, particularly in advanced hematologic disease settings. This field is now studied by several groups.

PRO research has the unique opportunity to push forward patient matters such as the discussions on informed consent and joint decision-making in older patients and offers enormous potential to improve the quality and results of our care.

Patient-Reported Outcomes (PROs)

Patient-reported outcomes (PROs) are one source to monitor cancer outcome. They include all parameters that are used to assess health outcomes from the patient's point of view. They provide a means of gaining insight into the way patients perceive their health and the impact that disease-related adjustments to lifestyle or treatments have on their quality of life.

PROs provide evidence of different dimensions of health from the point of view of the patient: Be it purely symptomatic (e.g. self-reported relevance or the response of a distressing symptom), more complex (e.g. the measurement of activities of daily living) or complex (e.g. health-related quality of life). They shed light on subjective treatment impacts or effectiveness, respectively, from the patient's perspective and are consequently of highest relevance in the discussion of diagnostic or therapeutic options with the patient.

The importance of PRO research was highlighted by the National Cancer Institute's Strategic Objectives: To ensure the best outcome for all, improving the "quality of life for cancer patients, survivors and their families" [1]. The US Food and Drug Administration (FDA) and the European Medicines Agency (EMA) followed with their draft guidance (Feb 2006) and Reflection Paper (July 2005) in emphasizing the major importance of PROs [2, 3].

PROs assess how people feel about aspects of life that are commonly believed to be important. But as for example no clear definitions for "health status", "quality of life", "health-related quality of life", and "functional status" are generally agreed upon, the optimization and development of assessing PROs are far from finished and will need significant further debate.

But for all that, the above mentioned directives are an important step towards further recognition of the relevance of the patient viewpoint, which in turn is on matters of highest subjective importance in the evaluation of a medical condition and/or therapy.

Recently, the message appears to be reaching physicians who are increasingly sensitive to the significance of psycho-social factors in the lives of their patients. More and more questionnaires that measure states of health and illness from the patient's perspective have been developed. To date, there has been less attention paid to measures for assessing older peoples' health in that fashion.

Despite methodological challenges and the scarcity of geriatric PRO research, there exists evidence that its assessment is feasible also in older hematological cancer patients. It has the great potential of providing valuable information and outcomes to further support/facilitate clinical decision-making. The recommendation of the most appropriate treatment for each individual patient after consideration of how alternative treatments might affect the individuals' PROs and survival during treatment and beyond has an outstanding priority.

Quality of Life

In the following sections we will review the existing research regarding the use of PROs for older patients with hematological malignancies. The main focus lies on health-related quality of life (HRQOL). HRQOL covers almost all sub-domains of PROs, namely symptoms (disease/treatment-related), functioning (physical, role, social), well-being (psychological), as well as global health QOL perception.

We use the term "Quality of life (QOL)" in many contexts, including not only healthcare concerns but also to evaluate the general well-being of individuals and societies. As said before, there is not one accepted definition of quality of life. Still, every one of us has a personal understanding of QOL and would argue that it is extremely important. QOL for many, may stand for general life satisfaction, including health, employment, safety, communication, education, and recreational activities. For matters related to health care, the term "health-related quality of life" (HRQOL) has been agreed upon [4]. Beyond quantity of life and economic cost, HRQOL resembles one specific measure to weigh the burden of an illness or its therapy.

Although length of survival has long been considered the most important factor when evaluating treatment options, the impact of illness on quality of life has received increasing recognition. Results indicate that its relevance subjectively increases with increasing age [5].

Oncologists have used scales to quantify cancer patients' functional capacities for treatment evaluation and planning for quite some time [6] and HRQOL assessment has been focused on for a while. The systematic assessment of HRQOL using standardized, self-administered questionnaires evolved to be one major aspect of an anticipated beneficial impact of newer therapies [7].

HRQOL is thought to be multidimensional and subjective. To measure it, we need tools that are comprehensive and are capable to meaningfully capture changes.

A definition of HRQOL is found as: "The extent to which one's usual or expected physical, emotional and social well-being are affected by a medical condition or its treatment" [8]. HRQOL measurement thus requires the patient's perspective and the capture of physical, emotional and social well-being [9].

We become aware of HRQOLs subjectivity when for example individual patients with the same health status report considerably diverse impairments in HRQOL. There are unique differences in expectations, internal values and coping abilities [10] and possibly many further inherent personal traits such as resilience. Obviously, HRQOL should – if at all possible – be reported by the affected individual.

With respect to HRQOL's various dimensions, the "Patient-Reported Outcomes Measurement Information System (PROMIS) Cooperative Group" aims to create an assessment system for self–reported health. It has set up a framework of self-reported health to develop computer-based standardized questionnaires that consider the various dimensions of HRQOL [11]. Instruments are organized into subordinate domains beneath the broad physical, mental, and social health headings. Each of these components again encompasses multiple subcomponents (e.g., the mental health component is comprised of affect, behavior, and cognition). These sub-domains are then further divided (e.g., negative affect is comprised of anxiety, depression, anger, experience of stress, and the negative psychosocial impact of illness). The modules that have been developed can be accessed at the respective internet site (PROMIS, www.nihpromis.org) for research or clinical practice.

Assessing HRQOL

While survival time has been the standard indicator of treatment effectiveness, there is now a stronger recognition of the fact that time without quality is of disputable value. How to best measure HRQOL may always be a challenge and create debate.

A number of validated and reliable questionnaires for assessment of HRQOL [12] are available. They may support our notion that time added – by new therapies for example – is of adequate value to justify them. To examine the value of therapies that do not add time to life but do improve its quality is another important aspect. As Cella put it: “Only a careful evaluation of patient-reported HRQOL can allow us to evaluate the trade-offs between symptom relief and toxicity” [13].

There are different types of PROs and the same is true for HRQOL measures. But generally, they include generic health status instruments, generic illness instruments, and, the disease-specific instruments.

Generic health status instruments assess the level of functioning in various domains. They are employable in all people and populations with or without the burden of a disease. To name examples: the Nottingham Health Profile (NHP) [14] or the Short Form-36 (SF-36) [15].

To investigate the HRQOL of individuals with any medical condition, generic illness questionnaires are applied. They can be used to compare different illnesses, levels of severity, or types of interventions. In addition to measuring the general health status, these instruments typically assess the individual’s perception of the functional impact of the illness or disability. One example is the copyrighted questionnaire “Functional Assessment of Chronic Illness Therapy (FACIT)” [16]. A list of all scales that are currently part of the FACIT Measurement System is available at the respective homepage (www.facit.org/FACITOrg/Questionnaires).

Disease-specific measures investigate functioning and/or wellbeing in aspects of life that are thought to be affected in individuals with specific illnesses, specific types of treatment, or specific symptoms. They are tailored to assess in detail aspects of HRQOL in light of specific diseases and are also likely to be more sensitive to specific treatment-related changes in HRQOL.

It has become more and more common in HRQOL research, to combine generic and disease-specific instruments in order to cover all details that may impact HRQOL. One example is the European Organisation of Research and Treatment of Cancer EORTC QLQ-C30 questionnaire. It has been developed to assess the quality of life of cancer patients. It is a copyrighted instrument, which has been translated and validated into 81 languages and is used in more than 3,000 studies worldwide.

Presently QLQ-C30 Version 3.0 is the most recent version (www.groups.eortc.be/qol/eortc-qlq-c30). A modular approach was adopted for disease specific treatment measurements. It is supplemented by more specific modules for e.g. Breast, Lung, Head & Neck, Oesophageal, Ovarian, Gastric, Cervical cancer, Multiple Myeloma, Oesophago-Gastric, Prostate, Colorectal Liver Metastases, Colorectal and Brain cancer which are distributed by the EORTC Quality of Life Department.

HRQOL in the Older Patient

As mentioned frequently in previous chapters, the median age at diagnosis of patients with hematological malignancies is currently around 70 years. Both the median age of patients and the proportion of elderly cancer patients are rising even further. The special aspects of an older patient's subjective estimation of HRQOL are therefore of great importance. Notwithstanding this, older patients are under-represented in cancer trials and studies. This raises the question how – for example – comorbidities, frailty or social support impact upon treatment options as these factors significantly interact with many older patient's HRQOL.

As Johnson et al. (2010) stated in their review, there is contradictory evidence as to whether older people with cancer have better or worse HRQOL than younger patients. Some studies reported that it is cancer rather than age that impacts upon HRQOL. Others reported that older cancer patients have similar or even better HRQOL when compared to non-cancer patients. Further aspects include the assumption that increasing age is associated with decreasing health and HRQOL and – possibly of major importance: Differing expectations on that what is individually defined "quality of life".

The (European Organisation of Research and Treatment of Cancer) EORTC Quality of Life (QOL) Group reported in this respect that responses to their questionnaires varied with age: substantial differences were seen in responses to physical function, role function and fatigue. Owing to these facts, the EORTC QOL Group developed a questionnaire specifically for Elderly Cancer Patients (QLQ – ELD15). The module has been proposed to address potential deficiencies of the QLQ system for cancer patients who are elderly. Developmental data suggested that older patients do have different concerns and may need a specific module. The final report assessing the applicability of the QLQ-ELD15 for use in older patients with any type of cancer or hematological malignancy is expected to be completed soon [17]. The system will hopefully enable the collection of reliable, valid and clinically important information on HRQOL outcomes in older patients.

Obviously, there is no single best HRQOL questionnaire for every application nor is there agreement upon a gold standard. A scale that may be advantageous in one clinical setting is inappropriate in another. Generic and disease-specific questionnaires have advantages and disadvantages. Together, they can provide comparability across types of cancer and sensitivity to specific issues or symptoms relevant to a certain disease or treatment.

Estimating Patients' HRQOL

Sometimes in the treatment of elderly patients it is not possible to obtain a self-reported PRO (e.g. due to cognitive impairment). In these cases, a proxy or care-giver may be asked to estimate values in HRQOL questionnaires. The few studies that have been performed investigating the reliability of results point towards an agreement between the patient's assessment and that of the care-giver. Certainly, we need to be careful when interpreting results to take into account a number of potential biases [18]. Results on the accuracy of judgments made by the treating physicians are not so consistent.

As discussed above, the concept of quality of life includes different dimensions or aspects that play an important role in the perception individuals may have about their lives. The relative importance of each aspect is different for each person and depends on the perspective from which quality of life is considered. For example health care professionals appear to underestimate the impact of symptoms on the quality of life in some instances: In one recent study, Efficace presented to patients with chronic myeloid leukemia (CML) and to their physicians a list of 74 HRQOL relevant items and asked them to indicate the importance of each aspect on a four point scale to identify the "top ten" items concerning the HRQOL of CML patients. While both patients and physicians agreed about the relevance of fatigue, their opinions differed about the meaning of symptoms like dry mouth, trouble in concentrating/remembering things, problems of urinating frequently, drowsiness, and skin problems: patients tended to see these problems as having a greater impact on their lives [19]. This aspect is an example of the adverse impact on HRQOL of the treatment (and not solely the diagnosis) of a hematological malignancy and how the ranking in the subjective importance of these events varies. Clearly, further research will have to pick up these findings and investigate them in more detail as adverse events in hematologic therapy certainly have great importance in long-term treatments such as in CML, as symptoms may undermine the treatment commitment. While this study illustrates the challenges we have in correctly evaluating adverse events, one encouraging result of this study was that physicians appear to be increasingly sensitive among other things, to the relevance of psychosocial factors in the lives of their patients.

Using HRQOL Data

There are several ways to use information regarding the impact of an illness or medical condition on HRQOL. Typically, clinical trials that compare different treatments include a HRQOL analysis as one means of determining a possible general clinical benefit, especially when relevant treatment-related side effects are to be expected. Compared to a control therapy, the alternative treatment option may be associated with a longer or shorter survival with better or inferior HRQOL.

Improved aspects of HRQOL may be strong enough factors to outweigh a possibly shorter survival. The latter has been proven as one of the major aspects for elderly patients with hematological cancer, especially its rapidly progressing forms such as acute myeloid leukemia [5].

Because HRQOL information can provide a detailed assessment of disease and treatment effects, and their overall impact on the individual's daily life, it can be used as a planning tool for assessing the need for further treatment, rehabilitation or palliative care. In particular, the HRQOL assessment may reveal anxiety or depressive symptoms, or a complaint of pain or dyspnea that may initiate patient-physician communication about medical, psychological or social interventions to improve the patient's well-being [20].

A number of methodological recommendations regarding study size, statistical prerequisites and further aspects of correct conduction of HRQOL studies have been published in detail elsewhere and need consideration prior to planning a HRQOL study [21, 22].

A very relevant and interesting finding of research in the field of patient-reported outcomes has been the evidence that single PROs have an independent prognostic role for several clinical outcomes. For example, several studies have shown baseline QOL parameters to be independent prognostic factors in different malignancies [23] underscoring the assumption that QOL scales add prognostic information to clinical measures and predict survival [24]. Patient ratings of physical symptoms (i.e. fatigue), physical functioning and global health status/QOL have repeatedly been the best predictors of survival. In other words, the patients' experience of disease-, and treatment-related impacts on life can provide clinically relevant information on prognosis. This in turn may facilitate more informed treatment decisions.

In this context, Oliva et al. reported a study on elderly AML patients in which QOL physical functioning was of prognostic relevance, yet somewhat surprisingly, did not correlate to the physician-assessed ECOG performance status [25].

The most recent work, however, in this field has been published by Efficace et al. [26], investigating in detail the question of whether baseline patient-reported symptom severity independently predicted overall survival in a heterogeneous hematologic population, mainly with advanced disease. The main finding of this study was that, indeed, PROs can provide additional prognostic information in the setting of advanced hematologic disease. Drowsiness emerged as an independent predictor of duration of survival. Granted, this is one of the pioneer works, and future longitudinal studies will have to investigate the prognostic value of PROs in homogeneous cohorts of hematologic patients to identify which type of PRO is prognostic in specific patient groups.

While the item "fatigue" has been shown to be prognostically relevant in several different malignant diseases, so far only hypotheses have been proposed to explain the mechanisms underlying the association between patients' reported health status data and duration of survival [27]. Fatigue is a patient-reported outcome and multi-faceted concept including both mental and physical components whose critical domains have not been sufficiently standardized and for which several scales have been developed [28]. Despite these shortcomings, most researchers believe that the further investigation of this extremely debilitating symptom observed in many if not all cancer patients will be fruitful for optimizing patient care.

Similarly, the examination of nearly 200 patients with advanced myelodysplastic syndromes (MDS) and acute myeloid leukemia (AML) above the age of 60 years showed that single dimensions of the EORTC QOL questionnaire C30 were highly predictive for outcome. This effect was most pronounced in the patient groups treated not with a primarily curative intent. The degree of prediction equaled functional parameters of a comprehensive geriatric assessment (CGA) [29].

In more detail, about 25 % of the patients in this study were allocated according to their physicians' recommendations or own wish to only receive best supportive care (consisting of transfusions, cytoreduction with hydroxyurea, and antibiotics) and approximately 38 % to either disease-modifying agents (such as hypomethylating agents) or standard induction chemotherapy (two-thirds of the latter proceeded to allografting). A third of the patients was diagnosed with MDS, two-thirds with AML and the median age was 71 years. Of all patients, 67 were impaired in activities of daily living (ADL) and only slightly more than 50 % had a performance status (Karnofsky Index) of above 80. Initial results of an in-depth geriatric and quality of life assessment differed significantly among the different treatment groups, with patients treated intensively being markedly younger and significantly less often affected by geriatric symptoms. Among variables which appeared to be of prognostic importance in univariate analyses, impaired independence (ADL) and increased fatigue (≥50 by EORTC QLQ-C30) remained highly predictive for overall survival in the entire patient group (irrespective of treatment) beyond the established, disease-related risk factors such as poor risk cytogenetics/IPSS and bone marrow blast count ≥20 %. Further, these parameters differentiated convincingly between high- and low-risk patients treated non-intensively, with those with a higher score in fatigue and ADL impairments having shorter overall survival.

Capturing changes in HRQOL to guide individual clinical care is increasingly important to clinicians. For instance, a brief multi-dimensional HRQOL questionnaire might be administered at every chemotherapy visit. The treating physician can then review the current HRQOL for indications of problems and compare it to the HRQOL from the previous visit. This may be of benefit in consultations where there is not always sufficient time to ask detailed questions about HRQOL.

In this context, Detmar et al. asked 273 patients to fill out the EORTC QLQ-C30 questionnaire before they had a consultation with their physicians; half of the physicians received the results of the questionnaires before the consultations. These patients had the impression that the questionnaires enhanced the physicians' awareness of their problems; the physicians, on the other hand, stated that the questionnaires facilitated communication, gave helpful information about the patients' symptom experience and helped to detect psycho-social problems and unexpected symptoms (e.g. sleep disorder). Moreover, a constant use of questionnaires may allow the physician to follow the development of the patients' clinical status and receive helpful information for future decisions.

With respect to data published on older leukemia patients, HRQOL has been shown to be significantly affected at the time of diagnosis. Again, fatigue was the most common, distressing, and persistent symptom in these patients. Further, it has been shown that the subjective estimation of general HRQOL was stable or slightly improving during the initial 6 months. Only fatigue appeared refractory during the same time frame and there was little improvement beyond the first half year [30].

When looking at first data on the arrangement of PROs of older leukemia patients under different therapeutic approaches, it has been noted that:

- Patients highly appreciate the opportunity to communicate PROs;
- Results do not comply necessarily with our (the physician"s) expectations nor with more objective measures of functionality;
- Results do not comply with the general question of potential curability of the leukemia (reflecting also treatment intensity); and
- PRO assessment-tailored interventions may be able to alleviate some limitations in functionality or HRQOL.

Decision-Making in Light of HRQOL

Patients have become more outspoken with respect to their wish that prolongation of life irrespective of its quality is not what they will opt for. When considering intensive, life-prolonging treatments or end-of-life decisions, it is critical to consider what makes life worth living for each individual that we are discussing therapeutic options with. Frequently, the discussion about an intervention not solely focuses on toxicity or survival time, but also on symptom palliation and toxicity. The importance of a careful evaluation of PROs/HRQOL is obvious. Again, as an example, given the palliative nature of even intensive therapy in 85–95 % of older adults with acute myeloid leukemia, this presents an ideal group with whom issues related to the treatment decision-making process and HRQOL should be explored. Intensive induction chemotherapy is known to result in a small chance for long-term disease free survival, but is associated with high up-front morbidity and mortality. The ability to offer guidance based on knowledge of how previous leukemia patients have made similar treatment decisions and the outcomes of those decisions may be helpful.

Some patients are willing to consider intensive and potentially toxic treatments despite slim chances of survival. Medical issues do not always constitute the sole factors considered. In one series, intensive therapy was more likely to be accepted among patients with a positive sense of social well-being or children living at home [31].

In the decision for either striving to live and seeking active treatment over death (even if associated with a poor HRQOL characterized by pain, immobility, and extreme dependence on others), psychosocial variables, including religiosity, values, and fear of death contribute significantly to the decision-making process. With respect to older adults with leukemia, Sekeres et al. performed an analysis of decision interviews with respect to treatment intensity. Overall, 97 % of patients agreed with the statement that quality was more important to them than length of life, regardless of their choice of therapy [5]. Baseline scores within the HRQOL questionnaires and prevalence of depression were similar for those choosing intensive treatment and those opting for non-intensive therapy. Yet, both groups were significantly compromised compared to the general population. According to their results with 20 patients treated intensively and 13 patients treated in primarily non-curative intent, the effects of treatment on a leukemia patient's HRQOL were limited to the time he or she was in the hospital. Thus, patients may be informed that they can expect their subjective HRQOL and ability to function to improve once they leave the hospital, and that it will be similar to their pre-treatment scores.

Taking again leukemia as an example, we have to consider that with aging, our organ reserve may decrease, comorbidities may develop, and the functional status may be affected. When additionally burdened with leukemia and the effects of therapy, the individual may develop multiple symptoms like pain, fatigue, and depression.

Therapeutic intensity and therefore treatment-associated strains and burden range from the one extreme of sole best supportive care to the other of intensive chemotherapy possibly followed by allogeneic stem cell transplantation. Thus, acute leukemias may be considered exemplary for the heightened incidence as well as the challenging decision-making process required prior to the treatment decision in many if not all malignant diseases in older people.

The results of treatment are generally inferior to those seen in younger adults, and long-term outcome of the older leukemia patient has not significantly improved in the past two decades. Novel non-intensive treatment options have slightly broadened the therapeutic spectrum and have raised hope for improved survival at proper HRQOL. In this context the importance of being able to estimate how parameters of HRQOL and functionality will be affected during the initial 6 months after diagnosis is comprehensible (for both patients and their physicians).

A longitudinal investigation of the development of HRQOL and parameters of a geriatric assessment in older patients during days 121–273 post treatment initiation revealed that only 41 % of all 200 patients initially interviewed were capable of responding during the given time frame. The majority of patients with a second assessment had received induction chemotherapy (66 %), while the remainder had undergone primarily non-curative treatment.

With respect to results of subsequent assessments, some changes reached statistical significance for those treated intensively with induction chemotherapy: first and foremost, a decline in the functional independence (instrumental ADL) was noticed. Still, this group reported a significant increase in emotional functioning. The non-intensive groups displayed a marked improvement in global health/QOL and emotional functioning with a tendency towards improved fatigue and dyspnoea. Yet, none of the reported changes reached statistical significance. The cohort that received best supportive care showed an improvement in their role function but a decline in cognitive functioning as well as increase in dyspnoea and pain. Again, differences within the group did not reach statistical significance. When comparing the different treatment groups with each other, only instrumental ADL differed significantly at the time of a subsequent assessment.

Finally, putting results in terms of proportions of patients that experienced an assumed clinically relevant change in results over time [32], in each treatment group, about 1/3 of patients experienced a relevant decline of over 10 points in global health/QOL [33]. In light of the sparse data covering this extremely relevant patient-centered topic, this study must be seen as a first approach to clarify the subjective and objective impact of treatment on elderly leukemia patients.

There are several possible approaches [13, 32] to interpret HRQOL data reflecting the following questions: Are observed differences in values clinically significant? What is the meaningful pattern of change that deserves clinical attention? Does a significant difference between treatment groups transfer to single-case interpretation? A lot more research will be required before we have clear and reliable data about clinical significance and the clinical value that goes along with the changes that we measure.

Assessment result-directed individual interventions may improve the individual care of the older patients. This has been demonstrated as a successful approach in other clinical settings such as perioperative intervention [34]. To improve patient fitness levels, functional capacity, and quality of life as well as reduce mortality and morbidity is a very attractive concept. However, its impact on outcome needs to be defined in adequately powered studies.

Furthermore, data indicated that the subjective estimation of HRQOL does not necessarily correlate with more objective functional measures – a phenomenon possibly attributable to a response shift or re-evaluation of internal values in light of a life-threatening disease. Data will need validation in much larger cohorts, yet they supply us with relevant information on patients' major issues and may stimulate further discussion and research in this field.

Most patients report that frequent (e.g. weekly) re-assessment aids in focusing discussions with their health care team. Providers found temporal changes in patient responses over time to be useful. Providing HRQOL information routinely to the hematologist can thus improve patient-physician communication [35]. Also, even if not sufficiently investigated, there is the implication that communicating HRQOL may have a positive effect on some aspects of HRQOL by itself.

Psycho-Oncological Interventions

Measurements and interpretation of reactions/adjustments to stress factors such as the diagnosis and treatment of a malignant disease are complex. The development of valid and reliable instruments to measure the patients' perspective of their illness and treatment was made possible by the demonstration of their psychometric properties by psycho-oncologists.

Psycho-oncological interventions are the other aspect of tremendous importance not only to the older patient. They tend on the one hand to influence in a direct way the illness or the treatment related symptoms, on the other hand they try to improve the illness coping. Important target variables of psycho-oncological treatments are, among others, the improvement of illness- and treatment related symptoms like pain, nausea or sleeping disorder, reduction of anxiety, hopelessness and depression, improvement of self-efficacy, of social integration and communication between family members, improvement of cooperation with the physicians and help in case of problems with the body image and sexuality, etc.. The patient-related psycho-oncological offers include counseling and information, patient education, supporting talk, crisis intervention, and symptom oriented treatment like relaxation or imagination.

To decide which older patient may benefit from psychosocial interventions, screening-instruments can be helpful to identify the psychic stress or even disorder, beyond the impression of the responsible physicians and nurses.

A number of international intervention studies confirm the effectiveness of psycho-oncological interventions especially on the different dimensions of HRQOL. Most of these findings examined behavioral therapeutic intervention which aimed to reduce side effects or distress and emotional problems and to achieve better illness coping, better social support or psychosocial well-being.

There are few studies which examined the effect of psychosocial interventions especially for patients with hematological malignancies. Mantovani et al. [36] assessed the impact of three different psychological interventions on HRQOL of elderly cancer patients which had solid tumors or hematological malignancies, and with symptoms of anxiety and/or depression. The study showed that the combination of psychopharmacological treatment with either social support for patients and their relatives carried out by volunteers or social support plus structured psychotherapy yielded the best results in terms of quality of life in the long-term treatment of elderly patients with advanced cancer – with almost equal effectiveness.

To improve psychosocial outcomes for patients with hematological cancer, further research investigating potential interventions by psycho-oncologist is needed.

Conclusions

The assessment of HRQOL is easily feasible as an array of validated questionnaires is now available and one specifically for older patients is underway.

In the future, we will need to include HRQOL as an end point in clinical trials, use HRQOL as a tool for assessing the efficacy and tolerability of treatment, and capture changes in HRQOL status during treatment. We need this information to evaluate the need for further assessment, treatment, rehabilitation, geriatric or palliative care, and to aid in decision-making in patients who are faced with intensive, possibly life-prolonging or even curative treatments, and end-of-life decisions. Thorough information can help patients make informed treatment decisions and may help them better cope with the disease, its treatment and decisions they had come to.

References

1. The NCI strategic plan for leading the nation: To eliminate the suffering and death due to cancer (2007). http://strategicplan.nci.nih.gov/pdf/nci_2007_plan.pdf.
2. Administration. UFaD. Guidance for industry. Patient-reported outcome measures: use in medical product development to support labeling claims. In: Administration UDoHaHSFaD, editor. http://www.fda.gov/downloads/Drugs/GuidanceComplianceRegulatoryInformation/Guidances/UCM193282.pdf2009.
3. Reflection paper on the regulatory guidance for the use of health-related quality of life (HRQL) measures in the evaluation of medicinal products. www.ispor.org/workpaper/emea-hrql-guidance.pdf.
4. Bergner M. Quality of life, health status, and clinical research. Med Care. 1989;27(3 Suppl): S148–56. Epub 1989/03/01.
5. Sekeres MA, Stone RM, Zahrieh D, Neuberg D, Morrison V, De Angelo DJ, et al. Decision-making and quality of life in older adults with acute myeloid leukemia or advanced myelodysplastic syndrome. Leukemia. 2004;18(4):809–16.
6. DA Karnofsky AW, Craver LF, Burchenal JH. The use of nitrogen mustard in the palliative treatment of carcinoma. With particular reference to bronchogenic carcinoma. Cancer. 1948;1:634–56.
7. Wagner LI, Wenzel L, Shaw E, Cella D. Patient-reported outcomes in phase II cancer clinical trials: lessons learned and future directions. J Clin Oncol. 2007;25(32):5058–62. Epub 2007/11/10.
8. Cella DF. Measuring quality of life in palliative care. Semin Oncol. 1995;22(2 Suppl 3):73–81. Epub 1995/04/01.
9. Aaronson NK. Quality of life: what is it? How should it be measured? Oncology (Williston Park). 1988;2((5):69—76, 64. Epub 1988/05/01.
10. Testa MA, Simonson DC. Assessment of quality-of-life outcomes. N Engl J Med. 1996;334(13): 835–40. Epub 1996/03/28.
11. Cella D, Riley W, Stone A, Rothrock N, Reeve B, Yount S, et al. The Patient-Reported Outcomes Measurement Information System (PROMIS) developed and tested its first wave of adult self-reported health outcome item banks: 2005–2008. J Clin Epidemiol. 2010;63(11): 1179–94. Epub 2010/08/06.
12. Kirkova J, Davis MP, Walsh D, Tiernan E, O'Leary N, LeGrand SB, et al. Cancer symptom assessment instruments: a systematic review. J Clin Oncol. 2006;24(9):1459–73. Epub 2006/03/22.
13. Cella D. Psychosocial interventions for cancer. Washington, DC: American Psychological Association; 2001.
14. Hunt SM, McEwen J, McKenna SP. Measuring health status: a new tool for clinicians and epidemiologists. J R Coll Gen Pract. 1985;35(273):185–8. Epub 1985/04/01.
15. McHorney CA, Ware Jr JE, Rogers W, Raczek AE, Lu JF. The validity and relative precision of MOS short- and long-form health status scales and Dartmouth COOP charts. Results from the Medical Outcomes Study. Med care. 1992;30(5 Suppl):MS253–65. Epub 1992/05/11.
16. Webster K, Cella D, Yost K. The Functional Assessment of Chronic Illness Therapy (FACIT) Measurement System: properties, applications, and interpretation. Health Qual Life Outcomes. 2003;1:79. Epub 2003/12/18.
17. Johnson C, Fitzsimmons D, Gilbert J, Arrarras JI, Hammerlid E, Bredart A, et al. Development of the European Organisation for Research and Treatment of Cancer quality of life questionnaire module for older people with cancer: The EORTC QLQ-ELD15. Eur J Cancer. 2010;46(12):2242–52. Epub 2010/06/29.
18. Sneeuw KC, Sprangers MA, Aaronson NK. The role of health care providers and significant others in evaluating the quality of life of patients with chronic disease. J Clin Epidemiol. 2002;55(11):1130–43. Epub 2003/01/01.

19. Efficace F, Cocks K, Breccia M, Sprangers M, Meyers CA, Vignetti M, et al. Time for a new era in the evaluation of targeted therapies for patients with chronic myeloid leukemia: inclusion of quality of life and other patient-reported outcomes. Crit Rev Oncol Hematol. 2012;81(2):123–35. Epub 2011/03/26.
20. McLachlan SA, Allenby A, Matthews J, Wirth A, Kissane D, Bishop M, et al. Randomized trial of coordinated psychosocial interventions based on patient self-assessments versus standard care to improve the psychosocial functioning of patients with cancer. J Clin Oncol. 2001;19(21):4117–25. Epub 2001/11/02.
21. Cheung YB, Goh C, Thumboo J, Khoo KS, Wee J. Variability and sample size requirements of quality-of-life measures: a randomized study of three major questionnaires. J Clin Oncol. 2005;23(22):4936–44.
22. Olschewski M, Schumacher M. Statistical analysis of quality of life data in cancer clinical trials. Stat Med. 1990;9(7):749–63.
23. Efficace F, Bottomley A, Coens C, Van Steen K, Conroy T, Schoffski P, et al. Does a patient's self-reported health-related quality of life predict survival beyond key biomedical data in advanced colorectal cancer? Eur J Cancer. 2006;42(1):42–9.
24. Quinten C, Coens C, Mauer M, Comte S, Sprangers MA, Cleeland C, et al. Baseline quality of life as a prognostic indicator of survival: a meta-analysis of individual patient data from EORTC clinical trials. Lancet Oncol. 2009;10(9):865–71.
25. Oliva EN, Nobile F, Alimena G, Ronco F, Specchia G, Impera S, et al. Quality of life in elderly patients with acute myeloid leukemia: patients may be more accurate than physicians. Haematologica. 2011;96(5):696–702. Epub 2011/02/19.
26. Efficace F, Cartoni C, Niscola P, Tendas A, Meloni E, Scaramucci L, et al. Predicting survival in advanced hematologic malignancies: do patient-reported symptoms matter? Eur J Haematol. 2012;89(5):410–6. Epub 2012/09/19.
27. Coates AS, Hurny C, Peterson HF, Bernhard J, Castiglione-Gertsch M, Gelber RD, et al. Quality-of-life scores predict outcome in metastatic but not early breast cancer. International Breast Cancer Study Group. J Clin Oncol. 2000;18(22):3768–74.
28. Minton O, Stone P. A systematic review of the scales used for the measurement of cancer-related fatigue (CRF). Ann Oncol. 2009;20(1):17–25.
29. Deschler B, Ihorst G, Platzbecker U, Germing U, Marz E, de Figuerido M, et al. Parameters detected by geriatric and quality of life assessment in 195 older patients with myelodysplastic syndromes and acute myeloid leukemia are highly predictive for outcome. Haematologica. 2013;98(2):208–16.
30. Alibhai SM, Leach M, Gupta V, Tomlinson GA, Brandwein JM, Saiz FS, et al. Quality of life beyond 6 months after diagnosis in older adults with acute myeloid leukemia. Crit Rev Oncol Hematol. 2009;69(2):168–74.
31. Yellen SB, Cella DF. Someone to live for: social well-being, parenthood status, and decision-making in oncology. J Clin Oncol. 1995;13(5):1255–64. Epub 1995/05/01.
32. Guyatt G, Schunemann H. How can quality of life researchers make their work more useful to health workers and their patients? Qual Life Res. 2007;16(7):1097–105.
33. Deschler BPU, Germing U, Lübbert M. Arrangement of parameters of a geriatric and quality of life assessment in elderly patients with myelodysplastic syndromes and acute myeloid leukemia during six months of different therapeutic modalities. Haematologica. 2010;95:189.
34. Jack S, West M, Grocott MP. Perioperative exercise training in elderly subjects. Best Pract Res Clin Anaesthesiol. 2011;25(3):461–72. Epub 2011/09/20.
35. Velikova G, Booth L, Smith AB, Brown PM, Lynch P, Brown JM, et al. Measuring quality of life in routine oncology practice improves communication and patient well-being: a randomized controlled trial. J Clin Oncol. 2004;22(4):714–24. Epub 2004/02/18.
36. Mantovani G, Astara G, Lampis B, Bianchi A, Curreli L, Orru W, et al. Evaluation by multidimensional instruments of health-related quality of life of elderly cancer patients undergoing three different "psychosocial" treatment approaches. A randomized clinical trial. Support Care Cancer. 1996;4(2):129–40. Epub 1996/03/01.

19. Efficace F, Cocks K, Breccia M, Sprangers M, Meyers CA, Vignetti M, et al. Time for a new era in the evaluation of targeted therapies for patients with chronic myeloid leukemia: inclusion of quality of life and other patient-reported outcomes. Crit Rev Oncol Hematol. [illegible]

20. [illegible] Randomized trial of a [illegible] in addition to standard care to improve the [illegible] of patients with cancer. [illegible]

[illegible]

[illegible]

Chapter 19
Palliative Care in Elderly Patients with Hematological Malignancies

Ulrich Wedding

Abstract Treatment approach in older adults with hematological maligancies is often palliative. Even in curative treatment approach a high risk of disease or treatment associated risk of dying exists. Therefore palliative care should be an essential part of care for older adults with hematological malignancies.

Keywords Hematological malignancies • Supportive care • Palliative care • Quality of life • Prognosis • Place of death

Introduction

Whereas some patients with hematological malignancies can be cured, most patients will finally die of their disease or side effects of treatment. However, other than in patients with solid tumours, patients with hematological malignancies have not been in the focus of palliative care so far [1]. Burden of symptoms and the need for supportive care differ between patients with solid tumours and those with hematological malignancies.

In some patients with hematological malignancies, supportive care is paramount not "only" to treat symptoms but also to enable them to stay a life. In patients with severe bone marrow failure, the termination of regular transfusions, either erythrocytes or thrombocytes, will result in death within days or a few weeks, and the termination of antibiotics and other anti-infectious agents either given as prophylaxis or as therapy of infections, will result in severe infection, sepsis and death in multiorgan failure in a short term period.

After providing the definition of palliative care by the WHO and some epidemiological data, the following chapter addresses (1) places of death of patients with hematological malignancies and differences in palliative and hospice care between patients with hematological malignancies and solid tumours, (2) prognosis, (3) typical burdens of symptoms patients with hematological malignancies will face,

U. Wedding, MD
Department of Palliative Care, University Hospital Jena, Erlanger Allee 101, Jena 07747, Thüringen, Germany
e-mail: ulrich.wedding@med.uni-jena.de

U. Wedding, R.A. Audisio (eds.), *Management of Hematological Cancer in Older People*, DOI 10.1007/978-1-4471-2837-3_19

focuses (4) on medical and other needs of the patients and suggests (5) some kind of approach to improve the care even when facing death.

For further details, a review by Epstein et al. is recommended [2].

Definition of Palliative Care

"An approach that improves the quality of life of patients and their families facing the problem associated with life-threatening illness, through the prevention and relief of suffering by means of early identification and impeccable assessment and treatment of pain and other problems, physical, psychosocial and spiritual:

- provides relief from pain and other distressing symptoms;
- affirms life and regards dying as a normal process;
- intends neither to hasten or postpone death;
- integrates the psychological and spiritual aspects of patient care;
- offers a support system to help patients live as actively as possible until death;
- offers a support system to help the family cope during the patient's illness and in their own bereavement;
- uses a team approach to address the needs of patients and their families, including bereavement counselling, if indicated;
- will enhance quality of life, and may also positively influence the course of illness;
- is applicable early in the course of illness, in conjunction with other therapies that are intended to prolong life, such as chemotherapy or radiation therapy, and includes those investigations needed to better understand and manage distressing clinical complications.

[http://www.who.int/cancer/palliative/definition/en/]

The term "with life-threatening illness" is important for patients with hematological malignancies as it justifies the integration of palliative care even in patients treated with curative intent with a high risk of mortality, either disease-or treatment-related.

Epidemiology

Epidemiology of hematological malignancies shows a typical age-associated increase of incidence and even higher mortality rates, as pointed out by Quaglia et al. (reference the Chap. 1). The older the patients are, the higher the likelihood that they die of their disease, as rates of cure decrease, due to the use of less toxic regimens and, the higher rates of resistant disease, as demonstrated most pronounced for patients with acute myeloid leukaemia (AML), see chapter by Klepin et al. (reference the Chap. 4).

Table 19.1 Major hematological malignancies, their median age at diagnosis, relative frequency of patients dying within a follow-up period of 2–8 years, and relative frequency of death in hospital, home, nursing home and hospice [3]

Diagnosis	Median age	% of patients dying	Place of death			
			In hospital	Home	Nursing home	Hospice
MM	73.0	63.4	64.5	15.7	12.0	7.8
DLBCL	70.4	51.8	64.5	14.7	11.3	9.6
MDS	76.0	74.9	70.9	15.8	7.4	5.9
AML	71.1	79.4	72.1	14.1	7.2	6.6
CLL	71.6	33.2	65.1	17.5	11.8	5.6
MPN	71.2	23.8	56.9	17.7	18.7	6.7
FL	64.5	22.6	61.5	19.6	10.8	8.1
HD	44.1	21.9	74.6	13.5	7.9	4.0
MCL	74.0	71.1	53.7	19.5	10.6	16.2
TCL	64.9	56.8	70.9	17.1	4.3	7.7
CML	59.2	21.7	72.7	9.1	11.4	6.8

MM multiple myeloma, *DLBLC* diffuse large B-cell lymphoma, *MDS* myelodysplastic syndrome, *AML* acute myeloid leukaemia, *CLL* chronic lymphocytic leukaemia, *MPN* myeloproliferative neoplasia, *FL* follicular lymphoma, *HD* Hodgkin's disease, *MCL* mantle cell lymphoma, *TCL* T-cell lymphoma, *CML* chronic lymphocytic leukaemia

Current Situation of Care

Place of Death

In a population-based trial, Howell et al. analysed the place of death of patients with hematological malignancies. 10,325 patients with a median age of 71 years were included. 47 % of patients died within the period of observation. 66 % of patients dying from hematological malignancies died in hospital, 15 % at home, 11 % in nursing homes, and 8 % in a hospice. The results for different kinds of hematological malignancies are summarized in Table 19.1. Short time from diagnosis to death was associated with in-hospital mortality. Of all deaths in the first months of diagnosis, 88 % occurred in hospital, compared to 72 % of those occurring in months 1–3, 62 % of those in months 3–6, 64 % of those in months 6–12, and 59 % of those above 12 months. Of all deaths, 14 % occurred in the first months after diagnosis, 13 % in months 1–3, 11 % in moths 3–6, 16 % in moths 6–12, and 46 % beyond month 12 [3].

In-Hospital Situation

Hematological malignancies where associated with higher death rates, higher in-hospital mortality and lower discharge rates in an acute palliative care unit compared to patients with solid tumours [4].

Providing Hospice and Palliative Care

Howell et al. performed a systematic review and meta-analysis to identify the frequency of patients with hematological malignancies that received palliative or hospice care [1]. Twenty-four studies were identified, nine could be included. All in all, patients with hematological malignancies were less likely to receive palliative or hospice care compared to patients with solid tumours. The following possible reasons were mentioned: (a) ongoing management by the haematology team and consequent strong bonds between staff and patients, (b) uncertain transitions to a palliative approach to care, (c) sudden transitions, leaving little time for patients, input.

In a further analysis, the authors report on the use of specialized palliative care (SPC) referrals in a population-based cohort of 323 patients diagnosed with acute myeloid leukaemia, diffuse large B-cell lymphoma or multiple myeloma over a 5-years period who died within 2–7 years after diagnosis. 48 % of them had at least one SPC referral. The following factors were associated with higher use of SPC: longer survival (>12 months vs. <1 months), multiple myeloma vs. acute myeloid leukemia. Patients dying not in hospital had a higher rate of SPC referrals. Forty-four percent of the patients included were 75 years and older [5].

Sexauer et al. report that there are about 70,000 deaths of patients with hematological malignancies each year in the US. Only 2 % of them use a hospice. They report a length of stay of 9 days in home hospice care and of 6 days in inpatients hospice care, with some of them receiving blood transfusion during hospice stay [6].

Prognosis

The majority of prognostic scores are based on patients, and disease characteristics when patients are newly diagnosed with a certain disease, for more details see the specific chapter for the different diseases in this book.

Other prognostic scores have been proposed to better adjust the likelihood of dying within a certain period after transition of patients to palliative care. They mainly included physicians, estimate of survival time, performance status, presence of symptoms, such as dyspnoea and cachexia, and some lab-results [7].

None of them focuses on patients with hematological malignancies in a palliative care setting.

Kripp et al. analysed factors associated with survival of 290 patients with hematological malignancies referred to an in patient acute palliative care unit [8]. The following factors were identified: (a) Eastern Cooperative Oncology Group (ECOG) Performance Status (PS): 0–2 vs. 3–4; (b) platelet counts: >=90 vs. <90 × 10 E-9/L; (c) Lactate-Dehydrogenase (LDH) <= 248 vs. 248 U/L; (d) opioid use: WHO level 0–2 vs. 3; (e) albumin >= 30 vs. <30 g/L; (f) packed red blood cell transfusion no vs. yes. According to the above mentioned factors, the authors suggested three different risk groups, see Table 19.2.

Age, comorbidities, or other items of a comprehensive geriatric assessment were not included in the analysis.

Table 19.2 Number of risk factors, frequency of patients, and outcome regarding survival in patients with hematological malignancies referred to an acute palliative care unit [8]

No. of risk factors	No. of patients	Median time of survival
0–1	48	440 days
2–3	120	63 days
4–5 (6)	78	10 days

The time of referral to palliative care is not a clearly defined and generally known point of time within the course of the disease, but varies widely from factors such as availability of service etc that are not patient- or disease-related. This limits the use of prognostic scores in the palliative care setting.

Burdens of Symptoms in Patients with Hematological Malignancies

The palliative care approach is more symptom-than disease-orientated. Symptoms in patients with hematological malignancies are common. Manitta et al. reported a mean number of symptoms of 8.8 in 180 patients diagnosed with hematological malignancies with a median age of 61 years, range 17–95 years. Most common symptoms were lack of energy 69 %, feeling worried 50 %, difficulty to sleep 41 %, feeling sad 41 %, drowsiness 41 %, dry mouth 40 %, pain 39 %, numbness hands/feet 38 %, shortness of breath 36 %, irritability 36 %, difficulty concentrating 34 %, cough 33 %, feeling nervous 33 %, lack of appetite 27 %. The mean number of symptoms was significant greater in those on treatment, those with poor performance status, inpatients, and those with advanced disease [9]. Age was not included in the analysis.

The prevalence and type of symptoms of patients with hematological malignancies in the palliative care setting varies according to the type of underlying disease. However data are limited. Following we report some data for patients with acute myeloid leukaemia, multiple myeloma, and for patients with malignant lymphoma.

Acute Leukaemia

Zimmermann et al. reported the symptoms of patients with acute leukaemia, mainly acute myeloid leukaemia, referred to a palliative care service. Two hundred and forty-nine were included. The analysis was not restricted to elderly patients. The patients reported nine physical and two psychological symptoms. Main symptoms reported lack of energy 79 %, feeling drowsy 56 %, difficulty sleeping 55 %, dry mouth 54 %, weight loss 53 %, lack of appetite 52 %, change in taste of food 51 %, pain 49 %, nausea 45 %, worrying 43 % [10]. Only 2 of 35 patients dying in the period of the study were referred to a palliative care service.

Stalfeld et al. reported the final phase of 106 adult patients with acute myeloid leukaemia, who died. Twenty-seven were treated with curative intent, 79 were in a palliative care approach. Forty-four percent suffered from bleeding, 71 from infection and 76 from pain in the last week of their life [11].

Multiple Myeloma

Palliative care needs of patients with multiple myeloma in advanced disease are often dominated by symptoms of the disease, especially pain, related to bone destruction, infections, bone marrow failure and renal impairment.

In the most recent recommendations for the treatment of elderly patients with multiple myeloma, palliative care approaches are mentioned in the appendix: "In the absence of effective antimyeloma treatments, counseling for patients and families provided by a palliative specialist is suggested. To relieve the disabling myeloma-related symptoms, low doses of cyclophosphamide, corticosteroids, or thalidomide may be used." And "Terminal care should include a multidisciplinary approach aimed at alleviating symptoms and addressing patient desires" [12].

The guidelines for supportive care in multiple myeloma recommend at several occasions the need to have an established collaboration with a specialized palliative care team as part of the supportive care for patients with multiple myeloma [13].

Validated instruments for symptom assessment and a structured assessment of quality of life of patients with multiple myeloma are available, as reported in a systematic review by Osborne et al., however, they are not validated in the palliative care setting [14].

Malignant Lymphoma

Palliative care needs of patients with malignant lymphoma in advanced disease are often dominated by symptoms of the disease, especially infections, bone marrow failure and local compression by enlarged lymph node masses. Specific recommendations for palliative care in patients with malignant lymphoma in general and in elderly patients especially are missing.

Medical and Other Needs

Hematological malignancies are a heterogeneous group of disorders with diverse clinical presentation, different treatment strategies and outcome regarding quantity and quality of life.

Palliative care focuses not only on physical symptoms, but most patients have psychosocial and spiritual needs as well. In addition, besides the patients the relatives are addressed. Giving them support helps them and helps the patients as the relatives are the most important caregiver for the patient and the most important persons patients are worrying about.

The maintenance of treatment, as continuation of anti-infective agents or continuation of support the blood transfusions prolongs life and improves symptoms in some patients with hematological malignancies, even in a very advanced stage. The step to stop this kind of treatments, to not start anti-infective treatment often implies a deterioration of the medical condition until death within a few days or a couple of weeks.

In a small cohort of patients with hematological malignancies treated in a palliative care unit, Cheng et al. reported that 87 % received blood sampling, 24 % granulocyte colony-stimulating factors, 14 % parenteral nutrition, 33 % red blood cell transfusions, 48 % platelet transfusion, and 90 % antibiotics within the last week of life [15].

A special problem is the broad range of the aim of treatment; cure can be possible, in some cases likely, in others unlikely but not impossible. In some cases, especially in acute leukaemia, all efforts are set to reach the aim of cure, but within a couple of days, the aim of treatment can become palliative, e.g. when bone marrow regenerates with blasts instead of normal cells after intensive induction chemotherapy, or when a severe sepsis occurs.

"They go for the cure. Nobody looks at the fact that most people going through only have a short time and so the dying is the most important thing to handle" are the words of a research participant, as reported by McGrath [16], suffering from AML.

A double message can help the patients and the relatives in such a situation: "Hope for the best and prepare for the worst". Cure can not be promised but hope can be supported, and on the other hand, the life-threatening character of the disease should be communicated.

Advanced directives are helpful and are a good instrument to raise the topic of the life-threatening character of the disease.

Situation in Patients with Acute Myeloid Leukaemia

In some patients cure can be achieved. As the aim of cure seams highly achievable, even in most of the elderly patients the aim of cure is followed initially, notwithstanding the fact that most of the patients will die of their disease within a couple of months. Regarding median time of survival, AML is not better and even worse than most solid tumour in the metastatic stage of the disease. In addition, the toxicity of treatment to achieve cure is substantially, implying that the patients have to have access to hematological care in an in- and out patient service.

In most of the elderly patients initially treated with an intensive induction protocol, the disease will recur within months after treatment. 2nd line treatment is hardly of curative intent again. Death is often caused by severe infection. Symptoms might be related to infections and bone marrow insufficiency, resulting in anaemia and thrombocytopenia.

Palliative Care Approach to Patients with Hematological Malignancies

Palliative Care addresses symptoms, and other needs of patients and their relatives, by providing care on different levels by a team of professionals with a common aim.

Structure of Palliative Care Services

The structure of palliative care services is highly influenced by differences between local, regional, and national health care systems. Overall, general palliative care and specialized palliative care services should be provided. Looking at patients with hematological malignancies, the general palliative care should be integrated into the hematological care provided to the patients, either by physicians, nurses, psycho-oncologist, and other professions. Thus, all care professionals for patients with hematological malignancies should have a basic training in palliative care. Part of this training should be the recognition of situations where specialized palliative care is needed.

Specialized care services should be available in all centres providing care for patients with hematological malignancies, including inpatient palliative care wards, inpatient consultations service, and outpatient home care and hospice services.

Burden for the Health Care Professionals

Health care professionals in patients with hematological malignancies often provide care for "their patients" over a long period of time during which they develop a close relationship to the patients and their relatives.

Shirai et al. analysed nurses'perception of adequate care for leukaemia patients in the incurable phase. The nurses identified the following topics as of major importance for a qualified care for patients with hematological malignancies in the incurable stage: (a) care for physical distress, (b) care for mental distress, (c) care for social distress, (d) care for distress related to decision making, (e) care for distress of family [17].

Barriers to Palliative Care in Patients with Hematological Malignancies

Patients, relatives and professional caregivers might avoid to take palliative care into account. They fear the finality, want to avoid destroying hope, etc. [18].

To rename the palliative care service to a supportive care service improved the use, physicians were much more willing to refer their patients [19].

Table 19.3 Special considerations for patients with hematological malignancies [20]

The high-tech and invasive nature of the treatments offered
Significant sequelae from treatment – quality vs. quantity of life concerns
The speed of change to a terminal event
The frequency of blood tests and the need for blood products
The possibility of catastrophic bleeds
Varied diagnostic groups with different prognosis and disease patterns
The fact that treatments can continue over many years
Close patient relationships with haematology unit staff
Clinical optimism based on a myriad of treatment options
Patients occasionally show positive signs of recovery when close to death
In some cases, there is no clear distinction between the curative and palliative phase; however, nurses noted that in the majority of cases there are clear clinical indications that the terminal stage has been reached

In addition, palliative care mainly developed for patients with solid tumours and might not be prepared for the special needs of patients with hematological malignancies.

In qualitative interviews, McGrath and Holewa identified 11 major factors associated with difficulties to involve palliative care into the care for patients with hematological malignancies, see Table 19.3 [20].

Special Offers of Care for Patients with Hematological Malignancies

As demonstrated by a report by Stockelberg et al., patients with hematological malignancies treated at home in a palliative care setting were in need for blood transfusions and chemotherapy [21]. In many countries, blood transfusions are not performed in a home care setting due to legal reasons, such as the fast access to a physician experienced in the treatment of acute adverse reactions.

Future Perspectives

There is a growing body of evidence that the integration of palliative care into active oncological care provides an improvement of the outcome for the patients, with some studies even reporting an improvement of survival [22], others an improvement of quality of life [23]. As a result, the American Society of Clinical Oncology (ASCO) recommends the integration of palliative care into oncological care [24]. The data for patients with hematological malignancies are much more limited, however, there is no reason to restrict the approach to patients with solid tumours. As the aim of treatment might be cure but only very few patients will be cured in fact, palliative care might even be involved in curative treatment approaches. This is in line with the WHO definition of palliative care, provided in the beginning.

References

1. Howell DA, Shellens R, Roman E, Garry AC, Patmore R, Howard MR. Haematological malignancy: are patients appropriately referred for specialist palliative and hospice care? A systematic review and meta-analysis of published data. Palliat Med. 2011;25(6):630–41.
2. Epstein AS, Goldberg GR, Meier DE. Palliative care and hematologic oncology: the promise of collaboration. Blood Rev. 2012;26(6):233–9.
3. Howell DA, Wang HI, Smith AG, Howard MR, Patmore RD, Roman E. Place of death in haematological malignancy: variations by disease sub-type and time from diagnosis to death. BMC Palliat Care. 2013;12(1):42.
4. Hui D, Elsayem A, Palla S, De La Cruz M, Li Z, Yennurajalingam S, Bruera E. Discharge outcomes and survival of patients with advanced cancer admitted to an acute palliative care unit at a comprehensive cancer center. J Palliat Med. 2010;13(1):49–57.
5. Howell DA, Wang HI, Roman E, Smith AG, Patmore R, Johnson MJ, Garry AC, Howard MR. Variations in specialist palliative care referrals: findings from a population-based patient cohort of acute myeloid leukaemia, diffuse large B-cell lymphoma and myeloma. BMJ Support Palliat Care. 2014. doi: 10.1136/bmjspcare-2013-000578 [Epub ahead of print].
6. Sexauer A, Cheng MJ, Knight L, Riley AW, King L, Smith TJ. Patterns of hospice use in patients dying from hematologic malignancies. J Palliat Med. 2014;17(2):195–9.
7. Maltoni M, Pirovano M, Scarpi E, Marinari M, Indelli M, Arnoldi E, Gallucci M, Frontini L, Piva L, Amadori D. Prediction of survival of patients terminally ill with cancer. Results of an Italian prospective multicentric study. Cancer. 1995;75(10):2613–22.
8. Kripp M, Willer A, Schmidt C, Pilz LR, Gencer D, Buchheidt D, Hochhaus A, Hofmann WK, Hofheinz RD. Patients with malignant hematological disorders treated on a palliative care unit: prognostic impact of clinical factors. Ann Hematol. 2014;93(2):317–25.
9. Manitta V, Zordan R, Cole-Sinclair M, Nandurkar H, Philip J. The symptom burden of patients with hematological malignancy: a cross-sectional observational study. J Pain Symptom Manage. 2011;42(3):432–42.
10. Zimmermann C, Yuen D, Mischitelle A, Minden MD, Brandwein JM, Schimmer A, Gagliese L, Lo C, Rydall A, Rodin G. Symptom burden and supportive care in patients with acute leukemia. Leuk Res. 2013;37(7):731–6.
11. Stalfelt AM, Brodin H, Pettersson S, Eklof A. The final phase in acute myeloid leukaemia (AML). A study on bleeding, infection and pain. Leuk Res. 2003;27(6):481–8.
12. Palumbo A, Rajkumar SV, San Miguel JF, Larocca A, Niesvizky R, Morgan G, Landgren O, Hajek R, Einsele H, Anderson KC, Dimopoulos MA, Richardson PG, Cavo M, Spencer A, Stewart AK, Shimizu K, Lonial S, Sonneveld P, Durie BG, Moreau P, Orlowski RZ. International Myeloma Working Group consensus statement for the management, treatment, and supportive care of patients with myeloma not eligible for standard autologous stem-cell transplantation. J Clin Oncol. 2014;32(6):587–600.
13. Snowden JA, Ahmedzai SH, Ashcroft J, D'Sa S, Littlewood T, Low E, Lucraft H, Maclean R, Feyler S, Pratt G, Bird JM, H. Haemato-oncology Task Force of British Committee for Standards in and U. K. M. Forum. Guidelines for supportive care in multiple myeloma 2011. Br J Haematol. 2011;154(1)):76–103.
14. Osborne TR, Ramsenthaler C, Siegert RJ, Edmonds PM, Schey SA, Higginson IJ. What issues matter most to people with multiple myeloma and how well are we measuring them? A systematic review of quality of life tools. Eur J Haematol. 2012;89(6):437–57.
15. Cheng BH,Sham MM, Chan KY, Li CW, Au HY. Intensive palliative care for patients with hematological cancer dying in hospice: analysis of the level of medical care in the final week of life. Am J Hosp Palliat Care. 2013 [Epub ahead of print].
16. McGrath P. Are we making progress? Not in haematology! Omega (Westport). 2002;45(4): 331–48.
17. Shirai Y, Kawa M, Miyashita M, Kazuma K. Nurses' perception of adequacy of care for leukemia patients with distress during the incurable phase and related factors. Leuk Res. 2005;29(3):293–300.

18. Fadul N, Elsayem A, Palmer JL, Del Fabbro E, Swint K, Li Z, Poulter V, Bruera E. Supportive versus palliative care: what's in a name?: a survey of medical oncologists and midlevel providers at a comprehensive cancer center. Cancer. 2009;115(9):2013–21.
19. Dalal S, Palla S, Hui D, Nguyen L, Chacko R, Li Z, Fadul N, Scott C, Thornton V, Coldman B, Amin Y, Bruera E. Association between a name change from palliative to supportive care and the timing of patient referrals at a comprehensive cancer center. Oncologist. 2011;16(1): 105–11.
20. McGrath P, Holewa H. Special considerations for haematology patients in relation to end-of-life care: Australian findings. Eur J Cancer Care (Engl). 2007;16(2):164–71.
21. Stockelberg D, Lehtola P, Noren I. Palliative treatment at home for patients with haematological disorders. Support Care Cancer. 1997;5(6):506–8.
22. Temel JS, Greer JA, Muzikansky A, Gallagher ER, Admane S, Jackson VA, Dahlin CM, Blinderman CD, Jacobsen J, Pirl WF, Billings JA, Lynch TJ. Early palliative care for patients with metastatic non-small-cell lung cancer. N Engl J Med. 2010;363(8):733–42.
23. Zimmermann C, Swami N, Krzyzanowska M, Hannon B, Leighl N, Oza A, Moore M, Rydall A, Rodin G, Tannock I, Donner A, Lo C. Early palliative care for patients with advanced cancer: a cluster-randomised controlled trial. Lancet. 2014;383(9930):1721–30.
24. Smith TJ, Temin S, Alesi ER, Abernethy AP, Balboni TA, Basch EM, Ferrell BR, Loscalzo M, Meier DE, Paice JA, Peppercorn JM, Somerfield M, Stovall E, Von Roenn JH. American Society of Clinical Oncology provisional clinical opinion: the integration of palliative care into standard oncology care. J Clin Oncol. 2012;30(8):880–7.

Index

U. Wedding, R.A. Audisio (eds.), *Management of Hematological Cancer in Older People*, DOI 10.1007/978-1-4471-2837-3

Q

R

S

T

MIX
Papier aus verantwortungsvollen Quellen
Paper from responsible sources
FSC® C105338

If you have any concerns about our products,
you can contact us on
ProductSafety@springernature.com

In case Publisher is established outside the EU,
the EU authorized representative is:
Springer Nature Customer Service Center GmbH
Europaplatz 3, 69115 Heidelberg, Germany

Printed by Libri Plureos GmbH
in Hamburg, Germany